SAY

ANARCHA

SAY
ANARCHA

A Young Woman,
a Devious Surgeon,
and the Harrowing Birth of
Modern Women's Health

J. C. Hallman

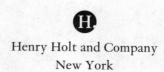

Henry Holt and Company
New York

Henry Holt and Company
Publishers since 1866
120 Broadway
New York, New York 10271
www.henryholt.com

Henry Holt® and Ⓗ® are registered trademarks of Macmillan Publishing
Group, LLC.

Library of Congress Cataloging-in-Publication Data is available.

ISBN: 9781250868466

Our books may be purchased in bulk for promotional, educational,
or business use. Please contact your local bookseller or the Macmillan
Corporate and Premium Sales Department at (800) 221-7945, extension
5442, or by e-mail at MacmillanSpecialMarkets@macmillan.com.

First Edition 2023

Designed by Meryl Sussman Levavi

Printed in the United States of America

1   3   5   7   9   10   8   6   4   2

Contents

Introduction

A Better Phantom

In August 2017, in the wake of the deadly Confederate monument protests in Charlottesville, Virginia, a consortium of local community boards and activist groups in New York City staged an event at the site of the Central Park statue of J. Marion Sims, the so-called Father of Gynecology. In less than twenty-four hours, an image from the protest was shared on social media more than 250,000 times.

J. Marion Sims was infamous for a yearslong series of experimental vaginal surgeries—begun in 1846 and conducted without the use of anesthesia—on approximately ten enslaved women in his backyard "Negro Hospital" in Montgomery, Alabama. The most consequential of Sims's experimental subjects was a young woman who has come to be known as Anarcha.

Sims was attempting to cure obstetric fistula, a horrific condition that is the result of prolonged obstructed labor. His true motive in this effort is one of the subjects of this book. More important, however, is Anarcha. Anarcha was the first woman that Sims saw, and she was subjected to upward of thirty experiments. After Sims claimed to have cured her, in 1849, medical text after medical text cited Anarcha as representing a crucial moment in the history of medicine and surgery. It was the birth of modern gynecology.

Criticism of Sims began with his contemporaries—his greatest critics were his assistants—but for decades after his death, in 1883, these voices were drowned out by enthused hagiographers who hailed Sims as a "savior of women." It wasn't until the late 1960s that a reevaluation of Sims's legacy began to creep into the mainstream. Activists, scholars, historians, artists, poets, playwrights, and journalists chipped away at his biographical facade. By 2017, Sims's legacy had become intertwined with broader reevaluations of the role of white supremacy in American history; with a long overdue indictment of the causes of racial health disparities, particularly in regard to maternal mortality;* with efforts to unwind vestiges of racist southern culture preserved in public monuments; and with tragic histories of medical experimentation performed on people of African descent.†

At the time of the protest of Sims's monument in New York, I had been immersed in a search for Anarcha—and in the Sims story—for almost two years. In 2016, I sold an article to *Harper's Magazine* about Sims's New York statue (one of a number of statues, busts, markers, and paintings created to commemorate him), and—I admit it—I wanted to cancel him. I delivered the piece in early 2017, and it remained in queue for publication at *Harper's* until Sims went viral. Almost immediately, New York mayor Bill de Blasio announced the formation of a ninety-day commission tasked with reconsidering the city's official policy on statues and monuments. This left just enough time to fact-check the article and publish it before the commission handed down its decision. The piece played a small backup role to the work of the community organizers and pro-

---

* The author of Sims's only full-length biography, Seale Harris, wrote of Anarcha and the other women who endured Sims's experiments, "[The] experiments brought them physical pain, it is true, but they bore it with . . . a grim stoicism which may have been part of their racial endowment or which possibly had been bred into them through several generations of enforced submission." This racist belief was espoused not at the time of Sims's experiments but a century closer to our own time, in 1950.

† The Sims story went viral in 2017, shortly before the world did. In the early days of the COVID-19 pandemic, when everyone (or so it seemed) eagerly awaited a vaccine, it wasn't clear that Sims's legacy would be particularly relevant. However, after the Delta variant surfaced in late summer 2021, Sims became more or less synonymous with vaccine hesitancy in the African American community. For a time, it was impossible to read a news story about hesitancy that did not mention Sims's fistula experiments alongside the more infamous Tuskegee syphilis study. Now, at a remove, it seems entirely appropriate to ask whether vaccine hesitancy might have been mitigated—and lives saved—had medical organizations whose own histories were twined with that of the doctor who had been called the "American Mengele" made a more robust effort to reckon with his horrific legacy.

testers who had been objecting to the monument for the better part of a decade, often with city officials working behind the scenes to tamp down enthusiasm for removing Sims's statue—or any statue.

It didn't work. The vote to remove the Sims monument was unanimous, and the statue came down in April 2018. By then, I was poring through the thousands of documents I had collected so as to enable a telling of Anarcha's story. In addition, I had spent ten weeks in Ethiopia, Nigeria, and Uganda to bear witness to the modern legacy of the Alabama fistula experiments. This legacy is described in full in the afterword of this book, but suffice it to say that Sims did nothing to ensure that a fistula cure reached the population that had provided him with his experimental fodder. A patient-centered model of care sparked by Anarcha and the Alabama fistula experiments—a model of care that has improved the lives of hundreds of thousands of African women—owes nothing to Sims. It is the accidental by-product of his lifelong effort to enrich himself. The treatment of obstetric fistula today is based almost entirely on fistula sufferers living communally, acquiring skills as they care for one another. This model was spontaneously devised by a group of enslaved women—teenagers, really—in a tiny clinic in Alabama in the 1840s. Today, hundreds of fistula survivors have followed in their footsteps to become nurses, nurse aides, doctors, activists, and community organizers.

The daughters of Anarcha are legion.

* * *

Say Anarcha is a book about a ghost—a ghost who has undergone periodic revision.

The first version of the ghost of Anarcha was Sims's own. He told the tale of his fistula experiments over and over; Anarcha's story was the pivotal anecdote in a fanciful narrative that brought him fame and fortune. For her part, Anarcha vanished: no record of her appeared to have survived, yet her memory was tugged along behind Sims's ascent into the medical firmament. For 170 years, the only evidence of Anarcha's existence was Sims's own suspect writings.

Somewhere along the line—it's unclear when—she became "Anarcha

Westcott." Sims's autobiography indicates that he first saw Anarcha on the "Wescott" plantation, a mile from his office in downtown Montgomery. But he never called her "Anarcha Westcott"; the application of her enslaver's surname to Anarcha did not appear in print until the second half of the twentieth century. It has since appeared, without caveat or comment, in numerous peer-reviewed articles debating Sims's legacy, in books of poetry that have given voice to her life, and in reputable media sources.

However, there was never anyone named "Anarcha Westcott." There is no document to suggest that Anarcha took the name of her former enslaver. "Anarcha Westcott" was another ghost, a name for a hole in history, the title of a story that could not be told.

Say Anarcha is a dual biography. It is a comprehensive retelling of Sims's life, a sandpapering away of layers of varnish applied by Sims himself and by successive generations of overly credulous apologists. It is a subversion of every aspect of a fraudulent narrative. More speculatively, *Say Anarcha* is an attempt to excavate the life story of a young enslaved woman who changed history, only to be forgotten by it.

This effort is twofold. First, it is the product of an exhaustive effort to find Anarcha, and her story as recounted here is a combination of extensive, direct evidence of her existence presented in concert with certainties, probabilities, inferences, informed speculation, and guesswork. It is, to my mind, the most likely story of Anarcha's life, but it is not the only possible story that lurks behind Sims's veil of obfuscations and half-truths, a deceitful fiction that has stood as factual history for almost two centuries.

Second, this archival scaffold of Anarcha's story is made more human and present with material drawn from a close reading of the fifty-five volumes of slave narratives compiled by the Federal Writers' Project (FWP) from 1936–38. A part of President Franklin Roosevelt's Works Progress Administration, the FWP recruited hundreds of interviewers to fan out across the South to seek out formerly enslaved people, ancient souls who sometimes claimed to be as old as 121 years of age, though few formerly enslaved people knew precisely when they'd been born. The interviews tended to follow a script. What did slaves wear back then? What did you eat? Do you believe in "conjure" and "haints"? The goal of the project was to produce an ethnographic trove of portraits that would push back against fictional caricatures of African Americans. There are good reasons to be wary of accepting every narrative at face value, however. The phalanx of interviewers included the likes of Richard Wright and Zora Neale Hurston—authors destined to be counted among literature's greats—but the ranks also included sons and daughters of the "Lost Cause." Some narratives stand out starkly from the rest for their emphasis on Black dialect and Black exoticism. Nevertheless, it was the hope of the FWP directors that the "composite autobiography" of the narratives would provide useful material for historians and creative writers.

Say Anarcha is an attempt to fulfill this lofty goal.

What this means is that the Anarcha presented here is yet another ghost, hopefully a better phantom. Anarcha truly lived—this can be stated unequivocally now—but she was always a symbol. She is a symbol in this book too. She is a symbol of the sisters she suffered with in Sims's backyard clinic, and she is a symbol of the countless hundreds of women, enslaved and not, who were experimented on by physicians before Sims, and after him. She is a symbol too of the women who fought to ensure that the products of her sacrifice would not simply serve the male medical establishment. Every woman living today owes a debt to Anarcha, and at long last the progress she represents has begun to escape the cloister of the so-called civilized world.

* * *

Elizabeth Lee, grande dame of local history in King George, Virginia, wasn't returning my calls. She wasn't answering my emails, either.

I discovered the first traces of Anarcha in 2015, in Alabama, where her name was recorded as "Anaka" and "Anarcky." ("Anarcha" itself is a specter, having appeared only in Sims's autobiography.) The search continued for years in archives, probate offices, public and private libraries, and privately held manuscript collections. I followed Anarcha from Alabama to Virginia, then to New York City and Connecticut, and finally back to Virginia. I knew she had lived for a time in Bowling Green, Virginia, but from there the trail went cold. It remained that way until I learned that her final enslaver had lived on a plantation called Alto, about twenty miles to the north, in King George.

If there was anyone who might know what happened in King George, I was told, it would be Elizabeth Lee.

Lee was writing a book of her own—perhaps I was not hearing from her because she feared that our research was in competition. (It wasn't.) I kept trying her contact information for another week, until I ran out of ideas about how to continue the search for Anarcha.

Full of trepidation—fearful that a yearslong quest would end in mystery—I set out for King George. I was desperate, but Anarcha felt very close at hand.

Lee was the president of the King George County Historical Society, an organization housed in a tiny room lined with shelves and cabinets displaying fragments of King George history. She wasn't there when I arrived, but it was the South: a kind woman promptly gave me her address.

I knocked on Lee's door. I was wrong to have feared that she was avoiding me. She was eighty years old, and worked diligently on her book every day. She didn't have much use for email and voice mail; my messages had never reached her.

She agreed to help me at once. I followed her back to the historical society, and we arranged some chairs in the center of the room. I told her the story of Sims, the experiments in Alabama, the enslaved women who had been used to usher in a new era in women's health. I mentioned Alto, the plantation that I believed was important to the very end of Anarcha's story.

When I said the name "Anarcha," Lee lifted her eyes and sat upright—and gooseflesh rose on the back of my neck.

"That name," she said. "Wait a moment . . ."

She rose to her feet—it was an effort—and pulled down from a shelf a loosely bound cemetery book, created by Lee herself. Working for decades to transcribe and combine a variety of ancient, hand-scrawled Virginia vital statistics records, she had created a comprehensive catalog of all the known cemeteries in King George County. There was just one

entry for the former Alto property: a single grave for Annacay and Laurenzi Jackson.*

I already knew that in Virginia the
unusual name Anarcha had a shortened
form: Ankey. Much
later, I learned that
Lee had transcribed
Anarcha's death record into a separate book, though she had not connected the death record of "Ankey Jackson," wife of "Lorenzo," to the
"Annacay," wife of "Laurenzi," interred on the Alto plantation.

Lee explained what had happened. Some
years before, a local man named Jim Pettry
had been hunting on land behind his home on
Eden Drive, which runs north-south through
Alto. A quarter mile deep in the forest, on a small, elevated wedge of land,
Pettry happened across a gravestone snapped off at its base, facedown,
mostly covered over with dirt and leaves. The area wasn't a graveyard;
the stone was alone in the woods. An amateur genealogist himself, Pettry
tipped the stone upright, leaned it against a tree, and wrote down what it
said on its face. That's what Lee had transcribed into her cemetery book.

At this point, I had known Elizabeth Lee for about ten minutes. I was
a complete stranger. In two minutes more, we were in a car, headed to Jim
Pettry's house.

Pettry wasn't home at first. I nearly got Lee's minivan stuck in a giant
mud puddle—but later in the afternoon, I caught Pettry at home. Lee
wasn't with me; she couldn't have managed the hike out to the grave.
Pettry agreed to guide me. It was only a few hundred yards behind his
house, but the forest wall at the edge of his property was a sharp cliff face
of foliage, like the barrier in a storybook marking the line between the
safety of home and the danger of the woods. Through the veil, the land

---

* The stone marking Anarcha's grave appears to have been placed long after she and Lorenzo died,
which would account for why the spelling of their names and the dates of their deaths differ from
earlier records. The stone itself is an ongoing mystery. Who created it, and how was such an ungainly
monument transported to a hidden and quite rugged piece of land?

was thick with shrubs and mud and creeks, and we climbed up sharp inclines from streambeds to narrow bluffs, and scampered over rotted, fallen logs. I was completely lost ten steps into the forest, and I have gotten lost again each of the half dozen times I have returned.

Pettry was a talker. Like a mountain man, he knew every snag and every turn of the streams, and while we walked, he pointed out the locations where he had shot a deer for meat. As we approached the grave, he began a long speech about a genealogical mystery he had been attempting to solve for years: the story of a distant relative, a man who had survived a mob's effort to hang him.

I was only barely listening as we arrived at the site. The stone still leaned against the tree where Pettry had propped it, and rain had been chiseling away at the granite for more than a century. I had to get close to make out the entirety of its text.

IN

Memory of

LAURENZI JACKSON

Died Sept. 28 1884

Aged 67 years

Also his wife

ANNACAY JACKSON

Died June 27 1869

Aged 48 years

Gone but not forgotten

I had found Anarcha, but I did not rejoice at this moment. After years of study, reading, and searching, there was still a great deal of work to do: verification in census records and documents of the Bureau of Refugees, Freedmen, and Abandoned Lands more commonly known as the Freedmen's Bureau. There was much more to learn about Anarcha's final years. As I read the stone over and over, clearing dirt and dead leaves from near its base, I recalled the moment when I'd first come across the story of J. Marion Sims, the craven and conniving physician who had been enshrined as a hero with biographical portraits sparkling with tortured, celestial imagery. Sims, one commenter claimed, was "the first bright planet that appeared in the dim light of [the] dawn [of gynecology]." Another asserted that among the luminaries of the professional firmament, Sims had "appeared as a comet, leaving a path of light that would forever reflect luster upon the medical art." The *Medical Record*, a prominent journal of Sims's day, stated it bluntly: "Then, like a meteor, appeared the genius of Sims!"

When I began work on Sims, I found it easy enough to scrape away at the facade of a false legacy. By way of contrast, Anarcha had fallen into the abyss of the past.

At Anarcha's grave site, I thought about facts. Facts tend to hide—they may even resist discovery. But with hard work, perseverance, and luck, the truth can be unearthed. Without Jim Pettry hunting in the woods, without Elizabeth Lee and her lifetime of devotion to primary sources, Anarcha might never have been found. Lee published her own book in 2021; she died not long after.

For a time, Jim Pettry and I stood reverently in the silent ache of the woods.

It was the end of the search for Anarcha, but it was just the beginning of telling her story.

In the whole of history, how many slaves' names are known to you? I can think of two.

—George Orwell, 1943

Say her name—Anarcha!

—Protesters, Fifth Avenue, Manhattan, 2016

Their Names

A complete list of all the formerly enslaved persons whose narratives contributed to the re-creation of Anarcha's story

Frank L. Adams • Rachel Adams • Will Adams • Frank Adamson • Fannie Alexander • Hannah Allen • Jim Allen • Lucindy Allison • Charles H. Anderson • Josephine Anderson • Mary Anderson • Nancy Anderson • Pernella Anderson • Sam Anderson • Frances Andrews • Samuel Simeon Andrews • Mary Anngady • Louisiana Anthony • Cora Armstrong • George W. Arnold • Stearlin Arnwine • Caroline Ates • Lizzie Atkins • Charity Austin • Georgia Baker • Henry Barnes • Mary Barnes • Spencer Barnett • Robert Barr • Robert Barton • Jasper Battle • Emmet Beal • Bob Beford • Frank Bell • Oliver Bell • Sophie D. Belle • Cyrus Bellus • Sarah Benjamin • Harriet Benton • Fannie Berry • James Bertrand • Charlotte Beverly • Della Mun Bibles • Arrie Binns • Ank Bishop • Boston Blackwell • Adeline Blakeley • Olivier Blanchard • Patsy Jane Bland • Irena Blocker • Henry Bobbit • Rias Body • Dan Bogie • James Bolton • Siney Bonner • Frank T. Boone • J. F. Boone • W. L. Bost • Nancy Boudry • Mary Wallace Bowe • Jerry Boykins • Rivana Boynton • George Braddox • Sam Bradford • Martha Bradley • Rachel Bradley • Gus Bradshaw • Wes Brady • Mack Brantley • Francis Bridges • Frank Briles • Della Briscoe • Della Britton • Susan Broaddus • Matilda Brooks • Sylvester Brooks • Anne Broome • Casie Jones Brown • Ebenezer Brown • Fannie Brown • George Brown • Hattie Jane Brown • Henry Brown • John C. Brown • Julia Brown • Liza Brown • Mattie Brown • Peter Brown • Sally Brown • William Brown • George Washington Browning • Vinnie Brunson • Robert Bryant • Alex Bufford • Belle Buntin • Jenny Butler • Marshal Butler • Dave L. Byrd • Sarah Byrd • Jeff Calhoun • Walter Calloway • Easter Sudie Campbell • Ellen Campbell • Sallie Carder • Richard Carruthers • Cato Carter • Joseph William Carter • Belle Caruthers • Susan Castle • George Caulton • Ellen Cave • Cicely Cawthon • Amy Chapman • Lewis Chase • Henry Cheatam • Bell Childress • Jeptha Choice • Lillian Clarke • Berry Clay • Henry Clay • Florida Clayton • Maria Sutton Clements • Joe Clinton • "Aunt" Clussey • Irene Coates •

Harrison Cole • John Cole • Julia Cole • Thomas Cole • Harriet Collins •
Tildy Collins • Sara Colquitt • George Conrad • George Conrad Jr. • Peter Corn •
Laura Cornish • Mandy McCullough Cosby • John Cottonham • Sallie Crane •
Hannah Crasson • John Crawford • Charles Crawley • Charlie Crump •
Richard Crump • Zenia Culp • Green Cumby • Mattie Curtis • William Curtis •
Julia Francis Daniels • Parilee Daniels • Charlie Davenport • John Davenport •
Aus Davis • Campbell Davis • Carrie Davis • D. Davis • James Davis • Jeff Davis •
Lizzie Davis • Louisa Davis • Minnie Davis • Mose Davis • William Henry Davis •
Jake Dawkins • Anthony Dawson • Mollie Dawson • Annie Day •
James V. Deane • W. S. Debnam • Sara Debro • Joseph Hammett Dell •
Jake Desso • Lizzie Dillard • Martha Ann Dixon • Douglas Dorsey •
Fannie Dorum • Tom Douglas • Alice Douglass • Daniel Dowdy • Willie Doyld •
Silva Durant • Esther Easter • Mollie Edmonds • H. H. Edmunds •
Mary Kincheon Edwards • Katherine Eppes • Louis Evans • Millie Evans •
Sam Everett • Robert Falls • Caroline Farrow • Lewis Favor • Gus Feaster •
Archie Fennels • Lou Fergusson • Frank Fikes • Orelans Finger •
Elizabeth Finley • Ellen Fitzgerald • Reuben Fitzpatrick • Angie Floyd •
Ida May Fluker • Charlotte Foster • Della Fountain • M. Fowler • Reuben Fox •
Orelia Alexie Franks • Carrie Nancy Fryer • Minnie Fulkes • Lucy Galloway •
William Gant • Delia Garlic • Leah Garrett • Ruby Garten • Gracie Gibson •
Frank Gill • Cora Carroll Gillam • Georgina Giwbs • Will Glass •
Peter Gohagen • Candis Goodwin • Arnold Gragston • Mary Ella Grandberry •
Charles Grandy • Austin Grant • Rebecca Jane Grant • Ambus Gray •
Alice Green • Esther Green • Happy Day Green • Henry Green • Isaiah Green •
George Greene • Pauline Grice • Fannie Griffin • Madison Griffin •
Sarah Gudger • Violet Guntharpe • Josephine Hamilton • Mamie Hanbery •
Eda Harper • Caroline Johnson Harris • Dosia Harris • Eliza Harris •
Rachel Harris • Marie E. Harvey • G. W. Hawkins • Tom Hawkins •
Ann Hawthorne • Charles Hayes • Eliza Hays • Emmaline Heard • Julia Henderson •
Ida Henry • Zack Herndon • Lucretia Heyward • John Hill • Louis Hill •
Marriah Hines • Adeline Hodges • Fannie Smith Hodges • H. B. Holloway •
Eliza Holman • Rose Holman • Joseph Holmes • Rhody Holsell • Rebecca Hooks •
Moble Hopson • Pauline Howell • Charlie Hudson • Annie Huff • John Hunter •
Emma Hurley • Ida Blackshear Hutchinson • Everett Ingram • Bettie White Irby •
Mary Island • Camelia Jackson • James Jackson • Maria Jackson • Martha Jackson •
Squires Jackson • Taylor Jackson • W. P. Jacobs • Tempie James • Ophelia Jemison •
Thomas Johns • Adaline Johnson • Fanny Johnson • Lizzie Johnson •
Marion Johnson • Mary Johnson • Randolph Johnson •
William I. Johnson Jr. • Abraham Jones • Betty Jones • Bud Jones • Charity Jones •

Edward Jones • Emma Jones • Estella Jones • Hannah Jones • Harriet Jones •
Taby Jones • Wesley Jones • Abner Jordan • Lucindy Lawrence Jurdon •
Tines Kendricks • Mary Kindred • Silvia King • Nicey Kinney • Preston Kyles •
Janey Landrum • Dave Lawson • Lu Lee • William Lee • Cinto Lewis •
Dellie Lewis • George Lewis • Hagar Lewis • Henry Lewis • Talitha Lewis •
Amos Lincoln • Abbie Lindsey • Mattie Logan • Kiziah Love • James Lucas •
Edward Lycurgas • Moses Lyles • Chanie Mack • Richard Mack • Anne Maddox •
Emma Malone • Mollie Malone • Charlotte Martin • James Martin •
Ishrael Massie • Beth Mathis • Ann Matthews • Hattie Matthews •
Rachael Exelina Mayberry • Bert Mayfield • Bob Maynard • Tom McAlpin •
Amanda McDaniel • "Curley" McGade • Jake McLeod • William McWhorter •
Charlie Meadow • Frank Menefee • Rose Mercer • Josh Miles • Harriet Miller •
Richard Miller • Harriett Millett • La San Mire • Mollie Mitchell • Sam Mitchell •
Patsy Mitchner • Adaline Montgomery • Fannie Moore • Jerry Moore •
America Morgan • Isaam Morgan • Patsy Moses • Claiborne Moss •
Calvin Moye • Mack Mullen • Hannah Mullins • Horace Muse •
W. S. Needham Jr. • Sally Neely • Virginia Newman • John Ogee • Jane Osbrook •
Wade Owens • Douglas Parish • Austin Pen Parnell • George Patterson •
Mary Anne Patterson • G. W. Pattillo • Martha Patton • Ellen Payne •
Elsie Payne • Harriet McFarlin Payne • Henderson Perkins • Amy Perry •
Simon Phillips • Spear Pitman • Sarah Poindexter • Sam Polite • Nelson Polk •
W. L. Pollacks • Levi Pollard • Irene Poole • Isaac Potter • George Pretty •
Robert Prout • Harve Quales • Doc Quinn • Mary Raines • Laura Redmoun •
Mary Reynolds • Caroline Richardson • Ida Rigley • Bowser Rimes •
Walter Rimm • Cornelia Robinson • Harriet Robinson • Sister Robinson •
Henry Rogers • Parthena Rollins • Gill Ruffin • Julia Rush • Mrs. Rush •
Benjamin Russell • Elizabeth Russell • Rose Russell • Sabe Rutledge •
Susan Dale Sanders • Eliza Scantling • Anna Scott • Janie Scott • Alice Sewell •
Will Sheets • William Sherman • Edd Shirley • Ben Simpson • Allen Sims •
Marrinda Jane Singleton • Richard Slaughter • Sarah Smiley • Berry Smith •
Gus Smith • John Smith • Jordon Smith • Lou Smith • Elizabeth Sparks •
John Spencer • Walden Squire • Kittie Stanford • Rosa Starke • Sam T. Stewart •
James Henry Stith • Simon Stokes • George Strickland • Amanda Styles •
Adah Isabelle Suggs • Salena Taswell • Cora M. Taylor • Cull Taylor •
Edward Taylor • Emma Taylor • Samuel S. Taylor • Dicey Thomas •
Omelia Thomas • Rebecca Thomas • Johnson Thompson • Laura Thompson •
Mary Thompson • Laura Thornton • Emma Tidwell • Phil Town •
William Henry Towns • Unnamed • Unnamed • Unnamed • Unnamed •
Unnamed • Unnamed • Unnamed • Unnamed • Unnamed • Unnamed •

Unnamed • Unnamed • Unnamed • Unnamed • Unnamed* • Neal Upson •
Charlie Van Dyke • John F. Van Hook • Lucinda Vann • Tom Vaughn •
Addie Vinson • Gertrude Vogler • Sweetie Ivery Wagoner • Clara Walker •
Henry Walker • Irella Battle Walker • Lilah Walker • John Walton •
Annie Whitley Ware • Henry Warfield • Eliza Washington • Ella Washington •
Lucindia Washington • Steve Weathersby • Easter Wells • Mary Mays West •
William Wheeler • Eliza White • George White • Julia A. White • Mingo White •
Anderson Williams • Andy Williams • Callie Williams • Charles Williams •
Charley Williams • Charlie Williams • Daphne Williams •
John Thomas Williams • Lou Williams • Louella Williams • Mary Williams •
Nancy Williams • Rose Williams • Wayman Williams • Willis Williams •
Wash Wilson • Willis Winn • Mrs. George Womble • Maggie Woods •
Henry Wright • Dink Walton Young • Narcissus Young • Teshan Young •
Tobe Zollicoffer

---

* I have indicated the number of times I relied on information from an unidentified formerly enslaved person; it is possible that two or more of these pieces of information come from a single source.

On Sources

Say Anarcha is a comprehensively researched work of speculative non-fiction. In printed form, the almost five thousand notes and sources on which the story draws would be significantly longer than the book itself. Readers who wish to engage with the book's research—or scrutinize the author's narrative choices, in real time—are encouraged to consult a comprehensive online accounting of sources, an "illustrated bibliography" that includes traditional citations and offers direct access to primary source materials, presented in partnership with Thomas Jefferson University in Philadelphia, and available at AnarchaArchive.com.

BOOK ONE

One

The night the stars fell—Anarcha born—Westcotts come from
South Carolina—Anarcha's parents, the Westcott plantation—
Anarcha's first trace—The sky rent in half

Early in the morning of November 13, 1833, three enslaved men in Talbot County, Georgia, moving north through dense woods after escaping their master, caught a glimpse of light and motion in the sky above, through a thick canopy of leaves. The men paused—perhaps it was patrollers. Not by chance, it was a very dark night, and the men had been reckoning their passage north by feeling for moss on the trunks of trees. At first, the movement was only a few bright wisps streaking silently through the element. The men continued north for several hours. By then, the heavens seemed to have ripped open, and the stars and the planets were leaking down to Earth like pitch from a torch.

How could they not have taken it for a sign? Stars told of weather, they told of when to plant corn and cotton, and though surely there was a star strung for each of us on a silver thread, to dream of stars was bad luck, and even a single falling star signaled death. Now, hundreds of sprangles peppered the ground like hail, lighting half the world like the sparkles of a million firebugs. A hissing started up, or reports like that of a child's popgun, and sometimes there came much larger explosions as fireballs nearly as wide as the moon burst in great flashes overhead and left behind fearsome streaks of prismatic light. It was beautiful and awful. On Sundays, many slaves were subjected to sermons delivered by white preachers—*don't steal, obey your masters*—and the vision of the stars falling thick as a mist recalled snippets from Mark and Matthew about the shaking of the Kingdom of Heaven. The first star would fall when the third trumpet was blown, Revelation warned, and the fifth trumpet would signal the sweep of the dragon's tail, and a third of the host would be cast down from the sky. Isaiah too claimed that the end times would begin when rotted stars fell to Earth like sour leaves from the fig tree.

The event was witnessed across the nascent United States. In Buchanan County, Missouri, a dance frolic in a slave cabin was interrupted by a messenger who warned that those who hoped for the mansions and the bright lights of Fellom City should say their prayers now, because the whole world was about to be crisped like cracklings. In Texas, a revival meeting had just reached the fever pitch of raining brimstone when a star shot from its place like a skyrocket, and then another came loose, and another, until the whole of the yonder zigzagged with trickles the color of fish blood. Most of those watching understood that the stars burned up in the sky, but some claimed that they burst only twelve feet from the ground, or hit barns to set fire to chaff and straw, or covered fields like a sheet, or like snow. In the ensuing weeks, there were reports of odd substances discovered: material like hot egg whites, lumps of soft soap, or boiled starch that evaporated when you put flame to it. It was recalled that an inflamed paste had fallen on Armenia in the year 1810, and that viscous matter had descended from the sky in India and Lusatia in the eighteenth century.

A soldier in Washington's army once witnessed a star fall and came upon the gelatinous mass as it was still sparkling.

In the Georgia forest, one of the three escaped men fainted in fear. His companions did not leave him. They carried him back to their master and none of them ever attempted to escape again.

The meteor storm of 1833, by dint of its peculiar intensity, inaugurated a fifty-year-long public obsession with comets and falling stars. News of the event, registering as far away as Europe, was joyously florid. Stories claimed that the blue cope of the beyond rained down a thick shower of flame, the breadth of the firmament shifting with phosphoric lines and luminous bodies. Rushing balls of liquid fire trailed festooned tails that bathed the land below in a mellow glow. The heights of the azure sprinkled dashes of light like a shower driven against a windowpane. Larger projectiles came shooting out of the zenith, firing down the concave sky to lose themselves against the dark expanse. Woodcut illustrations printed in the following days depicted the event as a firework as broad as the sky was wide, an umbrella of shooting stars, a portentous bouquet of light.

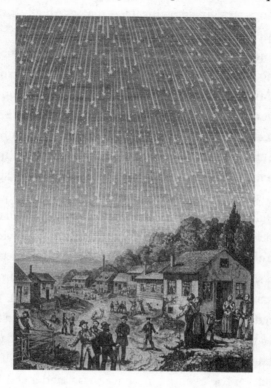

For astronomers, the event was as remarkable for the hints it offered about the cosmos as it was for the dual response it elicited in the public: admiration and delight in some, astonishment and fear in others. Telescopes directed toward the spot from which the phenomenon seemed to emanate—near the star Algieba, in the sickle-shaped neck of the constellation Leo—revealed nothing apart from the fact that the center of the storm was rotating along with the slow whirl of the celestial sphere. The science of astronomy, it was admitted, could not yet explain why the event appeared as falling stars at all. Some argued that it was matter ejected from volcanoes on the moon. Others claimed it was the ignition of gaseous matter in the atmosphere, as mysterious as the will-o'-the-wisp. The widespread discovery afterward of gluey substances—star jelly—seemed to confirm a commonly held belief that comets were transparent gelatin because actual stars could be glimpsed telescopically through their tails. Several astronomers proved susceptible to the pull of prophetic imagery: a particular meteor aimed at the star Capella was described as leaving behind it a long, straight, glowing trail that gradually twisted into the shape of a serpent drawing itself up in the sky.

Even without the falling stars it had been an auspicious night, cosmically speaking, with Orion and the dog stars Sirius and Procyon rising in the southwest, and Saturn and Jupiter shining wondrously in the southeast. The event began at around 2:00 a.m. and ended with the light of dawn. One observer counted 8,660 meteors in fifteen minutes, and later estimates put the display at a total of more than 200,000 falling stars over a period of several hours. In many places, the event was surreally silent. Some smelled sulfur, others onions. In certain counties it rained, leading to the conclusion that while stars lay in the devil's jurisdiction, God had intervened to spare the world from flame. Most could cite no such salvation, and the shrieks and prayers of enslaved families—some wryly remarked that slaves fell to their knees just as the stars had come tumbling down—woke their white masters. On one plantation in Tennessee, the master gathered his slaves together and began telling them who their true mothers and fathers were, and to whom their relatives had been sold— you see, the master too believed it was Judgment Day.

The intensity of the event in Alabama was evidenced by the release, one hundred years later, of "Stars Fell on Alabama," a jazz standard first recorded by Guy Lombardo and since covered by Billie Holiday, Frank Sinatra, Louis Armstrong, and many others. A book was published at the same time the song was released, *Stars Fell on Alabama*: a fancifully ethnographic account of the state's quirky subcultures, by Harvard-trained writer and temporary Alabama resident Carl Carmer. In 1984, future *New York Times* editor and Alabama native Howell Raines praised Carmer for his central image, even though Carmer had spent little time describing the night the stars fell. Until 2009, Alabama drivers could purchase "Stars Fell on Alabama" license plates.

* * *

Anarcha was born on the Westcott plantation in Montgomery, Alabama. In 1833, she was seven years old, perhaps a year or two younger or older—not many slaves knew their own age, and often they were told it was none of their business. In time, the falling stars would come to serve as a chronological reference point. Families would recall that a man was already a grandfather at the time the stars fell, or that a boy had achieved a good size when folks thought the world was ending, or that a girl had been born that very day, or just after it, so even though she didn't see the stars falling she could claim as provenance a moment that embodied the strangerest days of slavery times, when there were far more stars in Heaven than there had ever been since.

It's possible that Anarcha spent her earliest years in her mistress's house. But if she didn't, then her first glimpse of the falling stars was through cracks in the roof of her family's cabin, which at night appeared as blue splinters wide enough to permit her to count the stars as she lay on her tick mattress and drifted off to sleep. That night, the flashes overhead were bright enough to wake the sleeping. Alternately, one of her brothers—Manuel or Ben, but not Joe, Joe was too young, only five or six—was sent to feed the sorrel horses and the bay steed when they were heard to be stirring, and Manuel or Ben came running back into the cabin, waking everyone and asking their mother, Sue, if the stars would climb back into the sky.

Anarcha left her first trace in the estate inventory of her first owner, David Westcott, who died in 1828. Westcott had been born in 1760, near Charleston, one of five children and two sons, and he remained unmarried until well after his father died, leaving the family saddled with a twenty-one-year lease to build and operate a toll road over a swamp. What but the road and three sisters kept Westcott in South Carolina? He was past fifty when he traveled to Goose Creek, just north of Charleston, and met Eliza Railey, an Irish maiden with a thick brogue. He began to concoct a plan to venture west and chart his own future. He first went to Alabama after the toll road lease expired, when statehood was a plan but not a certainty. Published pamphlets bragged of the Alabama territory's navigable rivers, which enabled commercial intercourse, and of the green seed cotton that grew in the north and the black seed cotton that grew in the south. In 1818, annual bale production stood at fifty thousand, with the potential for five, six, or ten times as much! The Louisiana Purchase of 1803 had made necessary the construction of a federal road from Washington City to New Orleans, and eight years later a treaty was signed to permit white settlers to open inns along the parts of the road that ran through the Creek Nation, smack in the middle of the Alabama territory. These Indians were not nearly so plentiful as had been made out, the pamphlets claimed. At best, ten thousand of them controlled eight million acres, and the most warlike among them had been "pacified" a few years prior. Even now, one pamphlet promised, amalgamation was in the process of succeeding where the missionary system had failed. The fate of the Creeks was the destiny of all savage tribes amid civilization: total annihilation.

David Westcott headed farther west, to New Philadelphia, a village four miles south of Fort Jackson with a few hotels and a slave market. It promised to become a sizable town and would serve as the territory's seat of justice. He bought slaves and the first of what would be many tracts of land, and hired an overseer to begin the process of establishing a cotton plantation. He returned to Charleston and married Eliza on March 13, 1817. He was fifty-six. Eliza was sixteen. Their son Samuel was born in 1819, the same year Alabama became a state. Westcott sold his final two hundred acres and left South Carolina for good. By then, New Philadelphia had combined with two other villages and taken a new name: Montgomery.

Eliza was eighteen and pregnant again when they joined a thick caravan of sulkies, carts, and Jersey wagons, all trailing long lines of slaves, the vacant countenances of the most degraded among them contrasting with the rare slave couple that walked arm in arm, flowers in the girl's hair. All but the occasional failed pioneer were headed west, lured by the promise of black earth and profits. Congress had allocated $10,000 to road improvement projects in the new territory, but in many cases the topographical engineers who had been tasked with improving what had formerly been animal paths had limited their work to carving blaze marks onto trees so at least you knew you were headed in the right direction. Food was plentiful at inns: turnip soup, bacon, roast beef, turkey, and chicken, with sweet potatoes. But beyond the region of bread—heading west from Columbus, Georgia, was like leaving the known world—the diet turned to eggs, broiled venison, and cakes of Indian corn.

The Creeks were called Creeks because of creeks, as many as fifty of them over seventy miles, with steep banks of slick red clay. Mud rose halfway to the axles of the carts and wagons, and left horses and oxen as uncertain of how to take the next step as of how they should extricate themselves from the last. One mile of corduroy road over swampland—boards and logs laid across the mud, sometimes partly or entirely submerged—was like twenty miles of decent travel.

Trees towered primordially in the west, oaks and nut-bearing hickories, their trunks dividing close to the ground and climbing hundreds of feet into the air. Even magnolias soared over sixty-five feet. Of the shrubs that competed for sunlight, there were stands of woodbine, jessamine, buckeye, bay laurel, and crow poison. Deer took shelter in stands of bamboo and fed on grasses that grew twenty feet high in spots. There was iris and wild rose and giant hydrangea, and in clearings ground flowers grew so thick the earth looked upholstered with satin. Hateful Spanish moss dripped off of everything.

The Creeks kept slaves, too, and from the road, travelers might spot an enslaved woman skinning an otter next to a rawhide tent, or glimpse a warrior with a blade of hair standing atop a shorn skull like the plume of a centurion's helmet. Voyagers sometimes ventured off to witness the violent games the Creeks played in broad, cleared fields, but mostly the Indians remained out of sight, their fires shining through the black walls of the forest at night. The wagons continued on, step by step, in lantern light. Here and there, a blacksmith, a tavern, and a few log huts constituted a village, but often twenty miles passed with nothing more than a house that doubled as a drapery or grocery. Finally, the pioneers came upon the alien sight of the columnar edifice of a refined plantation house, and not long after that the town of Mount Meigs, with a post office and pleasant homes shaded by chinaberry trees. The federal road veered south from there, but some miles farther on was Montgomery, a metropolis of more than six thousand souls.

It's possible that Anarcha's parents, Jerry and Sue, having been gifted to the Westcotts as a traditional wedding present, traveled with them from South Carolina, Manuel suckling at one of Sue's breasts and Samuel Westcott at the other, as the wagon wheels strained through the road's deep runnels. For most of the way, Jerry and the other men pushed from behind, David Westcott stepping down to walk whenever the road climbed uphill. Eliza remained in the leather chair that her husband had fitted into the wagon to ease her mobile confinement. They arrived in Montgomery in 1820, a slave-built house having been made ready for David Westcott's young bride.

Additional slaves were purchased on the auction block in Montgomery, or from drivers who traveled through Alabama at the end of every December, their product of chained and freezing men and women shuffling forward like turkeys, sold door-to-door alongside mules and horses. The Westcotts' slaves cleared land, planted corn and cotton, burned brush, killed hogs, split rails for fences, and added onto the quarters for additional slaves who were purchased with loans secured by the collateral of themselves. The cabins formed a semicircle, all their doors visible from the Westcott porch. They had no window that was wide enough to put more than your head through.

The women were mostly kept pregnant—it was another thing the plantation grew, and that was why the children of *negro slaves* slaves were called their increase. There came to be several enslaved families on *and their increase* the Westcott plantation, Robbin and Lucinda, who had Rachel, Anna, George, and Jacob, and Bet whose husband died who had Mary and Isham and Minden and Charles, and Jerry and Sue who, after Manuel, added another Mary and Ben and Anarcha and Joe. There was Frank and Notice, who could have no children, and Tom and Ann, who could have no children, and there were others, Jonas and Silvey and Edy and Fran, and beyond the work in the fields there was the work of the spinning wheels, and the cotton gins, and the beehives that David Westcott could buy on credit because now he grew cotton, and cotton was king.

Eliza Westcott, who would soon be Anarcha's second owner, established a meetinghouse on their property for a Methodist congregation in 1821. That same year, she gave birth to the second Westcott child, William. For the house, she ordered rosewood furniture from New Orleans, bought a carriage for trips into town, and purchased from shops—on credit against the harvest, always on credit—mahogany sofa tables, and maple chairs, and cherry bedsteads, and featherbeds and washstands and wardrobes and bureaus. Eliza established a nursery for children, white and black alike, and she kept having more children herself: David Jr., who died in 1824, the same year he was born, and then Priscilla, and then Susannah. Eliza was twenty-seven years old, with four children under ten, when David Westcott died at sixty-eight years of age. She would never remarry, and David Westcott left behind no will to indicate how his possessions should be divided.

They had said, those pamphlets, that Alabama would be the most healthful state in the union. It was a lie. There were chills everywhere, yellow fever and typhoid and malaria. Dr. Hugh Henry, of Montgomery—there were already several doctors in town—was sent for when David Westcott fell ill, but the powder he prescribed did no good, and neither did the bleeding, and when David died Eliza had no idea how many acres she now owned. She became administratrix, and the court assigned a clerk to visit the plantation to count everything: the fifty-four sheep, the stock of hogs, the twenty-four cattle, the six hundred pounds of bacon, and the 250 bushels of corn, just harvested. In addition, there were monies that David Westcott had been owed—the note on James Pritchard for $3.75, the note on Josiah Palmer for $38.62½, and the note on Edward Mills for $400.00, which would be satisfied with the work of a slave named James. There were also the monies he owed, often to the same people, these debts paid off with the sale of bedsteads, a shotgun, a gold watch that was worth $100.00 but brought only $91.00, sheep that went for five head for $8.75, and yoke oxen that sold for as much as $28.50. Last, the clerks of court went cabin to cabin in the slave quarters, counting the heads on the Westcott plantation in 1828, not bothering with ages. This was how Anarcha left her first trace in the world, as the fourth of five children of a family whose valuation amounted to more than fifteen percent of the total Westcott wealth.

> *1 Negro Man Gerry and his Wife Sue, and their Children Manuel, Mary, Ben, Anaka and Joe —————— 1500 00*

Anarcha spent her first three years in the nursery. She knew her mother only because Sue arrived in the mornings and afternoons from the fields, to let her daughter suck. The mothers came at ten o'clock and two o'clock, sometimes stopping at the cabins on the way back to the fields for hoecakes for the men. During the cotton harvest, women were required to pick two hundred pounds per day, and men were required to pick three hundred pounds per day, but some among them could pick two rows at once, as many as five hundred pounds in a single day. They worked from sun to sun, from can to can't, woken in the morning by the horn of the overseer, or the slave driver, and the horn might be blown again throughout the day, as a signal of distressing news, to warn of rain, or in patterns that called certain slaves to the house. At the end of the day the cotton was weighed by candlelight, and those who hadn't picked enough continued on in the light of a burning pine knot.

Children were not sent to the fields until they were approximately ten years of age, but they were put to work caring for children younger than they were as soon as they were large enough to pick them up. Anarcha was neither tall nor portly, but she began helping in the nursery not long after David Westcott died. She was too young to remember it, but the horn blew wild that day, and all worked stopped and remained stopped for some time, and afterward another overseer was hired, and more slaves were purchased, as more hands were needed to make the plantation function. Anarcha helped care for her brother Joe, and for the missus's daughter Susannah, rocking her cradle when she was crying, and sometimes it was her job to be a playmate for the missus's other daughter, Priscilla, or to keep flies off the missus with a fan made of turkey feathers sewed onto a cane. Children had a variety of jobs: minding the crows off the corn with paddles, or keeping the cattle from wandering too far off because there were bears in the woods, or gathering pokeberries for dying clothes, or collecting chestnuts and walnuts that the missus put into sacks and sold, or hunting hens' eggs or turkey eggs, and you got a tea cake for every turkey nest you found. At night, Anarcha fanned the little missuses with a mulberry branch until they fell asleep—you could feed mulberry leaves to silkworms, also from the woods—and then she walked back to the quarters, where she climbed in beside her sister Mary on a trundle bed that pulled out from under her mother's one-footed bunk, nailed to two walls in a corner of the cabin. Her tick was stuffed with straw that was changed every summer, or with moss that you could use as long as you scalded it and buried it for a long time beforehand. She had a pillow stuffed with chicken feathers gathered one by one from the yard. On clear nights, she fell asleep with the stars shimmering through the splintered ceiling.

Conditions in Alabama were perfect for celestial observation on the night of November 13, 1833—little wind and no clouds, cool and the stars shining with uncommon brilliancy. Local newspapers regaled readers with the nocturnal grandeur of celestial bodies sparking across the firmament. Alabama was one of those places where it was also said that a fetid and fleshy matter fell from the sky. Unique to the state was a belief that the falling stars had carved great cracks in the floor of the forests that made escape from plantations treacherous.

Anarcha woke near three o'clock to the flashes overhead, or to her brothers returning from the stables where the horses were running wild, and the Westcott slaves gathered in the horseshoe-shaped yard among their cabins. At first, the young boys—Anarcha's brothers, and George and Jacob and Minden, and others who had come since—were chided by the adults for darting about to try to catch the falling stars. It was only the children who weren't afraid. Pigs raced and chortled in their pens, and chickens ran headlong through the yard and broke their necks on fence rails. Some of the adults took to their knees in case this was the end.

The Westcotts joined their slaves outside. Eliza was now thirty-two. She had survived the death of her husband and a son, and she would manage the plantation until Samuel and William, now fourteen and twelve, came of age. She believed God was giving her strength. In 1829, she helped organize Methodists in Montgomery, first forming an association, and they were now acquiring full possession of a church downtown. Wouldn't she too have suspected that the show of meteors was the wandering stars of Jude, the trampled host of Daniel?

Anarcha saw the sky rent in half that night. At seven, or five, or nine, she was a child but nursed the new babies and children as they appeared, though she did not know where they came from. An old slave, Pheriba, had been purchased for $175 to give medicines and catch babies. The missus called her Doctor Woman. But when the children asked Pheriba where babies came from, all the old woman would say was that she found them in the woods. They hid inside stumps, or in the hollows of trees. The children hunted for babies, but all they ever found, once, was a sleeping fawn left behind by its mother. Pheriba told them they didn't dig deep enough. That's when Anarcha knew it wasn't true. Likewise, on the night her elders were fooled by a false apocalypse, Anarcha knew the stars weren't falling because you could see some of them, behind the others, fixed and shining in their regular places. Still, on that night, she witnessed the burning meteors leaking down to Earth. She stood beneath a hole opened in the vault of Heaven, under a mute rainfall of light.

Two

SIMS WAS WORKING IN THE DEADHOUSE AGAIN, ALONE, AT NIGHT. IT WAS 1834, he'd recently turned twenty-one years old, and he was near to completing his second term of courses at the Medical College of South Carolina in Charleston. The single candle he'd brought for light was resting on the still stomach of a cadaver he'd taken note of earlier in the day. There was something odd about the specimen's tracheal artery. After lectures and dinner, he'd told the dissecting room supervisor not to wait for him and set to tracing out the vessel's peculiar distribution. It was March, and it was cold, but Sims worked well into the night, occasionally looking up from the corpse's flayed neck. The candle and the moonlight seeping in through the open windows and louvers rendered the bodies spread throughout the room down to shapeless outlines, like dormant ghouls. At one moment, Sims slipped and knocked his candle to the floor. The room went completely dark.

The dissection chamber stretched off the college's main building on Queen Street, semidetached to offer the various departments respite from the effluvia rising from the bodies. Above the classrooms was a museum collection of wax anatomical figures from Florence, on display with a range of morbid specimens bobbing in sealed bottles of spirits. As well, the school had recently acquired one of French doctor Louis Auzoux's famous dissectable manikins. It had elastic ligaments, and parts fashioned from cork and clay, and obstetrics professor Thomas Prioleau was fond of using it in his lectures to demonstrate craniotomy, embryotomy, cesarean section, and the various ways that enthused doctors could cause injuries during birth emergencies. Sims had little interest in birth emergencies, and he mostly avoided Prioleau's class. What could Auzoux's papier-mâché tell you about how the parts of the body moved, or what it felt like to put a blade to them?

For that, you needed flesh. You needed mettle too, for the atmosphere of the deadhouse, for the smell and the presence of the bodies at night. They were all slaves, the bodies, most of them decapitated, the heads having been removed to the phrenological collection. Charleston had long been a seat of medical innovation, but until recently it had not been a place of medical education. There was no school such as could be had in Philadelphia, and in fact several of the professors in Charleston had studied at the University of Pennsylvania with Benjamin Rush himself. After two decades of discussion, the Medical College of South Carolina had launched in 1824 as partner and counterpart to Philadelphia, and a good part of its appeal was a steady supply of anatomical material. Doctors all over the world struggled for clinical research subjects; some were reduced to grave robbing, and worse. South Carolina boasted of plentiful specimens acquired at far less expense than at any other institution in the country.

Sims had forgotten his matches. At an instant, in the room's chill and dark, he recalled the story of another student working late in the same dead room, two years before, having rigged a body upright to practice on an inguinal hernia. The rigging was precarious, and when the student jostled the specimen's leg by mistake, the body was yanked from its perch by its own weight. It fell on top of him. Sims imagined that he would have let the corpse fall to the floor, but in fact the student caught the body and calmly replaced it on the table.

That was what was needed, Sims thought. Mettle. Throughout his life, Sims spoke and wrote grandiloquently of the masculine resolve exhibited by true men, of the courage that was the defining characteristic of the male sphere. Surely, Sims thought of his night in the deadhouse as an opportunity to exhibit a dose of manliness that he had been heretofore lacking. Stories he'd been told when he was young had left him with a fear of mad dogs and runaway slaves in the woods. There were headless ghosts in the woods too, herds of headless horses and cows, headless men who sauntered by and brushed your elbow, and headless women who lingered in black mourning dresses. Even though Sims knew that stories of spirits were often nothing more than masters dressing up to frighten their slaves, the visions scared him. In the dark dissecting room, as he threaded his way through the row of headless bodies, he screwed up his courage and found the exit in the dark.

* * *

James Marion Sims was born in 1813, in the home of his mother's parents, bordering a huckleberry swamp near Heath Springs, South Carolina, a place once famous for an intensely cold mineral spring that bubbled up through clear sand and was said to cure constipation. Sims was named for the Swamp Fox, Francis Marion, the South Carolina general of the Revolution who in the Cherokee War of 1759 followed orders to raze native communities. Promoted during the rebellion and tasked with harassing the British in the South, Marion pioneered guerilla warfare, executed slaves found to be assisting the enemy, and is today credited as a forefather to the US Army Rangers and the Green Berets.

In 1780, the British dispatched Colonel Banastre Tarleton to dispose of Marion. Tarleton failed, and thereafter he camped near Hanging Rock Creek, two and a half miles from Heath Springs and the home of Sims's grandparents. Sims's grandfather was arrested as a spy and sentenced to death, and as a boy Sims heard many times over the story of how his grandmother, pregnant with child, sneaked into the British camp to confront Tarleton, on the ruse of selling fruit and eggs. If her husband was to be executed, she proclaimed, then she too should be executed, along with their child. Tarleton relented. Four months later, General Cornwallis surrendered at Yorktown.

Sims's father, John Sims, was also descended from Revolutionary stock, his grandfather having witnessed Braddock's defeat near Pittsburgh. John Sims fought briefly in the War of 1812 and later organized a local militia, but he never settled on a particular career, bouncing from sheriff to store owner to tavern and hotel operator, acquiring along the way a reputation as a handsome rapscallion with a too-strong affinity for cockfighting and billiards. Sims was the oldest of his mother's seven children. He was often left in the care of cruel schoolteachers, and when his father wished to move a dozen miles north, to the city of Lancaster, Sims and his siblings were left behind for a time with an overseer and the few slaves his father had managed to acquire.

In their parents' absence, Sims and his siblings saved their sixpences to pay a slave named Cudjo to visit their home on Saturday nights. Born in Africa, Cudjo was barely four feet tall, but he had a remarkable physique and a tattooed face, and he earned his fees with horrific ghost stories of witch doctors and cannibals and human sacrifice. Where could Sims's fears have come from, he would later recall, if not from the poisonous imagery of tales that were punctuated by the storyteller's fire eating and by the frightening knocks that he applied to his own head with a stick?

In Lancaster, at age eleven, Sims caught a glimpse of a daughter of Dr. Bartlett Jones, perhaps the most important man in town. He promptly fell in love. Theresa Jones was eight years old. It was said that her grandmother had been the first sweetheart of local son Andrew Jackson, who'd been robbed of the presidency in 1824 by Yankee chicanery. Could a girl of such quality ever return the affections of a boy of such humble origins?

Sims's father had fallen into debt to Dr. Jones. John Sims had overexerted himself to win a fox-hunting wager and contracted pneumonia. The cost of the treatment and the supplies that the Sims family purchased from Dr. Jones—he operated a dry goods business, in addition to his medical practice—meant that the only time Sims ever saw Theresa Jones was when he was sent as an errand boy to pay off his father's debts.

Dr. Jones was a renowned surgeon. He too had attended medical school in Philadelphia, and carried on a wide practice, riding a jig to appointments from Salisbury to Camden, a range of more than a hundred miles, always accompanied by a black boy named Cupid. The Jones family owned many slaves—more than forty—and it was said that Dr. Jones could bring men back to life, disembowel them and put them back together again. His name was preserved in medical books for having twice successfully removed stones from men's bladders, and he had restored vision to many who had been blinded for years by cataracts. It seemed foolhardy to hope that a man who was practically a saint would permit his daughter to marry a boy whose only ambition to date was to work at Stringfellow's store for three hundred dollars per year.

Worse, the women of the Jones household were known to marry well. Theresa's mother had once encouraged one of her daughters' friends to glimpse, through a parlor-door keyhole, the larger-than-life figure of General James Blair, who had arrived to visit with Dr. Jones. Blair was six foot seven and weighed 350 pounds but was wholly muscular, a man of true physical prowess. He wasn't a real general—though he'd distinguished himself in 1812—but he was a real congressman, having served a term in the Seventeenth Congress in 1821, and he would be elected again in 1828. Entranced by his bulk and his power, the girl who spied him through a keyhole declared at once that she would marry him. In fact, she did.

Blair was one of the day's great duelists, once shattering a newspaperman's arm over an untoward comment published during an election season. Sims had met Blair himself when the huge man stopped by the Sims family home on his way to settle another dispute with a politician who had publicly rebuked him. Despite the imminent confrontation, Blair took note of the Sims family's eldest son, and he later arranged for James Marion Sims to be offered a spot at West Point, so that Sims could carry on the military legacy of his namesake. However, Sims was small for his age—tiny, even—and not in particularly good health. He declined the offer.

For his part, Sims was as awed by the "Waxhaw Giant" as the girl who married him. That was the problem—for what could his chances be with Theresa Jones if women of the Jones household could so easily pluck their mates from among the ranks of warriors and politicians, men destined to be honored with likenesses in marble and bronze?

Sims and Theresa both attended Franklin Academy, a school in Lancaster cofounded by Dr. Jones. The girls studied downstairs, separate from the boys, but there was ample opportunity for Sims to take measure of his love. Despite the boys who gave Theresa their attentions as she grew into young womanhood, she seemed fond enough of him. Still, he was afraid to announce his feelings.

In his quick visits to the Jones home, Sims stole glances at Dr. Jones's library of Greek and Latin texts. The physician made a hobby of the study of classical poets in their original tongues. It seemed an act of providence, then, when Franklin Academy hired an instructor who looked and talked as though he had stepped straight from the world of Dr. Jones's books. J. F. G. Mittag was the first teacher to recognize in Sims anything other than a predilection for mediocrity. And as with Sims himself, the contrast that Mittag offered to men like General Blair could not have been more perfectly devised.

Mittag spoke nine languages, including French, Greek, and Assyrian, and he knew the sixteen sacred maxims of the Chinese empire. He was a trained phrenologist, a licensed attorney, and a prolific portraitist. Yet for all this he was a financial failure, reduced to teaching at Sims's school. The practical inhabitants of Lancaster failed to appreciate Mittag's classical intellect, and publicly he was regarded as a coward because he rejected the chivalric sentiment of the day. The man was lonely, and perhaps this was why he took a liking to Sims, a boy as unremarkable as he was diminutive, and who was completely uncertain of what he should do with his life.

As Sims ascended through puberty, Mittag became more confidant than teacher. Sims confessed to his mentor that he was afraid of manhood. He feared the rough world and worried that he lacked the intellect and resolve that would be required of him when he was pitted against the opposition that surely awaited him there. Sims's father wanted him to be a lawyer; his mother thought him suited to the study of divinity. The boy wanted neither, but he had no ideas of his own. In this, Mittag was a peculiar role model, in that he was a dreamer who dabbled in everything. He'd advocated for a railroad that would stretch from the Bering Strait to Cape Horn, and he'd imagined a device based on the properties of the newly discovered element selenium that would permit the transmission of images across great distances. Voices could be sent abroad as well, he said, via electricity, and he was sure that men would one day fly because our nighttime dreams told us it was possible. True men of vision, Mittag told Sims, were never appreciated in their lifetime. Hence, a man should be concerned less with honor in his own day than with the honor of posterity. Write books that tell your story, he advised, and put your name to inventions that will create the world of the future.

Sims was grateful for Mittag's kindness, but anyone could tell he was a bit of a crank. Mittag helped him write his Greek lessons and encouraged him to further his studies, but when Sims decided to attend South Carolina College, in Columbia, it was due less to Mittag's prodding or to any desire to please his parents than to Theresa's decision to attend a high school for young ladies in Barhamville, a mile past the Columbia lunatic asylum. On Sims's last visit to the Jones house before heading to college, Theresa's mother made a point of showing him a snuff box that Theresa's grandmother had received as a gift from the White House. Justice had been restored with Andrew Jackson's election in 1828, and one of the first things the president did from the Oval Office was write a note to his old love. Theresa's mother's motive in sharing the snuff box couldn't be clearer: Sims, she wanted him to know, was neither monied nor well-bred enough for her daughter.

* * *

South Carolina College's Steward's Hall suffered from bad everything— bad bread, bad butter, bad meat and eggs—and not long after classes started, Sims and a dozen or so of his classmates left their assigned rooms and moved uptown to board close to Isaac Lyons's oyster saloon, where over the course of two years Sims ran up a tab of $200. He weighed 108 pounds when he went to college. He didn't swear, gamble, or drink. Attempts to acquire the last of these skills confirmed that he had a weak liver, and on one occasion just two tablespoons of Madeira wine left him stumbling back to the boardinghouse. Six months into his studies, desperate for home, Sims arranged for a friend to answer roll call for him at prayers. He fled to Lancaster and told his mother that he wished to become a merchant's clerk after all. His mother would be dead within a year, of bilious fever, but she was still strong enough then to tell her son he was a fool and send him back to school.

Sims's housemates played pranks on one another at home, the worst of these resulting in confrontations and accusations, and even Sims once came close to demanding satisfaction with pistols. The Pedee brothers taught Sims and a few others to play whist, and games were held twice or thrice weekly, some of the young men learning to cheat by covertly communicating instructions to their partners with creative recitals of nonsense quatrains. In classes, Sims was undistinguished. His professors were old and equally uninspired, and Sims spent much of his time doodling his name in textbooks that were filled with the notes and signatures of the students to whom the books had previously been assigned.

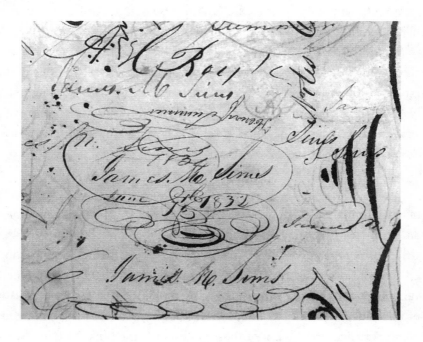

He made sure to see Theresa occasionally, if only to remind her that he existed. She had grown into a beautiful young woman, now even less likely to return his love. His feelings for her never wavered. He made friends, Dick Baker and Hamilton Boykin and James Thornwell, who was studying law and who was small and frail like Sims but shined in the debates of the Euphradian Society. Sims was a listless member of the group. Once, he watched Thornwell expertly dispense with an opponent in an exchange over the slavery question. Slaveholding states were being unfairly maligned as cruel, Thornwell argued. Slavery was simply honest capitalism that offered fine training for the future service we all would perform for the master of the hereafter. Slaves might be degraded in life, yes, but were they not realizing the limited potential God had given them, and thus being provided with a proper fitting to shine as stars in the firmament of eternity?

Greatest among Sims's college friends was Rufus Nott. "Rufe" knew of Sims's longing for Theresa, and one night in May 1831 he proposed that a number of the housemates sneak out to Barhamville to give the girls of Theresa's school a hellish serenade with toy trumpets and drums. The school's superintendent met the ruckus with a shotgun. Rufe suffered two bits of bird shot in his forehead, and another that he gnawed out of his upper lip.

Rufe was following his brothers on the physician's path. Altogether, five Nott brothers would become physicians, and a sister would marry one. As it happened, the most successful of the brothers, Josiah Nott, attended to another bit of gunplay that occurred during Sims's college years. Shortly after graduation, two of Sims's friends—both fine young students, tall and handsome—took to feuding over a dinner plate of trout. Grave words were exchanged, but honor was preserved with a solemn challenge issued in writing. Prominent Columbia citizens were secured as seconds and advisers. Josiah Nott was chosen as surgeon for a duel that would be fought on May 29, 1833, at Lightwood Knot Springs, ten miles northeast of Columbia.

Sims was impressed by the older Nott brother. He had attended South Carolina College in 1822 and then taken up the study of medicine, first in New York, then in Philadelphia. He was now working with a partner to open a medical school in Columbia. He hoped to offer public lectures in anatomy and surgery. In this, however, Nott was pitted against the president of South Carolina College, who had been instrumental in the formation of the new medical school in Charleston. If Nott's new school did not succeed, he'd said, he would further his studies in Paris and then perhaps move to Mobile, in the new state of Alabama. In Philadelphia, Nott had worked alongside a promising young Mobile physician named Henry LeVert, whose medical school thesis on sutures made from silver, lead, and gold—mysteriously, metal wire produced less infection in animal trials—had earned him publication in a respected journal immediately upon graduation. LeVert had told Nott that the streaming hordes of South Carolinians relocating to Alabama made it an excellent business proposition for a physician. LeVert planned to open a hospital there, and he believed it would be extremely lucrative.

Additionally, Nott was a champion of the recently articulated theory of polygenesis. There was not one Adam and Eve, he said, but many. How else to explain the vast gulf between whites, who were responsible for civilization, and the dark races that were doomed to extinction? Beyond economic opportunity, Henry LeVert had offered Nott vivid descriptions of the plentiful races to be found in Mobile. Not only did the licentiousness of black girls enable white women to retain their virtue, there was an endless supply of ethnographic stock—white, black, red, and many mixtures in between. Mobile would provide Nott with the opportunity to pursue theories he had about the physical, moral, and intellectual differences among the types of mankind.

The duel was fought at ten paces, which sealed its outcome. One of the young men was shot through the abdomen and lingered barely twenty-eight hours before expiring in great pain. The other was hit in the right thigh. The ball entered four inches below the lower trochanter—a knob where the muscle grabbed the bone—and came out two inches below the groin. The young man's thigh doubled in size as blood accumulated inside the leg. Luckily, the femoral artery remained intact. Nott had the young man carried ten miles back into town, but he did not set the bone for almost two weeks for fear of rupturing the artery. Then he had a stroke of genius. He modified a second double-inclined plane for the student's sound leg, to keep his pelvis square as he healed. This worked perfectly, and the young man was up on crutches by July 31 and left town a few weeks later. Nott would publish on the case and begin to make his name.

* * *

Sims graduated and in December 1832 returned home, where his father was now a widower with seven children. For a month, lovesick for Theresa, Sims took no steps at all toward advancing the course of his life. At last, his father demanded that he visit Mr. Howard to begin an apprenticeship in the law. Sims refused. He had, in fact, come to a decision about his future, but he had done so by default rather than inclination. If he must choose a path worthy of a college graduate, he told his father, it was clear that as a man of neither stature nor position, he was better suited to a career as a doctor than as a lawyer.

His father raged. What honor or reputation, he cried, was there to be found in jouncing around the countryside, a box of pills in one hand and a squirt in the other? It did not need to be stated aloud that John Sims had never dug himself clear of the debts he owed to the most famous doctor in Lancaster. Bartlett Jones had died a year earlier, months after performing yet another heroic operation, and he'd had himself buried in grandiose fashion: fully clothed, on a bed, without a coffin. The man was dead and gone—nevertheless, Sims's father snarled at the suggestion that his son would pursue the profession of the dead father of the girl he loved. There was no science in medicine, John Sims insisted. His son offered nothing by way of response—he wasn't sure his father was wrong—but he held steadfast until his father suggested that he visit Dr. Churchill Jones, Theresa's uncle, the only remaining physician in town.

Churchill Jones was called Dr. Church to avoid confusion with his better-liked brother, and though a fondness for drink often left him unfit for his duties, Sims was impressed by the high regard that his skills as a surgeon inspired in the surrounding country. Dr. Church was no teacher, and he had no medical books of his own, but Sims found himself drawn to the tools of the trade. The surprisingly heavy amputation saw with a ring for your finger like the trigger of a gun. The raspatory like the sharpened mallet of a dark knight. The curved bistoury that folded like a pocketknife and which you could pinch with the very ends of your fingers. And the blunt curettes with handles of bone or ivory. All of them were engraved with the initials of the smiths who had fashioned them, and some of them were named for the doctors who had invented them.

Fixed now to a path, Sims set to absorbing what texts on anatomy and practice he could find on his own. The months of study in Dr. Church's office were dull and trying—without instruction, the medical books were incomprehensible—but the opportunity to observe Dr. Church performing operations verified that surgery, if not the drudgery of a physician's daily rounds, offered a chance for distinction and prestige. Sims had begun to suspect that J. F. G. Mittag was right about dueling: it was a waste of important lives. Yet Josiah Nott's role in the duel at Lightwood Knot Springs had stayed with him. It seemed that a surgeon could make a career of preserving and protecting the lives of honorable men while simultaneously acquiring a bit of honor for himself. More to the point, perhaps a man who was neither physically distinguished nor markedly capable with words could use a career in medicine to earn the affections of a girl like Theresa Jones.

To that end, several months after beginning work in Dr. Church's office, Sims crafted a letter to Theresa. He had loved her since they were both children, he wrote. He was still young, and he was poor, it was true, but now his life now had trajectory and promise. Were his feelings returned? If so, he should like to have the chance to speak with her very soon about an important matter.

Sims's brother delivered the letter. The boy reported back that Theresa read it without visible anger, yet the missive was met with silence.

A torturous month passed before Sims and Theresa joined a party of young people visiting her brother-in-law's house in Cooterborough for tea. They walked home together, alone. It was a beautiful, moonlit night, and they strolled down the road that wended past Mr. Locke's blacksmith shop. They paused under an impressive old locust tree. At last, Sims broke the silence. Theresa was seventeen now, he said, old enough to contemplate weighty matters. Surely, she knew what his note had hinted at. Now he wished for an answer—would she marry him?

Her voice trembled. No, she would not.

Sims walked her home and said goodbye, and from there he settled into an oscillating haze of sadness and anger. At first, he contemplated getting drunk—he settled on a cigar, which made him sick—and then he contemplated suicide. At one moment, he felt sympathy for Theresa: He was a no-account fool, lacking in purpose and direction. How could she possibly love him? In the next moment, he cursed her name: Theresa was venal, desperate to sell herself—like all women. She had preferred Sims well enough when he was a boy, but now that she was beautiful she preferred tall North Carolinians, mature men with fortunes and positions and everything girls loved.

For weeks, Sims defied his fears and stayed out late at night, observing Lancaster from the woods that surrounded it. If mad dogs, runaway slaves, or headless ghosts had sucked him into the swamps and made a monster out of him too, it would have been a more welcome fate than the humiliating limbo of life without Theresa. He contemplated running away—south, in the opposite direction of runaways. He begged his father for $100 to head to the frontier, to Alabama. Josiah Nott's school had not succeeded; he would move to Mobile, as he'd planned. Perhaps Sims should follow him. John Sims told his son he was crazy and refused to provide the sum. The family didn't have the money anyway. He advised accepting his fate and carrying on with his studies.

After three months, a chance encounter with Theresa's cousin suggested there might have been a terrible miscommunication. The cousin knew nothing at all of Sims's proposal. But she knew that Theresa had been miserable for some time, and that she loved Sims as much as he loved her. The following morning, in an equal daze of uncertainty and hope—the precise date was July 23, 1833—Sims wandered into town for the first time in many days. He happened upon Theresa, walking alone. At last, he learned the truth: Theresa had refused him in order to obey her mother. She regretted it at once. Then and there, Sims and Theresa formed a secret pact. Innocent flirtations might come and go, they agreed, but they would remain true to one another as Sims completed his medical education. Surely, once he was established, Theresa's mother could no longer deny the fate of their love. In the meantime, Sims's brother would carry letters between them.

Reinvigorated, Sims enrolled in medical school. His meager training with Dr. Church did not suit him for study in Philadelphia immediately, but materials for the Medical College of South Carolina in Charleston boasted of their well-supplied deadhouse. It was precisely what a newly motivated student, anxious to pursue surgery, could best avail himself of. In his application, he lied and said his preceptor was Theresa's dead father. J. Marion Sims was accepted for study.

86 Sims, J. Marion, *A.B.* | do. |Lancaster Dis. |Dr. B. C. Jones.

* * *

In November, he booked a stage for the journey south, anxious for his first glimpse of the ocean. Charleston was a town of forty thousand, ten times the size of Columbia and completely dwarfing poor Lancaster. The stage rolled in from the west, passing alongside the infamous Charleston Workhouse, a structure of brick and stone that loomed up from an acre of land like a European castle, or a prison. With castellated walls and turrets pocked with suspicious portholes, it might once have been a fort to keep out invaders. Now, it served the opposite purpose: it was the city's municipal slave pen, simultaneously a place for local slave owners to send their slaves for punishment and a holding yard for brokers to stable their product until the weekly sales. It was said that inside the walls of the Charleston Workhouse, no distinction was made between male and female slaves as they were hung to be beaten with an array of whips and paddles, all cunningly designed to inflict punishments that did not result in the scarring that could drain the value of an investment. However, the women—particularly attractive mulatto wenches, some nearly indistinguishable from white—were frequently reduced to spasms and insensibility from the first blow. Sims marveled at the workhouse's huge external door, studded with large nails, and judged it wise that it had been positioned at the edge of town. Despite the stone walls, he caught the shrieks and sobs of a man being flogged just at the moment the stage trundled past.

Downtown Charleston had a welcoming, European flavor, with narrow brick streets of a dusty color and grand, cathedral-like churches that rang the hours. Sims took lodging at Miott's Hotel and at dusk walked Society Street, where in the days to come he would find board at Mrs. Murden's. His time in Charleston would be marked by Mrs. Murden's affinity for reading aloud the horrible news of the day, stories of runaway slaves and murders and shipwrecks. Sims had never seen homes like those of Charleston. Stairs curled up from the street to elevated entranceways, and wrought-iron fencing sectioned off private gardens with calf-high hedges that formed quaint walkways. Palm trees lined the avenues, orange trees and evergreens surrounded the homes, and ivy snaked along everything. One Charlestonian—a doctor, Sims noted—was the owner of an impressive home with a two-tiered piazza with Italian columns and a front door flanked by pilasters and topped with a handsome half-circle transom.

There had been recent slave insurrections, stemming from the conditions at the workhouse. There were many soldiers in town. A strict police presence and a citizen patrol jailed slaves if they were found wandering after sunset. That first evening, it had grown dark by the time Sims turned back toward Miott's. The streets were abandoned and melancholy. A patrolman, spotting Sims from afar, crossed the street to gauge at a distance whether his face was white or black.

Sims slept in on his first morning in Charleston and rose to strange news: the night had been interrupted by a phantasmagoric display of shooting stars. Witnesses claimed that for hours the sky had squirmed with the brilliance of a hundred thousand burning lights. After one meteor passed near, a group of observers claimed that their skin had been left diffused with a lambent glow, and some rejoiced in a belief that the shower obviated the need for a thunderstorm to clear the air of disease. Newspapers told an amusing story: an old slave from Baltimore, driving a cart as the stars began to crumble and fall, took it for an omen and continued on to Jones Falls. The falling water would save him from falling fire.

It's all over with the white folks now, the man said.

Sims slept through the whole thing. He was oblivious, but he didn't care. It was November 13, 1833—his first day of medical school.

Three

*I*T TOOK THREE DAYS TO GATHER ENOUGH WOOD TO HEAT THE VAT OF WATER that was required at hog-killing time. The hogs were herded together and knocked on the head with the butt of an ax and then stuck with a very sharp knife. Their legs were tied and they were dragged into the boiling water for three minutes, until the hair and the dirt could be scraped away. Then they were butchered, and the adults gave the hogs' bladders to the children of the Westcott plantation, who took them to the river to wash them. They used the bladders as noisemakers, marching through the yard and squeezing the organs to produce a sound similar to that which followed the crack of whips carrying more than a mile from neighboring plantations.

The Westcott children and the Westcott slave children played games together when they were young, all wearing nothing but long homespun shirts, split up the side and made of the ducking or osnaburg cloth that sacks were made from. They played Pretty Pauline, and Fox and Geese, and Green Grow the Willow Trees, and No Boogerman Tonight, and Mollie Bright, and Walking to Jerusalem, and Bugger Bear, and Wolf on the Bridge, and Holly-Golly, and Sheep-Meat, and Jack-o-Maringo, and Old Molly Whoop Scoop.

The boys played marbles until their fingers wore off, Seven-Up

Marble with one marble in the center of a large circle and four at the corners, and you lagged in from about fifteen feet. The marbles were made of clay that was molded by hand and baked in the sun, or India rubber when they could find it. For other games, they made balls out of tightly wrapped rags, sometimes with a rock inside. They played Town Ball and they played Anti-Over, one boy heaving a ball over the Westcott house to a crowd of boys gathered on the other side.

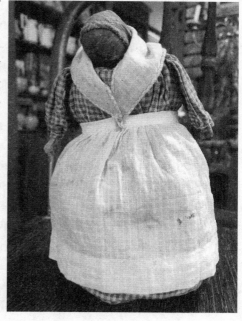

The girls played with hoops from the missus's worn-out dresses, and they made frog houses and mud people by mixing dirt and clay with an egg they stole from the hens. They made dolls from corncobs and rag babies from cotton waste, a roll of linen or a walnut for a head and leftover scraps for pants or skirts that were fitted onto forked sticks for legs. They watched doodle-bugs, with fat bodies and faces like shears, dig meticulous homes in the dirt. The girls—Anarcha and Rachel and Anna and Mary, and Priscilla and Susannah Westcott alongside them—made hats from hickory leaves and decorated them with wildflowers, and they made pins from pine needles and rosebush thorns. They wove long willow branches into stick horses, and the willow grove close to the river became their horse lot.

For a time, there was little distinction between the white and black children on the Westcott plantation, but after David Westcott died—after Anarcha was born—Samuel and William Westcott began wearing small cotton suits, and store-bought shoes, and under their pants they wore cotton drawers. They watched as their former playmates Isham and Minden and Charles and Manuel and Ben were allotted their first supply of grown-up clothes—cotton and linsey-woolsey shirts, jean pants for summer, wool for winter—and were sent to work in the fields alongside their parents.

Some of the children did not realize they were slaves. But Anarcha always knew it and she knew it best from the food. The young children were fed in the nursery, and there was a very large wooden bowl, and the children all gathered around it at once with wooden spoons to shovel up potlikker, or boiled beans, or onions and poke salad, or cornmeal dumplings, or milk and mash, or meat and ashcakes, or bread and molasses syrup. They ate collards in greens time, potatoes in potato time. On Sundays, the slave children were brought to the Westcott family dinner, and the first time Anarcha sat with them, she was asked what she would like to eat and she thought of lye hominy, which her parents ate and which she had tasted once and it was delicious, grown-up food off a wooden plate that was her own, no fighting with her sister over the scrap of meat that was sometimes found in the big wooden bowl. So she asked for lye hominy, and the Westcotts laughed—even Susannah and Priscilla laughed—and they gave her chicken and sweet potatoes on a real plate, a china plate, though she wasn't given a knife and she ate with her wooden spoon.

The Sunday dinners looked like generosity but they weren't generosity. They were a chance for the missus to observe the young slaves, to make sure they were neither stunted nor sick beyond the skills of the Doctor Woman, Pheriba. If they were ill with worms or chills or rheumatism or whooping cough, Eliza Westcott would give them doses of castor oil or bluemas or calomel, or camphor mixed with whiskey that you rubbed on the head, or just a single drop of a mixture called Number Six, it was dangerous to take any more than that. If a slave was still sick after Pheriba's treatments, and after the missus's treatments, she sent a servant into town to fetch Dr. Hugh Henry, who lived in a big new house and owned many slaves and many acres, in Montgomery and nearby, and who was considered an honest and industrious man, his credit good for all engagements. Dr. Henry rode horseback to the plantation, his saddle pockets stuffed with little bottles, and sometimes he poked them all full of medicine, just in case. Other times, he produced his scarificator and a cupping set. The scarificator was a little box machine with twelve blades that shot out of thin holes, powered by springs, and Dr. Henry would clamp it to the back of your neck and pull the trigger to release the blades, and they bit you like a snake. The cupping set was like a tea set, but all the glasses were of different sizes, and Dr. Henry would withdraw the scarificator and apply a cup to the wounded area, and he let you bleed until the cup was full or until minutes passed, and he stood there watching the minutes pass on a big watch on a chain that he fished out of his pocket with two fingers.

When Anarcha was very young—before the stars fell—she once asked Susannah or Priscilla Westcott for fifteen cents, just to see what money looked like. Slaves made money sometimes, her father worked Sundays to earn money for things they weren't apportioned—church clothes and whiskey—and others made charcoal to sell, or carved utensils, or they sold vegetables from the gardens they were allowed to work at night, and some slaves made a piece of money by diving into the Alabama River to retrieve things from riverboats that burned and sank. Others made money by selling snakes and terrapins to the sailors of those same boats, to control cockroaches. One man stole an old copy of the Blue Back Speller and taught himself to read and write—at the risk of losing a thumb or forefinger—and he made money by forging the notes that you gave to patrollers when they found you wandering at night.

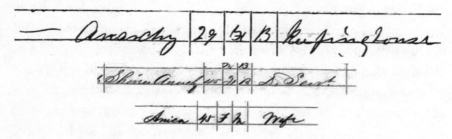

In later census records of Alabama, a few Anicas and Anachys were described as "Keeps house" or "D. serv^t." or "Wife," and surely this would have included cooking, but Anarcha was not a cook—she never learned to cook when she was young. But there were times, after she was too old to be brought to the Westcott house on Sundays for good food, when she carried meals in from the kitchen, a freestanding building erected a short way off from the house to prevent the spread of fires. She carried to the dining room the biscuits and the coffee that slaves coveted but were afforded only on holidays. One morning, knowing that no one had counted or could count the huge stack of waffles that she was bringing to the table, Anarcha stole one, a single waffle, crisp and delicate and melting inside her mouth, as luscious as a fulfilled promise. It was at this moment, when she compared the waffle to the goobers, and the whippoorwill peas, and the crackling bread, and the parched-corn-and-okra-seed coffee that she now ate and drank daily, to the raccoon and the opossum on which the slaves would feast in the quarters if the missus gave the men a pass to hunt after sundown (the coon more delicate, and the hair didn't stink up the meat), that she realized she was a thing that was owned, an object like the wooden spoon that she had clutched to her chest when she walked up to the Westcott house on Sundays, or like the two coins that Priscilla Westcott dug out of the pocket of her dress to show her money, though she wouldn't let Anarcha touch them.

By then, she had been allotted a cotton checked dress and a matching sunbonnet, a balmoral petticoat and linen pantalets, and a pair of brass-toed brogan shoes that were so hard you had to rub them with tallow or fried meat grease just to get them onto your feet, and even then it was better to go barefoot. Rather than cook, Anarcha became a helper to Pheriba, though she wasn't allowed to help catch babies. When the time came for the babies to arrive, the children were told only that the mother had broken a leg, and no one was allowed to go into the sickroom off the kitchen when the babies came because Pheriba had important papers spread on the floor that couldn't be disturbed. Anarcha was asked to bring water or chunks of fire and sometimes, inexplicably, an ax. She fetched things from Pheriba's cabin that she knew were good for stopping bleeding. A salve of soot and sugar, a gourd stuffed with cobwebs, a little jar filled with lint from worn-out felt hats. In this way, Manora came to Harriet, and Ann came to Louisa, and Richard came to Hester, and Nancy came to Anarcha's mother, Sue, and Minerva came to Betty.

Pheriba had no husband and no children and she lived alone in a cabin set just down from the quarters, and Pheriba's cabin was where the Westcott slaves went first if they fell ill or had miseries in their backs or their heads, and it was where the children went every morning for a daily dose of bitters—whiskey mixed with tree barks. Pheriba's cabin was smaller than the others, with a dirt-and-stick fireplace at one end rather than the middle, where everyone cooked with spider pans and iron contraptions to suspend pots over the open flames. She had shelves of jars filled with dried herbs preserved in whiskey: wild cherry bark, pennyroyal, butter-fly root, and spice bush bark. She had rolls of string, and sometimes the string was knotted and soaked in turpentine and tied around joints for rheumatism, or around the skull for neuralgia, and the string was also used for the little bags of asafetida that all the children wore around their necks for protection. Pheriba had mallets for pounding bark and leaves and garlic and mustard to make poultices, and every day she sliced an onion and laid it out in her cabin to keep illnesses away.

There was a large sack and a hoe that no one was allowed to touch, and sometimes Pheriba went into the woods to gather herbs—hoarhound, mint, goose grass, and chamomile. Anarcha began to learn the cures that Pheriba said no white doctor in Alabama knew anything about. For fevers, use teas of elderbush, slippery elm, feverweed, or devil's shoestring, or wrap the feverish person up in cabbage or ginseng leaves, and if it gets worse mix ashes with shavings from the hoof of a hog and make a tea from that. Tea of life everlasting, also called rabbit tobacco, was good for colds, as was boneset, scurry grass, rats' vein, and lye, but lye tea had to be weak or it would do more harm than good. Cow manure with water and salt was also good for colds. Sheep-waste tea was good for stomach ail-ments and constipation, but you could also use snakeroot, peach leaves, jimsonweed, and peppergrass. Sassafras in springtime would purify the blood, and dogwood and cherry bark mixed with whiskey was also good, and belladonna would leave you cleaned out better than anything, if it didn't kill you. If a girl gets the whites or has cramps, crush some egg-shells, parch them, and make a tea, and if the cramps are very bad take strips of slippery elm bark and insert them in her vagina. If somebody got burnt, kill a hog and spread its grease over the wounds to take the fire out of them. For mumps and corns, use marrow from a hog's jowl if willow ashes don't work. Poke root for smallpox, tobacco smoke for earache, cornmeal and lard for bruises. Devil's shoestring was also good for toothache, and for pain use either a poultice of tansy leaves or pour urine over a hot brick and apply it through flannel to steam the misery away. Lastly, when you think that someone might be dead, take a slice of bread, butter it, and lay it over their lips. If the butter melts, they're not dead yet.

The more Anarcha worked for Pheriba, the more Pheriba told her of what she knew of runaways and the woods. There were slaves who ran off and were wild like wildmen, with wild hair and wild beards, and there were tales of families who found caves underneath their masters' houses and dug tunnels to them and made homes right beneath their masters' feet. Not far from the Westcott plantation, a slave man had prepared a cave for his wife right before she was going to be whipped. He brought her pine straw and pine logs for furniture, and a stove with a pipe that ran out through the ground, and then he ran off too, and they lived there for seven years, having free babies in the woods. Pheriba had sometimes taken them food and matches, but now they were gone, and the cave was empty. There were white people in the woods too, she said, poor whites who lived far back in the hills, far away from any town and living as mean as any slave, and at harvest time, when hands were needed, poor white people worked alongside the field hands for pay, and some of them were more generous than any master. Others had gizzards instead of hearts, and they worked as patrollers and overseers and were viciously cruel, and some picked up slave babies that were abandoned at railroad stations when the mother was purchased and her new master didn't want any babies, and the mother was forced to put her baby down beside the tracks and climb aboard. Poor whites snatched up that baby, took it to the hills, and raised it till it could be sold for money.

Sometimes, Pheriba grumbled about the ways the devil made mean-ness, but it was just talk—she didn't believe in anything she couldn't put in her stomach. It made sense to put mullein leaves in with the baby water when you washed them, she said, and sometimes tying a copper around a little one's neck might help with teething, but using the hind foot of a mole, or a grasshopper nest, or wood lice or a rattlesnake rattle or alligator teeth or nine black bugs for the same purpose was just devilment. Even so, Pheriba was among those who thought that the night of the falling stars was a harbinger, a sign, and she read into it rumors of a coming war: sons against fathers, daughters against mothers. After the night of November

13, 1833, sitting around the fire, Pheriba would look up at the stars in the sky and spot signals there of a coming time when wagons would run without horses and when the peoples of all nations would return to the homes they'd come from.

Pheriba made money catching babies, both for herself and for the missus who gave her passes when slave women on nearby plantations came close to their time. Pheriba took a horse and a little wagon on the day she caught the baby, and then she would return every day for seven days thereafter to check on the mother and the infant. By now, Anarcha knew the mothers didn't have any broken legs, and she'd figured out that the babies were buried inside of the women and not inside of any stump, but all Pheriba would tell her about catching them was that babies came out the same way they went in. Pheriba let Anarcha blow the horn to call the mothers in from the fields for the suckerling babies, and she taught her how to nibble a baby's fingernails and toenails instead of cutting them, though it wasn't true that this prevented them from becoming thieves. Give a baby a piece of fatmeat to suck on to prevent colic, she said, and if you didn't have any fatmeat, then dunk your finger into some potlikker and let them suck that instead. More cryptically, Pheriba explained that when a baby came, something else came with it. It wasn't a baby, and it wasn't alive, and it wasn't dangerous—but be sure to burn it and not bury it, because if you buried it dogs would dig it up and carry it around, and that would leave the child ailing.

Pheriba had lived on other plantations before the Westcott plantation, and she had visited even more plantations, and that meant she had seen stories and she had heard stories, and she told them both. Nursing children wasn't safe work like some field hands thought it was, she said. There was one mean master who got mad at his baby's nurse because she couldn't get the baby to stop crying, so the master hit the nurse on the head with a pair of fire tongs, and she died. Another nurse, a young girl, was carrying her master's grandson when she fell down some steps, and the man's wife and daughter cried to him, even though the baby wasn't dead or dying. But because his wife and daughter were crying, the master took a big board and hit the poor nurse on the head, and she died too. The master made the other slaves throw that girl's body into the river, though her mother begged him not to.

The Westcott plantation was a baby too, Pheriba said, and what she meant was that it wasn't yet old enough to be selling the babies it was growing, though soon enough it would be. There were bigger plantations, however, older plantations where the making and selling of babies was no different from and was maybe more profitable than the growing of cotton or sugar. Eventually, there were so many babies on these plantations they couldn't have a regular nursery. Instead, they built large shallow troughs or basins that sat out in the open and were sealed at the bottom so that snakes couldn't get in. There was one such trough on the Blackshear place, in Arkansas, where it was said that money grew on bushes and hogs wandered in the woods with forks stuck in their backs for convenience. On one Sunday afternoon, after church, the Blackshear overseers and drivers gathered all the plantation's fine-looking boys and girls, eyeballing those who were at least thirteen years of age. They stripped them naked and locked them in a barn overnight. Sixty head of babies were thus produced, and they were kept in the large trough that had been built in anticipation and which stood under a large cottonwood tree a long way off from the fields where the slaves worked. One day, when they were working at the fields' far edge, a cloud rose up in the sky, and very suddenly it began to shower great sheets of rain, and it came down first on the cottonwood tree and took its time before reaching the fields. They ran back to the trough, but it was too late. The Blackshears never got a lick of labor nor a red cent out of any one of those sixty babies.

* * *

THE GREAT COMET OF 1835! DAY & GANT, 216 Main street, have just received, direct from England, a few copies of—"*Observations on Dr. Halley's great Comet,* with a History of the phenomena attending its return for six hundred years past; also, an elucidation of the cause of the comet's tail always pointing from the sun, &c. by R. J. Morrison, Esq. Cheltenham."—London: Sherwood & Co. Paternoster Row.   Price 25 cents.
October 14.   70

The next star that came loose didn't fall quickly to the ground. It shot slow toward the sun instead. This time white people knew all about it in advance, because they read about it in books, and before it could be seen with the naked eye, they watched it slipping across God's sky with special pieces of glass. No one was afraid this time except a plantation owner in Selma, who said it would be a shame if Hell's Comet hit the Earth and destroyed the handsome estate he'd managed to scratch together. It was 1835, and by September Hell's Comet shined brighter than Aldebaran or Antares. It was soon giving off a swish of luminous matter, and the tail curved in the sky as though it was driven by a big wind, and some said there were really two tails or that the star's tail was cleft, and that from night to night it swung back and forth like the pendulum of a clock. The tail glowed brighter and brighter until the middle of October, and then it grew dimmer and dimmer and vanished near the sun. Some wondered if it portended a departure or an arrival—and if so, of what?

By then, Anarcha had been leased to Rose Hill, the Lucas plantation in Mount Meigs, twelve miles east of Montgomery. She was nine now, or seven, or eleven, and it was as far from the Westcott plantation as she had ever been, practically all the way to Creek territory. Mount Meigs was smaller than Montgomery, but Rose Hill was much larger than the Westcott plantation, with perhaps fifteen hundred slaves and many babies, and there was illness near Mount Meigs, so there was need of servants who could nurse children and watch over sick people. Eliza Westcott arranged for Anarcha to go there and use what Pheriba had taught her until the time came for her to get married and have babies of her own.

Rose Hill was the first stop for the stage outside of Montgomery. A row of oak trees led up to the Lucas mansion house from the road, but Anarcha saw it only from a distance. There were two quarters. One was high up near the mansion, for the house slaves, the cooks and their assistants, the butlers with their teams of waiters and waitresses, the housekeepers with more maids than they could ever use, and fourteen slaves who worked for a white gardener from England who made $1,500 per year for growing flowers, pineapples, coffee bushes, and tea plants in greenhouses.

The lower quarters was for the Lucas field hands, and it was like a city itself, a row of cabins facing each other across a road that could fit a double team wagon and stretched for half a mile in a straight line. The day began before the sun came up, with loud bells that sounded from the Lucas house—the Lucas overseers and drivers used bells instead of horns—and for a time in the morning you could smell woodsmoke coming from the mud-and-stick chimneys, and sow bellies frying in the cabins, and the guinea fowl raised a ruckus near the edge of the forest, waking the roosters and the ducks, and sometimes in the mornings there was the sound of slaves being whipped for things they had done the day before. There were more beatings on the Lucas plantation than on the Westcott plantation, even for pregnant women. A hole was dug in the ground, and the woman was stripped of her dress so that it wouldn't be bloodied, and she put her baby in the hole, and then her back was lashed. It wasn't yet light when the overseer walked the road between the cabins, hollering left and right and picking ham from his teeth with a goose quill. The field hands gathered and marched off to their day of work.

The Lucas slaves made everything that on the Westcott plantation was bought from Montgomery stores. During the day, the quarters remained active with the work of the tannery and the blacksmith shop, and there was a house for the carders and spinners and the women who churned looms all night long. There was a shoe house, where there was a man who didn't do anything but make shoes for other slaves, and there were women who made candles from the tripe and kidneys of killed beefs. There were slaves that broke the mules for the treadmills that ran the cotton gins, and others that cared for horses or packs of dogs specially trained to chase after squirrels, possums, snakes, and runaway slaves. There was a house for sick slaves, and sometimes there were as many as twenty or thirty sick at a time, and Anarcha worked here making teas and preparing poultices, and she worked in the nursery as well, and no one on the Lucas plantation cared about papers laid out on the floor, and that was how Anarcha learned how babies came out, though she still didn't know how they went in. She also learned why Pheriba sometimes sent for an ax when a baby was coming. The Lucas grannies sometimes slid an upright ax or a piece of rusty tin under the cord bed when a woman was pushing a baby out. When the woman looked down and saw that blade pointing up at her it made her forget all about her pains, and all about her baby.

At midday, two dozen mothers walked in from the fields to let the babies suck. Food at Rose Hill wasn't as good as food on the Westcott plantation. The field slaves were given meat from sickly beefs, or from hogs that ate so many grasshoppers their meat was red, and there wasn't any extra allotment of food for children. On the Lucas plantation, there were far too many children for a wooden bowl of any size. There were too many even for a single trough, so there were troughs for children of different sizes, and they swarmed around the troughs not with wooden spoons but with mussel shells, and oyster shells, and cockleshells that their mothers brought in from the fields. They used these for spoons.

Every cabin had a corn-shuck mat out front, but the Lucas slave cabins sat right on the ground, and the floors were not plank but dirt, and there were holes in the walls big enough for dogs and cats to crawl through, and sometimes the chimneys caught on fire at night. There were usually two families in a cabin, but family on the Lucas plantation didn't mean what family meant on the Westcott plantation. Most of the Lucas slaves knew who their mothers were, but most weren't sure who their fathers were. Rose Hill was only one of many Lucas plantations. The quarters at the Lucas mansion were the largest, but there were others as well, and some-times the mothers married fathers from other quarters, and so they saw their husbands or their fathers only at corn shuckings, or at the Fourth of July, or in the few days after Christmas. Sometimes their father was a strong or portly man whose master hired him from plantation to plan-tation like a racehorse to father hundreds of strong or portly children. Sometimes their father had been sold away and was never heard from again. And sometimes—often, even—their father was an overseer or the master himself, Henry Lucas. The bright or yellow children that were fathered in this way didn't remain in the lower quarters but climbed up to the upper quarters and worked in the mansion. Pheriba had warned Anarcha that babies fathered by a white man could come out looking any shade from noon to midnight, but this was also true of even the darkest mother, and a girl could get whipped at the command of the missus if she birthed a black baby that looked too white at first. Regardless, many of the Lucas slaves didn't know whether their father was making their shoes or giving them orders, and so everyone they lived with was called brother and sister, and sometimes there were as many as three families to a cabin.

The field hands returned after sundown, walking slow and singing with tired voices, and the quarters again filled with the smell of wood and cooking, and there was music played with swamp quills and instruments made from gourds and horsehair, and if you stretched cowhide over a cheesebox you had yourself a tambourine. The singing was picked up from cabin to cabin, until the overseer came around at about nine o'clock, and then everything went quiet until the slaves got up again to talk amongst themselves in the dark, and if they talked about white people they talked about white horses instead in case the overseer or drivers were nearby, eavesdropping. They reminisced about the great frolic that had happened on the Lucas plantation ten years earlier, when a famous old French general who helped America escape from England came around on a tour of the country he saved. All the important white people in Alabama arrived, and for several days there was no work except for caring for the horses and carriages and omnibuses that white people took on rides around the countryside.

They recalled too the story of the slave on a neighboring plantation who had shot and killed an overseer and taunted his pursuers until they caught him. A judge in Montgomery had refused to impose the penalty of burning that man alive, because he said he wouldn't do that even to a dog. But that slave was burned alive anyway, and others saw him burned up and remembered it now and always would. They offered advice. If you were out on a pass to see your sweetheart or your husband on another plantation, and you came across a nicely dressed man on horseback who asked you about whether your master was good to you, gave you good food and good lodging, be sure to say yes, sir, Mr. Henry Lucas is good to all his slaves, he goes to Mobile every Christmas to buy us special clothes, and every Fourth of July there is a feast with food and lemonade spread out on the ground for everyone. Say these things because probably that gentleman is your master, Mr. Henry Lucas himself, and how would you ever know otherwise?

Anarcha learned quickly that the Lucas slaves had stolen cotton plants from the fields and planted them inside their cabins. They clipped off everything except the roots, which kept growing underground. If a girl got pregnant and she didn't want to be pregnant, then the cotton roots would be dug up and the girl would chew on them, and the baby would go away.

Pheriba would never have stood for most of the treatments of the

Lucas granny doctors. Even Anarcha knew that putting a horn on a spot of misery wasn't going to make it go away, nor was two lightning bugs in a whiskey bottle the best thing for pain. For whooping cough, the Lucas grannies chopped off the head of a land turtle and dripped blood from its head over sugar, and if someone fell into spasms, they threw cold water onto them or burned a piece of clothing just next to their body. In times of illness, they planted sticks of fat pine dunked in tar all over the quarters to kill the sickness in the air, and if a person was already foundered, they made them jump over the sticks that were already lit.

Lots of things were signs that someone was going to die: cows lowing at night, a bird flying into your cabin, a woodpecker rapping on your roof, and of course the sound of a screech owl, though if you quickly put a shovel into the fire you could make the screech owl stop screeching. The granny doctors said people with blue gums were poisonous, and if you ate a rabbit that was caught in a graveyard everyone would get sick. Cross two pieces of straw on someone's head for a nosebleed, and tie knotted string around a girl's waist for cramps. If you were sick and didn't want visitors, put a fresh-laid egg in front of your door.

The master had a cousin who was a doctor, Dr. Charles Lucas. Dr. Lucas lived right next to his cousin in a big house called Bright Spot. He owned many slaves too, and sometimes Anarcha was called to work for him when white people got malaria. Pheriba was right about white doctors. There were some who used herbs but didn't know a lot about them, and there were some who thought a bit of illness was a cure, but most of them gave you powders or put things inside of you with a squirt or took your blood, and sometimes it worked and sometimes it didn't. If a white doctor was called to a slave birth, he mostly stayed outside the nursery and called in instructions. The women did the work and caught the baby on their own, if it lived. Before Hell's Comet, the master had a son who was going to be a doctor, and he worked with Dr. Lucas for some time before he went to Philadelphia to study medicine. Anarcha had been on the Lucas plantation for almost a year when the sad news came that the master's only living child had died of a disease in medical school. It was some time after that—after Hell's Comet came and went—that Anarcha cared for another young doctor who had also come from Philadelphia and who had known the master's only dead child. The young man's name was Dr. Marion Sims.

Dr. Sims looked like a young boy. He was very small compared to other men, and he was a different kind of doctor, because he didn't believe in taking blood. It was said that he believed most things could be cured with a knife. Anarcha had never seen him, but she heard stories about him, and in particular she would have heard the story of Dr. Sims's first surgical success in Alabama—news traveled fast of what white doctors did with knives and scissors. A mean overseer on the Ashurst plantation had grown very ill. Hoodoo didn't work on white people, but, even so, the overseer was so mean that his meanness filled up his body with spiders and worms. Dr. Sims said they should put a knife into him. Otherwise he would die. So they stuck a knife in the belly of the overseer, and all the spiders and worms came seeping out of him, people said.

White people got malaria more than slaves did. When Dr. Sims fell ill, Dr. Lucas told Anarcha to care for him, to bring him water when he asked, and she cared for Mrs. Judkins too, and for Mrs. Judkins's son, who died. Dr. Sims refused when Dr. Lucas came around to bleed the malaria out of him. It looked like Dr. Sims would also die, but Pheriba had taught Anarcha cures for malaria. Tea of cow shucks and dog fennel would vomit it out of you. A bath of bitter weeds and then a wrapping would sweat it out of you. For Dr. Sims, Anarcha took some snakeroot that she had gathered in the spring when the sap was high, and she walked down to the blacksmith shop to sift around in the dirt until she found some iron chips near the anvil, and she brewed the chips with the root and some whiskey, which was a cure for consumption, though Pheriba said it would work for malaria too. She gave it to Dr. Sims when he was dreamy and talked about the woman he wanted to marry in South Carolina. He didn't know what he was drinking. After two weeks, another doctor came and gave Dr. Sims quinine, and his hair fell out. After that, he got well again, and the doctors believed it was the quinine that cured him, but Anarcha knew it was her tea that saved the life of Dr. Marion Sims.

Four

PROFESSOR PRIOLEAU ILLUSTRATED MOST OF THE LECTURES IN HIS PRINciples and Practice of Obstetrics course with diagrams and plates, but now he was again working with Auzoux's manikin on the demonstration table at the head of class. He had flipped it over and was attempting to twist it into an impossible position. Sims and his classmates climbed down from their desks in the amphitheater seating of the main lecture hall to observe more closely. Some took a genuine interest in what another of the college's professors, Dr. James Moultrie, had described as the pains that were inflicted on woman for her violation of the law given to her as a test of her obedience. Sims didn't fight through the crowd as Prioleau flailed with his model, attempting to bend its knees. At last, the professor gave up and described a "genu-pectoral" or "knee-chest" position that sounded painful even before you knew what it was meant to facilitate. Place a woman on her knees on the surface of an examination table, then lower her torso so that her chest also was pressed on the surface of the table. Her nates would be raised so high in the air that the only way to proceed with modesty intact for all would be to throw a sheet over her.

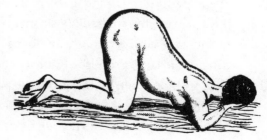

Most of Prioleau's lectures—descriptions of the condition of the gravid uterus, and the care to be given to women in the puerperal state—didn't stick with Sims. The man wasn't a surgeon, he didn't publish, and Sims had absolutely no intention of focusing his career on diseases of the female pelvis. Yet he would recall the way that Prioleau described the purpose of the genu-pectoral position. He shifted to a tone of high propriety and spoke not as though it was a procedure he had performed but as though it was one he had read about, perhaps in a European medical journal.

Gentlemen, Professor Prioleau said, if any of you are called to a case of sudden inversion of the uterus, place the patient in the knee-chest position and then introduce one finger into the rectum and another into the vagina. Push up, and pull down.

He mimed this motion on an invisible woman hovering before the eager students, vigorously pumping his hands like the coupling rods on the wheels of a steam engine.

If you do not return the uterus to its proper position by this means, he said, you will hardly effect it by any other.

Like most of his colleagues, Prioleau had studied medicine at the University of Pennsylvania. One day in 1806, one of his professors had prepared a batch of gas that was rumored to kill pain, combining nitric acid and the carbonate of ammoniac. The gas was given to a fourteen-year-old boy named Henry Latrobe, to breathe. The boy was affected in the most violent of manners, goose-stepping about the laboratory and laughing until he frothed at the mouth and tears rolled down his cheeks. Intrigued and knowing that such symptoms could not be counterfeited, the professor prepared another batch of nitrous oxide to give to his students, in doses of two and four quarts. One young man ran around the laboratory like a mad bull, striking at everyone he encountered. Another believed the gas made him incredibly strong, and the mouthpiece apparatus used to apply the concoction was removed from his face only with great difficulty. Years later, Professor Prioleau enjoyed reporting to his students his own reaction when he was given the painkilling agent.

I am in heaven! Prioleau called out. *Ye gods, stars, comets, meteors! Mahomet's a jackass! The Elysian fields are hell compared with this!*

Then he fainted.

Prioleau's medical school thesis was about another reported pain-killer, a plant called *Aralia spinosa*, or devil's walking stick, which in 1794 and again in 1801 had been used to cure rattlesnake bites. It was often confused with devil's shoestring, several plants of the genera *Vibrunum* and *Cracca*, which slaves had been known to use for toothache. Prioleau conducted an experiment on himself, adding alcohol to an infusion of the plant's inner bark to further extract its virtues. He drank several glasses of the mixture, which induced vomiting and headache, and later he snorted it in a powdered form, which produced the same purging but with fewer ill effects. He concluded that the bark could be used by slave owners as a cheap substitute for ipecac.

* * *

Even though Sims didn't witness it, the night of the falling stars marked a change in him. In Charleston, he diligently wrote letters to Theresa and anxiously awaited her reply. He enjoyed games of chess in the evenings with Mrs. Murden's four beautiful daughters, and he occasionally attended frolics with his college friend Dick Baker, who had decided on medical school as well. Nevertheless, the wantonness of youth was over, and Sims recognized that none of the faculty of the Medical College of South Carolina would serve him well as a role model.

Dr. John Holbrook's anatomy class had its uses, and the man had married well and owned an impressive thirty-three slaves. But his lectures were like sermons—and what could one possibly say of a physician who so abhorred pain that he couldn't perform surgery? Dr. Henry Frost wanted to change the name of his materia medica course to "pharmacologia," but Sims didn't particularly care whether roots were harvested in the autumn when the stalks were dry, or if seeds were gathered while still in their proper vessels, and everyone agreed the man's lectures were dull, oppressed by his own modesty. Moultrie's physiology course was a slog through the difference between organic and inorganic compounds, but Sims wished his father could have heard the man speak about the medical profession. On the one hand, Moultrie argued, history had shown that knowledge is power, and that medicine is knowledge. Physicians, therefore, were instruments appointed to forward the gracious plan of the Benevolent Author. On the other hand, doctoring was the most perfect embodiment of a broad range of sciences: mathematics, physics, botany, zoology, and the philosophy of the mind. Sims took special note of Moultrie's explanation for why American physicians had thus far made only limited contributions in the realm of medical invention. History had provided Europeans with far ampler opportunities for experimentation: their hospitals, armies, and cities all acted as incubators for innovation.

Dr. Samuel Henry Dickson taught practice of medicine, but far more valuable than his course was his brilliant introductory lecture, in which he defended slavery in an eloquent, musical voice. Slavery was an evil, Dickson allowed, but only insofar as it was poverty, and poverty was evil. Slavery was a condition of necessary dependence. Emancipation rested on the idea that the slave is a fallen creature. But he is not. The savage in his homeland is as insecure as the beasts he hunts, and the race as a whole could not be raised from destitution—was not civilizable—unless it was controlled by its white superiors. As with women and children, Dickson claimed, the slave should be denied rights because he was neither adequate to their exercise nor fit for their enjoyment. The change of residence from Africa to America was merely the swap of a white despot for a black one. What did the slave lose in the bargain but his natural insecurity and the certainty that his African life would be short and impoverished?

Dr. John Wagner's surgery course was by far the most helpful. It was said that Wagner had brought surgery to Charleston single-handedly, having studied in New York, Liverpool, London, and Paris. He spent a year as a dresser at Guy's Hospital, and three years studying with Sir Astley Cooper. To this day, Wagner kept in his office a bust of Dr. John Hunter, which Cooper had given to him on his departure. Wagner happily told the story of the tooth that Hunter had once extracted from the mouth of one patient to insert into the mouth of another. It was fully six years before the tooth fell out again.

In 1826, Wagner had offered a series of public dissections and demonstrations in Charleston. The college's collection of specimens was largely compiled from his efforts. He was known for a particularly heroic amputation of a man's arm at the shoulder, tying off an artery after an aneurysm.

His reputation was secured with a public operation for osteosarcoma of the lower jaw, in which more than half of a man's mandible was cut away. Wagner's knife work was likened to the graceful efforts of a sketch artist, and he was proficient with either hand, a fact made more remarkable still by his lifelong battle with rheumatism.

Sims had little interest in the doctrine of irritation and inflammation that launched Wagner's course, but he took painstaking notes on the lectures for a host of surgical procedures: modes of operating on clubfoot, amputation of the penis, types of sutures to be used, the uses of stomach pumps and feeding through the nose, extravasation of blood within the cranium, wounds and diseases of the globe of the eye and cataracts, and so on.

After his coursework, Sims spent almost every moment he could in the deadhouse, and the late hours not only afforded him the opportunity to acquire a comprehensive understanding of anatomy, they enabled him to reflect on the ways in which American physicians could distinguish themselves. Doctors required a steely nerve to confront the late-night ghosts of dissection chambers and the courage to approach their profession as though it was exploration into the unknown. Wasn't it foolish for doctors to experiment on themselves and their students when providence had organized itself such that American physicians—southerners, in particular—had a ready supply of experimental subjects close at hand? Slaves might need to be coerced into surgery, but surely ingenuity could find ways to advance the science of medicine in the absence of willing patients.

The profession, Sims now learned, was beginning to suffer from the spread of so-called medical ethics. A secret society, Kappa Lambda, had been launched in 1819 at a medical school, of all places, and the group's stated goal of fraternity among physicians was a front for motives that were antithetical to progress. First, responding to so-called quackery, the Kappa Lambda men hoped to restrict doctors' ability to advertise their services. But how, without advertising, could a physician earn enough to afford the leisure that would enable him to engage in the sort of thought and experimentation that would grow the scope of the profession? Second, the Kappa Lambda men claimed to be scientists, but truly they were men of a deceptively artful character. The society had been publicly exposed in 1831, but already it had metastasized to chapters throughout the country. The extent of its influence was unclear.

Long before the night Sims's candle was extinguished in the dead room, he had resolved to further his studies in Philadelphia, like so many other physicians. The University of Pennsylvania was beyond him, but there was a new medical school in the city, Jefferson College, where Dr. George McClellan had made a surgical name for himself. McClellan, it was said, was a true man. There were stories of his speed and dexterity, of the gowns that showed the red evidence of his skill and labors, and of the banter he conducted with his patients as he gouged and chiseled away at them. *Courage, my brave fellow! We wound but to heal! It will soon be over . . .*

Sims, Dick Baker, and Theresa Jones's brother Rush, following in his father's footsteps, applied to attend Jefferson College in the fall of 1834. Once again, Sims lied about having studied medicine with Bartlett Jones.

On one of their last nights in Charleston, Sims permitted Dick Baker to talk him into the most foolish of escapades. Fayall's Ballroom was throw-

ing a costume masquerade, and Baker proposed that they attend together with himself dressed as an aging country wagoner and Sims done up as the old man's daughter. They visited Baker's cousins to outfit Sims with a dress and earrings that were tied onto his ears and hung down to his shoulders. It rained horribly that day. They arrived at Fayall's only to learn that the masquerade had been canceled. Baker wasn't content to give up on his fun. He convinced Sims to attend the theater instead, a production of Edward Bulwer-Lytton's *The Lady of Lyons*. They were admitted

after the show began, and Sims would recall the gaze of the entire audience's opera glasses trained on him as a courteous gentleman insisted that
the young lady take his seat near the stage. For the rest of his life, Sims
remained grateful that he was not arrested that night for appearing in
public in women's clothes.

Five

AFTER GRADUATION IN SOUTH CAROLINA, SIMS REMAINED IN LANCASTER for several months before traveling to Philadelphia. He went back to work for Dr. Church and occasionally saw Theresa, while maintaining the secrecy of their pact. Not only would he complete his education before they appealed to Theresa's mother for permission to marry, he would demonstrate that he could earn a living equal to the status of their family.

Sims's college friend James Thornwell was now living in Lancaster. He'd given up his legal ambitions to attend seminary in Massachusetts, and by good chance he'd been assigned to the Presbyterian church that Theresa and her mother attended. Thornwell knew all about Sims's pact with Theresa, and he had agreed to keep it quiet.

J. F. G. Mittag was gone. Tired of being labeled a coward, he had permitted an argument over states' rights with one of Sims's former classmates to grow heated. When the young man challenged his former teacher to a duel, Mittag surprised everyone by accepting and seeking out the counsel of Camden's great duelist Chapman Levy. The duel was fought in Chesterfield District, and though Mittag was wounded in the thigh—his antagonist was unharmed—his courage would never be called into question again. Once he had healed, he embarked on a long overdue journey to London, Paris, Milan, Venice, and Rome.

General James Blair was gone as well. He had disgraced himself. The year before, the general had caused a row when he took offense at *Tele-graph* editor Duff Green's claim that South Carolina Union party members were Tories who had profaned the Union name. Blair accosted Green outside Gadsby's Hotel in Washington City on Christmas Eve, 1832. He struck Green on the head with a club and then broke the editor's arm as the man attempted to draw a dirk from his breast pocket. Blair paid $300 for the offense. Thereafter, it was unclear why Blair seemed to descend into madness. It might have been the slip in his honor, or the opium that had become his habit. He became agitated by religious subjects, and he once fired a pistol at an actress on a Washington City theater stage.

On April 1, 1834, General Blair and former Alabama governor John Murphy retired to Blair's lodgings at Mrs. Tim's on Capitol Hill, after the House recessed. Murphy read to Blair from some letters that were waiting for him. One was from his wife, the girl who had glimpsed him through a keyhole in Theresa's home. She pleaded with him to resign his seat and return to South Carolina. The huge man was moved to tears, and as Murphy attempted to find a kerchief for his friend, Blair took a last drink from a tumbler, produced a pistol from his desk drawer, and raised the barrel to his temple to place a period at the end of his sentence of existence. Members of both houses of Congress were still wearing armbands of mourning when Sims departed Lancaster for his second round of medical training.

* * *

In Philadelphia, Sims, Dick Baker, and Rush Jones fell in with a number of other southerners, taking lodgings in the spare rooms of Miss Edmunds's school for young girls on Sansom Street. Philadelphia was a modern metropolis of eighty-five thousand, with neatly ordered buildings and avenues and gas lighting that would soon be installed throughout the city. The fine ladies of Philadelphia strolled along Chestnut Street, and were rendered more beautiful still when compared to the women of Charleston. Miss Edmunds ensured that three or four pretty girls were present for every breakfast and every dinner, and at tea she sometimes told a humorous anecdote about having once been accosted by a sailor. Sims greatly enjoyed the story. It had been only Miss Edmunds's advanced age and ugliness that prevented the sailor from making violent love to her!

As in Charleston, most of the faculty at Jefferson College were impressive but not of much use to Sims. Dr. John Revere was the son of the famed patriot Colonel Paul Revere, but of what practical use were his theory and practice lectures about rheumatism, blistering, and the ability of an excitement of the mind to bring about death in delicate women? Dr. Samuel Colhoun was widely published, but the ongoing tedium of materia medica—use copper to adulterate an ounce of sulfate of zinc when used as an emetic, and so on—was made even worse by Colhoun's personal manner and harsh lecture style. Dr. Jacob Green's chemistry course was enlivened by his tales of having, at sixteen, invented a machine to verify Benjamin Franklin's electrical experiments—he'd nearly electrocuted himself—but Sims could learn nothing from a doctor whose preceptor had intentionally put him off surgery by forcing him to attend a particularly gruesome operation.

There were two professors, men of proper kidney, who rose above the rest: Dr. Granville Sharp Pattison and Dr. George McClellan.

Pattison had a rogue's reputation. He was from an affluent family in Glasgow, Scotland, but had performed poorly in his early studies and entered medical school at fifteen only because his family lost a significant portion of its wealth. In anatomy class, Pattison thrilled at electric currents applied to corpses to make them smile or thrash their limbs about. A famous anatomist soon employed him as the leader of a gang of student grave robbers. It took about an hour to rob a grave. After digging a tunnel under a gravestone to expose a third of the coffin, the thieves snapped the lid with a crowbar and removed the corpse with ropes. To keep a steady supply of cadavers available for anatomy courses, the bodies were salted and hung to dry like herrings, and reconstituted with water when the time came for their use.

Pattison completed his studies at twenty-two. Two months later, he was admitted as a member of faculty at the same college that made him a doctor. Ten weeks after that, the grave of the well-to-do wife of a wool merchant was found disturbed in the desirable middle portion of Ramshorn churchyard. Word spread of the desecration, and suspicion fell on Dr. Granville Sharp Pattison, of the College Street Medical School. A search team descended on Pattison's chambers and found him inside with two students and six bodies in various stages of dissection. A pan of human bones had been set on fire, and other pans were filled with hearts, livers, kidneys, and lungs. Ropes and dirtied digging utensils were found piled against a wall. One of the investigators stepped on a human ear; a jawbone was discovered in the pocket of one of the students. The head of the wool merchant's wife was found bobbing in a tub of bloody water—it was missing its jawbone and one of its ears.

Pattison was put on trial for violating the sepulchers of the dead and criminal abstraction of a corpse. He was acquitted—not because he was innocent but because the charges against him could not be proven. He sailed for Philadelphia not long after, and went on to become professor of anatomy at Jefferson Medical College.

McClellan might have been less colorful than Pattison, but he was the school's great surgical gun. He graduated from the University of Pennsylvania in 1819. The following year, he was performing much-heralded public procedures, an extraction of the lens in cataract surgery and, like Dr. Wagner in South Carolina, treating a case of osteosarcoma of the lower jaw in a young girl. Sims attempted to befriend McClellan. Welcomed at the McClellan home, he made a point of giving coins to the doctor's young son, another George McClellan, for gingerbread and taffy.

As it happened, both Pattison and McClellan had clashed violently with the University of Pennsylvania's Dr. William Gibson. By dint of becoming the first physician in the world to perform two successful cesarean sections on the same woman, Gibson was the undisputed surgical lion of Philadelphia. Despite his growing aversion to female health, Sims had begun to develop an interest in the science of reproduction. However, the grisly and oft-repeated stories of Gibson's cesarean case—four pregnancies in a young Irish immigrant—tested the gusto of every man who heard them. Sims was left confirmed in his decision to avoid the realm of women's medicine.

* * *

Mary R. was a rachitic dwarf—four and a half feet tall, doubly disabled by rickets and a fall that left her bedridden for two years as an infant. The twist of her femurs and her misshapen pelvis did not prevent her from marrying and becoming pregnant. The doctors who attended her first difficult labor—she was bled and given laudanum—were slow to recognize her physical abnormality. Perhaps, they thought, her birth was obstructed by a rectum engorged with hardened feces. A persistent fetal heartbeat posed a quandary. The baby was an imperfect being, but which posed the greater risk to the mother's life—cesarean section or craniotomy, in which the baby would be destroyed and extracted? The doctors debated until nature decided for them: the fetal heartbeat disappeared.

A surgeon struggled for a time with Botschan's improved craniotomy scissors. The vagina was too cramped to permit the usual drilling motion into the fetal skull. A trocar with a triangular head succeeded in making several holes, which permitted the scissors to break up the infant brain. Mary R. was permitted to rest for five hours—putrefaction failed to set in—and then the bulk of the infant's medullary substance was scraped out. Even great force failed to bring away the rest of the baby. Dr. Davis's osteotome was used to further cut away bone, but a simple crotchet proved a more effective tool to chip away at the frontal and parietal bones. Someone fetched a standard pair of tooth forceps. This proved effective in grabbing and twisting the bone until it broke. Soon, nothing was left of the baby's head but the base of its skull and its lower jaw. After thirty-three hours, a doctor reached into Mary R.'s vagina and managed to deliver the head, and from there the shoulders and hips came away in twenty minutes each. The umbilical cord was shrunken and black, and the placenta made a crackling noise when handled.

Mary R.'s second pregnancy proceeded much as the first, though this time the breaking up of the infant's head was eased by instruments that had been designed for the job in the interim—beaked forceps, with beveled joints and serrated jaws.

A cesarean was prescribed for her third pregnancy, and nine physicians total attended the procedure. Obstetrics was not Dr. Gibson's peculiar province, but given the dangerousness of the operation it was judged best to trust the work to Philadelphia's most experienced surgeon. The danger of cesarean section was cutting into the peritoneum, the bag that contained most of the internal organs. The peritoneum was the great bugbear of surgery. Even an accidental puncture was a death sentence. Infection soon followed, then death. No one knew precisely why.

As Mary R.'s water had not yet broken, a doctor poked a finger up through her vagina and cervix, attempting to rupture the amniotic sac and prevent fluid from spilling into the peritoneum. He failed. Gibson made an additional incision to drain the amniotic waters, and then he expanded the cut through the skin, between the abdominal muscles, and into the peritoneum and the body of the uterus. Assistants gripped the edges of the wound tightly to prevent wet knuckles of intestines from slipping out of the body. The child, a large girl, was found in breech position. She was not breathing when she was removed, but a massaging of the chest, a few breaths blown into her mouth, and several drops of brandy placed on her tongue revived her. Another finger was then poked into Mary R., this time in the opposite direction, down through her uterus and cervical os and into the rear of the vagina, to ensure that blood and fluids drained normally. The wounds were closed with three stout silken sutures, supported by adhesive strips and lint.

Mary R.'s fourth pregnancy was remarkable only in that Dr. Gibson was forced to cut through the scar of his previous incision. This time, the baby was not breech, and for a moment the uterus clamped around the baby's head, as though the womb itself was reluctant to relinquish the child it had cradled. Gibson's pioneering success was heralded in the *American Journal of the Medical Sciences*, Philadelphia's premier publication for physicians.

* * *

Sims's classmates at Jefferson gossiped freely about Gibson's feuds with McClellan and Pattison, both of which dated back more than a decade.

In 1822, McClellan had reviewed an essay Gibson published about fractures of the thigh. Gibson rejected the apparatuses employed by other physicians. Dessault's splints and Cooper's triangular frame were unequal to the task, he wrote. He proposed his own improvement. McClellan offered a twofold criticism. First, Gibson's conclusions were based on a single case. Second, his experiment had resulted in failure. Gibson responded with a

flood of pamphlets and handbills, some published anonymously. He suggested that the best use of his splint might be to break it over McClellan's
back. In response, McClellan published a thirteen-thousand-word essay
accusing Gibson of infirmity of purpose and weakness of nerve.

Gibson's feud with Pattison was even more dramatic. Pattison's arrest
for grave robbery in Scotland had hardly slowed him down. In 1816, he
was charged again for performing operations without consultation. In
1818, he seduced the young wife of an older colleague. In 1823, having
fled Europe for Philadelphia, Pattison fought a duel with the brother-in-
law of a medical school professor who had labeled him an ignorant hum-
bug.

The quarrel with Gibson had begun as soon as he landed in the United
States. Pattison announced that he had been the first to identify a thin
sheet of tissue that surrounded the male prostate gland. Another physician had announced a similar finding. No one was sure whether the
features were identical, and both men claimed credit for the discovery.

Gibson dismissed Pattison as no discoverer of anything—and declared
that furthermore his habits were inconsistent with the principles of honor.
To put the matter to rest, Pattison exhumed the body of a young boy. He
cut into the boy's perineum, only to find the prostate in an advanced state
of gangrene. Nevertheless, those in attendance agreed that the sheet of
tissue described by Pattison was present. The honor was his.

Another bout of published pamphlets ended with Pattison suggesting
that the episode provided ample evidence of the puny soul that animated
Dr. William Gibson.

The atmosphere of feud was still very much in the air during Sims's
studies in Philadelphia. He learned as much about surgery at Jefferson as
he did about the cutthroat nature of the medical profession. The secretive Kappa Lambda men were wrong about medical ethics, but they were
right about the arena of medicine: it was as vicious as a cockfighting pit.
It became clear to Sims that a young surgeon must not only learn how to
distinguish himself with innovations, he must also be prepared to defend
himself against volleys that would be launched against him as his fame
accrued.

Sims was unsure whom he should emulate—McClellan or Pattison.

He was honored that McClellan frequently invited him to assist in surgeries, including one case that caused a sensation. McClellan cut into a man's chest to remove a length of dead rib, and the procedure was performed successfully, without injury to the delicate fluid-filled cavity between the lungs.

By comparison, Pattison was the best lecturer on anatomy in the world, and the only danger of attending his riveting talks—the man's enthusiasm chained students to their chairs—was the stream of spittle that spluttered from his lips at peak moments of excitement. Lectures were valuable, Pattison raged to his charges, but the great essential of one's medical education was the solo dissection of the dead body. Such activity could not command too much of one's attention. Pattison was a rapscallion, but the students enjoyed the stories of his floutings of law and propriety, and in turn, Pattison took a father's pride in helping students out of the peccadilloes they sometimes found themselves accused of.

* * *

Among the southerners that Sims befriended in Philadelphia was a young man named James Lucas, from a town called Mount Meigs, in Alabama. Lucas's father, Henry Lucas, was a wealthy planter with fifteen hundred slaves on a plantation called Rose Hill. The young Lucas's preceptor was his father's cousin Dr. Charles Lucas, who lived nearby on a plantation called Bright Spot. Lucas reveled in telling Dr. Lucas's rags-to-riches story. Charles Lucas had come to Alabama a number of years before with only fifty cents in his pocket. His first consultation fee was $25, and for six weeks' attention on the son of a wealthy planter he earned another $600. He promptly invested in land and slaves. Dr. Lucas now made $15,000 per year and owned two hundred slaves of his own, a fine home, and a horse track, where thoroughbreds competed in best-of-three races of four passes around a mile-round track.

Lucas claimed that Alabama, and in particular the counties west of Montgomery—Lowndes, Autauga, and Marengo—was perfect for the new generation of physicians. Most doctors on the frontier were old, indiscriminate bleeders who bragged of not having read a medical book in twenty years. Of note, and assistance, to young doctors was a series of laws that had recently passed in Alabama, foiling the efforts of so-called botanical doctors, who promised cures with herbs. No one in Alabama knew anything of surgery, and excess of need was matched by excess of wealth. Annual cotton production in Alabama had boomed from twenty to sixty-five million pounds in a little more than a decade. Now they were overplanting, Lucas said, but even that was good for a physician. It meant the slave population was also booming. A forceps delivery of a slave baby could earn a physician as much as a hundred dollars—twenty dollars for natural delivery. Amputations and syphilis cures earned fifty dollars and forty dollars, respectively. Beyond medicine, physicians in Alabama grew wealthy as Dr. Lucas had: first with doctoring, then with slaves, cotton, dispensaries, and careers in banking.

Sims had been hearing of Andrew Jackson's treatment of the Alabama Creeks since he was a boy. Lucas made them sound almost romantic. The Indians had impeccable skill in ricocheting their arrows off the ground, he said. No white man could imitate it. The most famous Creek of all, Big Warrior, towered over most men and owned three hundred slaves. He died the same year as Thomas Jefferson, whose vice president, the scoundrel Aaron Burr, had been captured in Alabama in 1807. He was paraded through the Creek Nation on his way to trial. Two decades later, General Lafayette passed through Alabama on his famous tour; Lucas's father had feted the general at a Rose Hill gala. Notably, the general remarked that when he had fought in the Revolution, all the servants in America were black. Now, they all seemed to be yellow or white.

Like Sims, Lucas worked frequently in the Jefferson College deadhouse. Few noticed when, late in the spring term, Lucas failed to appear for several consecutive lectures. No one suspected it had anything to do with the autopsies he had performed. The students trusted Pattison, who had offered a warning that dissection was a filthy operation and could leave a student's health deranged. However, he'd assured them that the dissecting room of Jefferson Medical College had been constructed on such advanced principles of ventilation that breathing its atmosphere was like breathing the air of any other apartment.

Sims was fond of Lucas—the boy had roots in South Carolina. After he had been missing for several days, Sims called on him. He found Lucas gravely ill. Sims nursed his friend at night, but what did he know of nursing? For that matter, what did he know of any illness not susceptible to the knife? Sims had studied medicine for more than a year now. He could cut down on any artery in the body and tie a ligature around it, but the late nights beside his suffering friend was time to reflect on the fact that he had no clinical experience at all. He knew little of sickness and less of hospitals. He had no idea what Lucas was suffering from or what to do about it. Nevertheless, his dutiful thesis on croup had been approved, and he would soon receive a second diploma as a doctor of medicine.

When Lucas took a turn for the worse, Sims called on Dr. Pattison to attend to him. Pattison conducted a thorough investigation and wrote out a prescription.

What is the matter with him? Sims asked.

I thought you knew, Pattison said. Smallpox. He is going to die tonight.

Smallpox! Pattison explained that one of the bodies in the deadhouse had been a victim. Had Sims been vaccinated? Sims had no idea whether he had been vaccinated. He rushed to Dr. McClellan's house for a scratch and some virus. McClellan hurried Sims into his office and prepared his lancet. Then he paused: there was a mark on Sims's arm as fine as any fellow's in the college. The newly minted physician had completely forgotten that he'd been scratched for smallpox in 1831.

Lucas and two other students at Jefferson Medical College died of the outbreak before graduation.

* * *

The newspapers said that Halley's Comet had signaled the coming of Mithridates VI more than a century before the birth of Christ. There were hints of its return from the years 223, 399, 530, 855, 1066, 1230, 1305, 1380, 1456, and 1531. Johannes Kepler spotted it in 1607, but it wasn't until 1705 that Edmond Halley anticipated that it would return again in 1758. The comet was sighted once more on Christmas Day, 1758.

Stories about the return of Halley's Comet in 1835 had been appearing for years. Their frequency increased as Sims completed his studies in Philadelphia in the spring of 1835 and returned to South Carolina. Journalists thrilled in quoting Shakespeare—comets signaled pestilence and war—but surely, Sims thought, the predictable appearances of Halley's Comet amounted to the triumph of science over poetry and superstition. It was opportunity, as well. Men like Lubbock, Damoiseau, and Pontécoulant were being quoted all over the world with announcements of the specific date on which the comet would once again be glimpsed in the heavens.

He arrived home with a new set of surgical tools and copies of John Eberle's seven-volume *A Treatise on the Practice of Medicine*. These were the only medical books he owned. His father rented him an office on Main Street, and Sims arranged for a large tin sign to be printed with his name. He opened for business as the second physician in Lancaster. He visited Theresa often, but though he attended services with her at Thornwell's church and walked and rode with her, he could not yet claim her hand. He had no money. When Theresa's servant Annie overheard her mother announce that Theresa's affair with Lancaster's new doctor must end, Sims wrote a letter to Mrs. Jones. This time, Thornwell delivered the missive. The young preacher assured Mrs. Jones that Sims did not intend to disgrace Theresa by eloping with her. After ten days of crying and grief, Mrs. Jones at last assented to a union, with the unstated agreement that Sims make his fortune first. But how could Sims make his fortune when societies like the Kappa Lambda worked in secret to prevent doctors from advertising, purporting to quash epidemics of quackery?

Sims sat alone in his office for several weeks. His books remained sealed in a locked bureau. At last, the former mayor of Lancaster strolled in to ask Sims to visit his eighteen-month-old boy, who was ill. Sims had little difficulty with the diagnosis—the miserable toddler had the summer complaint, chronic diarrhea—but beyond cutting the boy's swollen gums down to the teeth, all he knew to do was consult Eberle's chapter on cholera infantum. He started with the powders and mixtures listed at the front. Nothing worked. He sent new leaves and prescriptions twice a day, but nothing affected the boy's condition. When Sims next visited, an old nurse had been brought in to care for the child. The inscrutable woman watched as Sims monitored the infant's pulse. At one moment, the child seemed to faint. Sims lifted it up, blew into its mouth, and shook it in a head-down position, as he had been taught. He continued until the old nurse touched his shoulder.

No use shaking that baby, the woman said. That baby's dead.

Sims's second patient, identical to the first, came two weeks later. This time, Sims tried cures from the end of Eberle's chapter. He cursed Dr. Church, who couldn't be consulted because he was visiting his sister in Tennessee. Again, none of the cures affected the child in the slightest. When Dr. Church returned, he confirmed that Sims's second patient would also die. So far, his effort to make his fortune had been limited to ten dollars that he had earned by sitting with a wealthy plantation owner suffering in the aftermath of a two-week frolic.

It was near the time that Halley's Comet at last appeared in the sky—some claimed a German shepherd dog was the first to glimpse it—that Sims pulled down the tin sign of his Main Street office and threw it into a well. First, he had failed to recognize the signs of smallpox and lost a friend. Now, two innocent babes had died in his care. He told himself that if he had any other career option, he would abandon medicine in an instant.

His mind turned again to Alabama. Perhaps Lucas had been right. Others believed so: Nott would be heading to Mobile the moment he returned from Paris. His friend LeVert was already there, having moved on from experimenting with metal sutures to the organization of his hospital. Another Lancaster friend, Ward Crockett, had already settled in Lucas's hometown of Mount Meigs. Even Theresa's brother Rush—and her mother—had spoken of following the great thrust of people leaving South Carolina for the frontier.

At first, the comet appeared in the sky like a nebula—a circular, misty object more like a fog than a planetary body. As it passed Earth, its tail spread out like a partially opened fan. It was now understood that its light was reflected from the sun. But the movement of the tail from night to night remained a mystery—was the force electric or magnetic? Regardless, it was when the comet was at its most brilliant that Sims decided to head for Marengo County, Alabama. His interest in medicine had resolved to a threefold preoccupation: procreation, to ensure the sustenance of important family names and dynasties; cancer, where quack doctors were making quiet fortunes; and the peritoneum, which for a surgeon was as much a wild frontier as the west. Too often, Sims thought, doctors timidly settled for animal trials where a braver man would press forward to human subjects. Alabama spelled opportunity.

So it was decided. Sims would travel to Alabama, establish a practice, and build a home, then return to marry Theresa and take her west. His father would accompany him—all Sims's siblings were in boarding school. They left on October 13, 1835, a month shy of the two-year anniversary of the night of the falling stars, and shortly before Halley's Comet reached perihelion. Their journey took three weeks, and every night they marveled at the light of the comet flying close to the sun.

* * *

For much of the bout of malaria that struck Sims in late 1836, he remained confused and delirious. Yet he recalled the name of the young servant who was present when Dr. Charles Lucas attempted to bleed him for the disease. It was a strange word: *Anarcha*. At least, that's how it sounded to his ear.

After Sims arrived in Mount Meigs, he sought out Dr. Lucas and James Lucas's father. He revealed that he had known the young Lucas in medical school, but he never let on that a better student and nurse might have recognized the symptoms of smallpox and saved the boy's life. Sims's classmates had asked him to deliver a memorial lecture about the three students' deaths at graduation. He refused. The boy who spoke in his stead gave a self-congratulatory speech. Homer sang of both warriors and physicians, he opined, and the mythical doctors Chiron and Machaon were favorites of the gods.

The girl, Anarcha, was probably mulatto. It wasn't always easy to tell. Sims had quickly learned from working among Alabama slaves that when the father of a baby was a master or an overseer it was often sold off, or not told who its parents were. It didn't matter in the end. Even one quarter black blood was effective immunity from malaria, so the girl made a passable nurse. Others were dying in the rooms around him, but Anarcha slept alongside Sims at night for two weeks straight. She brought him water when he asked for it, and sometimes when he didn't. If Sims didn't know better, he would have taken her insistence that he drink as evidence that there was medicine in the cup.

He hadn't liked Mount Meigs at first. It was a hotbed of activity for the recently formed Whig party that opposed Andrew Jackson. He described the village in a letter to Theresa as a promiscuous huddle of ginhouses, stables, blacksmiths, grogshops, and taverns. He once bristled at the sight of twenty white men, drunk and fighting in the street, with a free negro banjo player in their midst. Planning to press on to Marengo County, Sims spent several days exploring areas to the west, around Montgomery, where there were countless lines of cotton plantations of one thousand or two thousand acres. Each had a slave quarter, some small and some sprawling. The potential for the growth of medical knowledge in Alabama was apparent in how masters protected their investments from disease. There were cabins specially designated as hospitals where sick slaves were immediately sent, cutting them off from the rest of the population. Sims would later write publicly of the poverty, laziness, and filth—not to mention the cramped intellectual capacity and blunted moral feeling— that made slaves susceptible to afflictions like lice and infant lockjaw. But aggressive quarantining by conscientious masters had succeeded in stamping out diseases such as smallpox, syphilis, scrofula, and consumption. He was sure that surgical experimentation would lead to similar advances.

Lucas had been correct. There was opportunity in Alabama, but there were already accomplished physicians in Montgomery, and there were several in Lowndes County and Autauga County as well. Mount Meigs had only two: Dr. Lucas, who barely saw patients as he was often called to Tuscaloosa on bank business, and Dr. Childers, who had only recently settled in town but was already planning to leave the state. Soon after he arrived, Sims accompanied Childers to attend to a beautiful young woman dying of consumption. Childers bled her and told her she would now be well. But he knew the girl was doomed, and his lancet probably hastened her demise.

A few weeks later, Sims rode a day east from Mount Meigs to attend to a case of puerperal fever with another physician, Dr. Bronson. Bronson was educated but drank. He was drunk even as they saw their patient, who had fallen ill after giving birth six days earlier. It was here that Sims learned that to a great extent a doctor's job in consultation was to confirm for the patient and her family that absolutely everything was being done in accordance with principles handed down by the highest medical authorities. Bronson was incompetent. Sims was hardly any better. What did he know of puerperal fever? Yet for several days he stood alongside the drunk doctor and insisted that Bronson's course of action required no alteration.

The woman died the day after Sims left. Nevertheless, the same family called on him to visit a sick overseer. The case would give Sims his first chance to demonstrate his diagnostic skill and resolve. Over several days, Sims and several doctors from Pike County consulted on the man's mysterious wasting condition. Sims argued that there was pus in his abdomen, probably in his liver. It needed to be drained. The others advised against surgery. At last, Sims was permitted to plunge a bistoury into the overseer's flank. It was the happiest moment in his life when two quarts of pus squirted from the man's belly. The overseer was saved.

He wrote to Theresa frequently. He described a Christmas ball in Montgomery with one hundred Alabama girls that he avoided out of a sense of propriety and duty. He grew panicked when he received only two letters in three months. Had she forgotten him? He sent her worried notes, then frantic apologies. She claimed that she wrote infrequently because their relationship was still secret outside of the family. Rumors of their engagement, however, had followed Sims all the way to Alabama. He insisted that his betrothed write him at least every other week.

Sims resolved to stay in Mount Meigs. He bought out Childers for $200—his books, his medicine, and his patients. In January 1836, he purchased lumber to build a home, then traveled back to South Carolina to claim Theresa, but Mrs. Jones insisted that he wait until Christmas. He returned to Alabama just before another Creek uprising. Sims signed on to a volunteer corps, serving as an assistant surgeon under the command of Dr. Hugh Henry of Montgomery. Dr. Henry was no military commander, and the corps spent a miserable five weeks in the woods near Tuskegee. They saw no action, but Sims returned to Mount Meigs with more than a hundred new acquaintances upon which he might build a profitable practice.

Remuneration remained elusive. For the most part, his work was in the slave quarters; he prescribed as he moved from miserable cabin to miserable cabin. In early September, as he made rounds on a plantation down with fevers, he felt a shiver slide down his back. A chill laid him low that night. By morning, he was barely able to mount his horse for the return to Mount Meigs.

Dr. Lucas saw him the next day. After a careful examination, he called for the young girl Anarcha to bring him string, cotton, and a bowl. Sims refused to be bled. Dr. Lucas said he was a damned contrary fellow, and that Sims could die if that's what he wanted.

The fever raged in Sims's room, and in the rooms of others nearby—Mrs. Judkins and her son, who died of it. Sims drank everything Anarcha gave him. But it wasn't until a visit from one of his comrades from the Creek uprising, an Englishman and druggist from Montgomery, that the fever broke. The druggist gave him quinine. Sims's hair fell out—but at last he began to improve. By late November, he was well enough to travel, though he was haggard and nearly bald when he married Theresa in December 1836. Mrs. Jones gifted the newlyweds a pair of married servants as a wedding present. When they left for Alabama after the new year, Sims had his wife and his first slaves. Now all he had to do was keep them.

Six

Monsters—Raw Head and Bloody Bones—Westcott plantation—
Slave sales—The Westcott wedding—Rumors of Sims—
Field work—Comet of 1843—Rape—Dr. Henry—
Forceps delivery

*T*HERE WERE CREATURES IN THE WOODS. ESCAPED HOGS TURNED WILD, wild beefs you could hunt like deer, and there were bears as big as the beefs in the woods, and there were alligators in the bayou that would sometimes come up and take a woman's arm when she was washing clothes. Plagues of worms fell from trees in the woods, and there were panthers in the woods whose cries at night sounded like women screaming.

On the Lucas plantation, Anarcha heard stories of winged creatures that brought the devil's miasmas from the swamps, and of witches that flipped themselves inside out at night and flew across the countryside to turn milk into blood. The most frightening was a monster called Raw Head and Bloody Bones, which was a slave that had escaped, like the escaped slaves that Pheriba had told her about, but Raw Head and Bloody Bones was nine feet tall, with huge hands, and lived in an abandoned millhouse or in the well of an old brewery, and he would chase children who were out playing marbles after dark and bash in their heads and eat what was inside. Anarcha was thirteen or eleven now, and she would soon be returning to the Westcott plantation. She was old enough to know that Raw Head and Bloody Bones wasn't real—it was how parents kept their children away from the wagons of the speculators who sold slaves but also stole them when they had the chance. The fearful story kept the children inside at night, and the children were tasked with preventing fire from burning down the cabin when their parents went to meetings or frolics. Raw Head and Bloody Bones made the younger children tremble and cry themselves to sleep, and all you had to do to get them to behave was threaten to put them outside at night.

When Anarcha returned to the Westcott Plantation, Pheriba told her a story about Raw Head and Bloody Bones. Raw Head and Bloody Bones was always hungry, Pheriba began, hungry for the meat of children and cattle and sheep. One day, he came upon a farmer who had just killed a beef. *I want some meat*, Raw Head and Bloody Bones said. The farmer gave him a front quarter, and Raw Head and Bloody Bones ate the front quarter. He said, *I want some more meat*. The farmer gave him the other front quarter, and Raw Head and Bloody Bones ate the other front quarter, and then he ate both hind quarters as well. He kept gobbling up animals, hogs and beefs, until tricky Mrs. Rabbit invited him home for some lamb. Raw Head and Bloody Bones followed Mrs. Rabbit home and opened his mouth to demand more meat, but right then Mrs. Rabbit jumped down his throat with her scissors in her hand. She let out all his entrails and crawled back out of his mouth, and that's how the settlement was saved.

Pheriba scoffed at those who said they had seen Raw Head and Bloody Bones in the woods. That was just the skinned head of a beef that a master put on a stick, she said.

* * *

Anarcha was brought back to the Westcott plantation in late 1840, when the young Westcott boys weren't young anymore and it was time to divide the master's property among Eliza Westcott and her four living children. Of the twenty-nine slaves that David Westcott owned when he died in 1828, only seventeen remained, including Anarcha. Robbin was gone, Isham and Minden were gone, Fran was gone, and Anarcha's sister Mary was gone. Her father, Jerry, was gone too, though one day Pheriba put her dark arm beside Anarcha's lighter arm and told her she shouldn't be so sure Jerry was her father, even if he had acted like her father. Her mother, Sue, now married to another man, didn't say anything about it one way or the other.

Now there were eighty-six slaves on the Westcott plantation. There were many children, and some of these children were kept and some of them were sold, though the Westcott plantation was doing more buying than selling, and sometimes they bought from the speculators who arrived more frequently now with their cloth and their horses and their lines of chained slaves, once a month or once every few weeks. One woman who was bought from the speculator wagons had fits because her baby wasn't bought along with her, and another woman named Susan who was older than most was sold to the speculators directly from the fields. The speculator wagon rode down to the fields to put her inside, and Anarcha met them at the gate with Susan's last baby so she could let her baby suck one more time before she rode away with a bag over her head so she wouldn't know how to get back to her baby if she ran away.

The church that the missus had helped to found was open now in Montgomery, and sometimes some of the slaves would walk behind the Westcott carriage into town to go to church on Sunday. On the Lucas plantation, the slaves hadn't gone to church, but they had gathered in cabins at night to sing and get happy and pray into pots lowered over their heads so the overseers couldn't hear them, but in Montgomery a few got to sit inside, up in the gallery, and there was another service outside run by black exhorters who taught them to sing hymns because they couldn't read, either music or words. It was when Anarcha was in town that she witnessed the other way that masters put slaves in their pockets, which meant selling you and turning you into paper money that folded up and went into masters' pockets. Auctions were held right in the middle of Montgomery, near the big basin where everyone got their water. White people gathered around a small area where there was a curtain for a stage, and there was an overseer with a black snake whip in one hand and a pepperbox pistol in the other, and there was a man who cried the bucks and the wenches and told jokes to entertain the white people in gowns and tall hats who watched the auction like they were at a picnic. A slave woman always sold for more than a slave man, particularly if she was known to be a good breeder, and children that were part white always sold for more money too. Masters sold men that were unruly, and missuses sold women if they wanted a new dress. It was hard to sell slaves with lots of scars on them; that's why overseers dunked them into brine after whippings.

Barren women were sold to speculators who took them farther south, to sugar plantations in Louisiana. Slaves sold at auction were dressed up in fine clothes, and the overseer would take a meat skin and grease their faces and hands and feet just before they put them out to be sold, to make them look like they were well fed, and the crier would make people laugh and tell their ages and what they could do, field work or tanning or cobbling or nursing children. Buyers put on white gloves and examined the slaves for broken bones and whip marks, and they would look at their teeth to see if the crier was lying about how old they were. Anarcha watched as one buyer examined the teeth of a wench and then pulled down her dress to test the weight of her breasts and then lifted her skirts to examine her there too and joke about whether she had teeth down there as well.

On the Lucas plantation, there were stories of slaves being sold on other plantations. Once, there was a couple that didn't want the wife to be sold, so one day they tied up their master and poured boiling water down his throat. The master refused not to sell the woman, and later that couple was lynched together. On another plantation, a white woman, the master's daughter, married a slave man, and the master didn't like it, so he sold the man and sent him away. But the master's daughter found her husband, bought him back, and brought him home, and then she mixed his blood with whiskey and drank it so she could always say she had black blood in her.

Some slaves cut off their own hands so that they couldn't be sold. Others told their masters they better put them in their pockets or they would run away.

On the Westcott plantation, it was often a girl's first child that was sold away. Anarcha knew how babies were put into women now, she'd seen it on the Lucas plantation—sometimes a man with his wife, but also sometimes when an overseer would ring a bell in a pattern for a particular slave girl to come help him with something in the barn, and she went to the barn and everyone knew what it meant. Anarcha had seen babies coming out again too, helping the Lucas grannies as they let nature take its course or if nature took the wrong course they called for the white doctors. Babies on the Lucas plantation stayed on the Lucas plantation—there weren't

many that were sold away, not babies, anyway—but on the Westcott plantation girls had babies before they were married, and these infants were
sold, and then afterward they married another Westcott slave or perhaps,
with permission, a man on a neighboring plantation, and then a woman's babies remained, and that's why the Westcott plantation had so many
babies and young children. There were six births in the five months after
Anarcha came home, and then at last the Westcott family, thirteen years
after David Westcott died, divided up his property.

The overseer blew the horn to call all the slaves to the house, and the
missus was up on the porch with a man named Judge Bibb from the city
who was writing things down, and she told the gathered slaves one by
one to say their name aloud and then go stand by the person who was
their new master, and the man Bibb glanced at each of them and guessed
at their ages and wrote this down beside their names. Priscilla Westcott,
who was fifteen years old, got eighteen slaves. Susannah Wescott, who
was ten years old, got seventeen slaves. Eliza Westcott kept fourteen slaves
for herself. Samuel Westcott got eighteen slaves, and William Westcott
got nineteen, including Anarcha and her brothers Joe and Ben and her
mother. These are your masters now, the missus told them, and then they
went back to their cabins just like before.

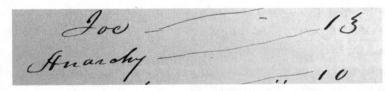

Samuel Westcott was twenty-one years old then, and William Wescott
was nineteen years old, and they were the real masters now and they had
been for some time. The young masters had had no father to raise them,
and there were twenty women on the Westcott plantation who might bear
children. There was Isabel who was thirty-five, and Jany who was twenty,
and Caroline who was twenty, and Harriet who was eighteen, and Mary
who was sixteen, and others, too. Of the eighty-six Westcott slaves, thirty-
one were children younger than Anarcha.

Priscilla Westcott got married in 1841, when she was sixteen, and her
wedding in June was a bigger celebration than any Christmas or corn

shucking. For days beforehand, the Westcott slaves were occupied with egg beating and butter creaming and sugar pounding and jelly straining and silver cleaning and floor rubbing and pastry making and peeping at Priscilla as she tried on her dress with its long veil and train. The tail feathers of all the peafowls were plucked to make wedding fans and to put into hats for the missus and Susannah Westcott. As the day approached, the slaves spread Marseille carpets and linen tablecloths throughout the Westcott house, and there were two silver candlesticks in every room, and there were four wine decanters and four nutcrackers and four silver ladles and six silver sugar tongs and a silver mustard pot and two silver fruit stands. In addition to wine, the missus bought liquor from Montgomery and champagne that had come from across the water, and the day before the wedding, they started the cooking of turkeys and chickens and the peafowls without feathers and good old ham as well.

On the day of the wedding, the guests arrived in carriages and sur- reys and buggies and on horseback, and the young women who rode up wearing long riding habits immediately went upstairs to the guest rooms to put on dresses with ruffles and lace and wide hoops. The celebration was to last three days, and the women brought with them trunks that held quilts and coverlets and their second-day dress and their third-day dress. For the ceremony, Priscilla wore a wreath of flowers on her head, and white people tossed rice at the newlyweds, and there was a band with a fiddle and an accordion, and on the first night there was waltzing and minuets but no dance contests as on other holidays, no slave fiddler call- ing figures to "Green Corn Dance" and "Cut the Pigeon Wing," telling the white dancers to promenade, or sashay, or swing corners, or change partners.

On the second and third days, the missus gave the white women a tour of the Westcott plantation, including the slaves themselves, and indicated how many increase each of the women had produced, and showed off the cabins, which the slaves had cleaned for this very reason, and pointed to the cabins' plank floors so that people knew the Westcott slave cabins had floors. The men occupied themselves with horse racing: the slave men set out a big oval track, and the masters and the young masters raced horses that weren't their buggy or wagon horses but were special horses bred for racing, and the one to win was the one who reached down at a full gallop and snatched the head off a goose that was tied to a post at the finish line. In one race, two masters bet a slave on the outcome, and now there was a man going to a new plantation when the wedding was over.

A whole army of slaves arrived with the guests, and they stayed in the Westcott slave quarters and it was very crowded for three days; some of the men slept outside. It was at such holidays and celebrations, late at night around fires, that slaves shared news they heard from the masters' mouths over dinner. This was also how stories of whippings and killings and Br'er Rabbit passed from one plantation to the next, and it was how Anarcha heard that there was a fearful doctor named Dr. Sims who was now swooping around the countryside, moving from plantation to plantation as quick as any inside-out witch or hungry runaway monster. In addition to pulling spiders out of overseers, it was said that Dr. Sims had a knife that he used on slaves' eyes or feet. He didn't make any teas or take your blood or give you scratches or powders, and it didn't matter whether you wanted him to fix you at all. Dr. Sims had moved to Montgomery, and behind his office for white people he had opened a hospital for plantation slaves and for city slaves, who were freer than most but not free. The slaves were frightened of Dr. Sims, and Anarcha surely didn't tell anyone that she had once cared for Dr. Sims and maybe she had saved his life.

It was also at celebrations—or perhaps at church, where a man might slide up next to a woman he liked and take her hand—that slaves met the men and women who became their husbands and wives. Every he thing, it was said, from a he king down to a bunty rooster, got excited about getting married. Girls poked dried chinaberries onto strings and wore them around their necks to charm the men they liked. An older man or the missus would notice a young couple giving attentions to one another, and the master would arrange a small ceremony. A new cabin was prepared, and the bride wore a blue calico dress, a man's shirttail for a head rag, and her stiff brogan shoes, and words were said by the master or someone else—*You're both good slaves, treat each other right, or by God I'll take you up and whip you* or *Dark and stormy may come the weather, I join this man and woman together / Let none but Him that make the thunder, put this man and woman asunder / I therefore announce you both the same, be good, go long, and keep your name*—and then the couple would step or jump over a broom for luck, and it was bad luck if you touched the broom, so the husband and wife stepped extra high over it, and if the luck didn't work and you wanted a separation you stepped back over the broom the other way. No slave got married out of the book the way white people did, and if the man and the woman didn't come from the same plantation it was understood that the increase would belong to the master who owned the wife.

Not all slaves were allowed to pick who they married. Missuses sometimes paid close attention to who the girls were to marry, and if a house servant got interested in the good-looking daughter of a field hand, there was a fuss and probably nobody got married. You could get whipped if you didn't like the man they married you to, and you could get whipped if you married someone without your master's permission. One master who ran a saloon grew enraged when one of his slaves got married when the master was on a drunk spell. The master discovered that his man was escaping at night to see his wife, so the master took up a big knife and he chopped off the wife's head and put a big weight around her body and made his slave throw her in the river. Then the master put the man in chains for a long time and whipped him.

On another plantation, a free black man named Tom Vaughn from the north saw a field hand he liked. Tom Vaughn worked on the insides of pianos, and he had come south looking for piano work. He forgot all about pianos when he saw that woman, whose husband had died. She had three sons already. Tom Vaughn let himself into slavery so he could marry that woman, and then he worked in the fields alongside her, and they had six babies of their own, all girls.

* * *

By the time Anarcha returned to the Westcott plantation, Pheriba had trained several of the young girls to help her with the children and the babies and the nursing, and *Anuaka* *500* the Westcott house slaves did not need another cook or maid. Anarcha worked in the fields until her blood came.

Women worked in one field, men in another, and now young mothers were carrying newborns to the fields in baskets on their heads and nursing them there until they could walk. They left the babies in old quilts shaped into pallets near the fence line and stopped to let them suck after weeding a row of corn or picking a row of cotton. They pulled fodder, built fences, and plucked the worms off the leaves of the crops, and if you missed a worm you had a choice: three lashes or eat it. Breakfast in the fields was fatmeat, molasses, and corn bread, and when the horn sounded at midday you stood up and if your shadow was right under you it was dinnertime—roasted corn, baked potatoes, boiled pork, and buttermilk.

During the cotton harvest, the horses worked the gins, and a squad of boys pulled the bull-tongue plow instead. The horses were given more rest than the boys. Sometimes, early in the morning, a runaway would burst out of the forest and run circles among those working the fields, attempting to confuse his scent with that of the others as dogs in the woods came barreling down on him. There were men who were so fast it was said they could grab onto the tail of a horse, let it run, and keep up just fine. The runaways had pepper in their shoes and a handful for the dogs' eyes if they got close, or they had rubbed onions onto their feet if they were barefoot, or doused them with graveyard dust or the smoke of lightwood splinters. There were pots hidden in the woods, near deep creeks. Runaways lowered them over their heads as though to pray, and then sank down in the water and breathed inside the bubble as they walked to the other side. The dogs lost their trail, and the runaway left the pot behind for the next runaway who came along.

Field hands sang a song about how the morning star rose and broke in your soul, and in 1843 a star appeared in the daytime sky and drew a nick in it. One morning in March, it appeared very close to the sun, a little bright swipe that hung just next to it, and early in the evenings a streak appeared behind it, growing longer and longer as the days passed and the star moved closer and closer to the horizon, pushing forward as though it had a place to go and a purpose for going there. White people said it was the longest falling star anyone had ever seen and some said that it might hit the ground, and at night the slaves talked about the masters discussing lectures on the star in Mobile and Huntsville. Even looking through their special glasses, it was hard to know whether the star-grazer star was a small one close by or a big one very far away, but if it was small and close and hit the Earth then it would probably break up and explode and make a show, and this might disturb the equilibrium and cause violent tempests or make the air bad to breathe, but no one was worried this time because it was said that people faced greater dangers every day—heat and cold, for example, which had always fought against each other for all of history but neither ever got the upper hand—and anyway big wandering stars had been following their courses for thousands of years and there was no indication that any of them would ever hit the ground. In the evenings, Anarcha looked up at the great line across the sky and knew that it was the same star that had appeared when she was a girl. Now it was return-ing, as though to deliver the message of its journey.

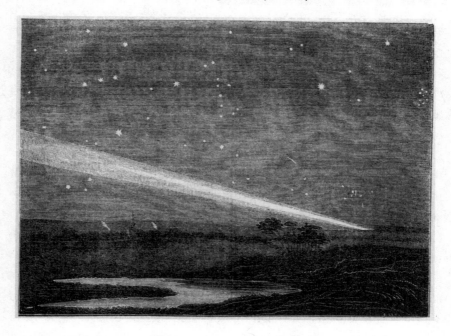

Two months after the star faded, Anarcha's blood came. There was no use hiding it, as it had come late to her, and William Westcott had already asked her if she was bleeding yet and he was watching her for signs. Some of the field hands had been giving her attentions in anticipation: John and Jim and Dick who belonged to Susannah Westcott, and Isaac

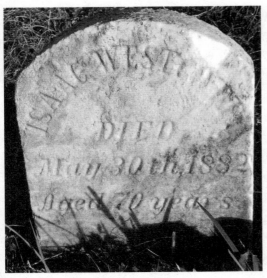

who belonged to William West-cott, and Jacob who belonged to Samuel Westcott. Anarcha didn't announce it when it did arrive, but she didn't hide it either, and it was some months before she flinched at a cramp and an over-seer saw her, or Pheriba noticed the difference and told the mis-sus. But no one was surprised one Sunday when an overseer came to the cabin after dark and told Anarcha to go to the barn to shuck corn. It was August 1844.

The corn was still growing. It would not need to be shucked for another three months.

It was dark in the barn and when the door shut behind her, Anarcha was grabbed from the rear, and she did not resist as her hands were tied to a sawhorse and someone pulled up her dress. A man shoved himself into her. A jolt flashed from that stabbed spot to her fingers and toes, her face and lips, every part of her fired and pained. She thought about stories that slaves visiting from other plantations had told. She thought about the woman who was suspended from barn rafters and whipped because she refused to be the wife of a man her master wanted her to make a baby with. She thought about the woman who gave her baby something to make it die before it got sold off. She thought about stories of women trying to escape with their babies—one who leaped perilously across a frozen river, jumping from floe to floe until she made it to Ohio, and another who was chased down by dogs that ate the breasts right off of her body. Anarcha could not say how long it lasted. She had never been whipped, and she did not scream like those who were whipped, and when it was over the man left the barn and someone else came in to release her hands, but she never saw either one of them and she did not know if it was an overseer, or a driver, or William Westcott, or a stud buck whose master had been paid to put a baby into her. It happened five more times, on the next five nights, and then a baby did begin to grow inside of her.

Anarcha had learned of other ways that women unfixed themselves—calomel and turpentine, or the indigo that was grown for dye, and Pheriba had a better recipe for cotton than just chewing a root: boil the seeds, scoop them out when they floated, and mix cornmeal with the likker to make a paste that you ate. There were many ways to make a baby go off to the same void that falling stars vanished into, but if you did it your master would whip you and put another one into you, and if he believed that you couldn't make babies he would put you in his pocket and you'd be off to Louisiana.

Slave women on the Lucas plantation and on other plantations worked in the fields when they were pregnant, and some knew the month they'd been born because that was the field their mother had been in up to an hour before giving birth—corn or fodder or cotton—and some women gave birth right there in the fields. On the Westcott plantation, women with growing babies did not work the fields. The Westcotts wanted portly babies, so pregnant girls were kept around the house, and even though Anarcha was not portly she was given the same food as the Westcotts to help make a portly baby. As she grew larger and larger, William Westcott praised her from the porch and told her that if she was a good multiplying woman she'd never have to work in the fields again. When the baby began to move inside her, it did not feel like her increase at all, it did not feel like anything that belonged to her—not even so much as her wooden spoon on the Westcott plantation, nor the mussel shell that she used on the Lucas plantation, nor the dress that she now wore on her back or the brogans on her feet. It was her baby but not her baby, and the only reason it kicked like it wanted to get out was because it didn't know any better.

She knew there was something wrong when the pains began and she spent all night in the sickroom off the kitchen and the baby didn't come, despite it trying hard to do so. The pains lasted all night. In the morning, Pheriba sent the girl named Mede that William Westcott had recently bought to fetch an ax. Pheriba positioned it under the bed where Anarcha lay, and she looked down at the blade pointing up at her. Nature refused to take its course. It refused that day, and it refused the second night too. In the morning, Pheriba called for the missus, and the missus called for Dr. Hugh Henry, and Dr. Henry arrived in the afternoon and tried calling in instructions from outside the sickroom, but nothing worked and then he came inside and by that time Anarcha was exhausted from the pain and from no sleep in two days' time, and the labor pains had mostly stopped, and the baby hadn't moved in some time either.

Dr. Henry and the missus spoke right there in front of her. He couldn't use ergot, he explained, because the baby was too large, which meant it was a mechanical obstruction—that's what he called the baby—and there was a danger that her womb was going to burst, and if that happened the baby would go backward into her stomach instead of out of her vagina. He suggested that bleeding would relax Anarcha's womb and birth canal and make delivery go easier, and the missus gave her consent because William Westcott wasn't anywhere near that sickroom, and Dr. Henry pulled out his big scarificator box to suck her blood, and they turned Anarcha onto her side, and he pressed the cold box against her neck, and she felt the twelve blades bite and slice into her, but just barely, and they drained twenty ounces of blood into a cup, and it felt like her soul leaking out of her, like the light of a star falling farther and farther away, and if it relaxed her birth canal it didn't matter because her baby, which wasn't her baby, was too big for a canal that was either stiff or relaxed.

There were two surgical options left, Dr. Henry explained. Both were expensive, and neither could he perform himself. One was that the baby could be cut out of Anarcha. She would die, but the baby might live. That was $150. The other was that they could wait a little longer, and then the baby could be pulled out of her with tools. Anarcha would probably live, but the baby would most likely die. That was $100, with an additional $20 if the placenta needed to be delivered as well. For either, Dr. Henry said, he would ride back into town to fetch Dr. Marion Sims, who had trained in Philadelphia and had proved himself to be the best doctor in Montgomery for working with the newest procedures and instruments.

The missus stared at the ground. Go fetch Dr. Sims, she said.

The name, perhaps, poked a hole in Anarcha's delirium. In an hour's time, Dr. Sims arrived in a flourish, impatient and annoyed. He looked at Anarcha, but if he recognized her he gave no sign of it. Dr. Sims was much smaller than Dr. Henry, but he moved and talked like a master, and he turned Anarcha's head and looked at the fresh wounds of her bleeding and mumbled something about barbarity. Then he dug into his bag for an implement that struck Anarcha—though she was barely awake now, listing in and listing out—as familiar. Eliza Westcott smoked a pipe, and sometimes when Anarcha had been very young the missus would call her to the house and tell her to go inside for a red coal, and Anarcha would go inside and pluck a small red coal from the fireplace with a pair of fire tongs, which was also an implement that cooks used to put things into fires and take them out again. Anarcha brought the red coal for the missus, and she used it to light her pipe on the porch, and the implement that Dr. Sims produced from his bag and held up in the air was exactly like that pair of fire tongs, as though it was no baby or falling star he was going to pull out of her but a blazing sun too dangerous to touch. They were talking about blood and bleeding now, all of them down between her legs, the missus and Pheriba and Dr. Sims and Dr. Henry, but Anarcha didn't know whose blood and whose bleeding, and wouldn't any woman half crazy with pain, half conscious from exhaustion, find her mind slipping back to the stories of witches turning themselves inside out at night and wonder whether she too was being turned inside out? She wanted to speak. If the baby came out alive, she wished to say, let it lay for twenty minutes and then cut the cord. Grease hog lard on a scorched rag and put that on the belly button, and don't wash that baby for a week. But she couldn't speak, and she could barely move. She felt a tugging inside of her. Then it felt like something snapped. Then it all went dark, and she never laid eyes on that baby once, and she didn't know if it came out looking black or white, or even if it lived.

Seven

ALABAMA PLANTATION OWNER R. R. MOSELY'S SLAVE SAM CONTRACTED syphilis in 1840. It took a year of medicine to cure it.

A year later, a rising commenced on the right inner portion of Sam's jaw. The lesion resembled a gum boil, but it was so stubborn Mosely suspected it wasn't a gum boil at all but an effect of the syphilis cure. A doctor pronounced it a gum boil and lanced it, but it refused to heal. A short time later, the same physician examined Sam again and found that most of the teeth on the right side of his jaw were now loose, barely fixed in their sockets. The doctor cut down to Sam's jawbone and found it diseased, coated with a film similar to brain matter. Sam insisted the rising didn't hurt, but he was a house slave and the growth now stretched disturbingly across the entire front portion of his lower jaw. It had the unsightly appearance of a fleshy, lopsided beard.

Sam was next sent to a surgeon. At the first touch of the doctor's knife, he leaped from his seat and refused to submit to any additional cutting.

Mosely was left in a bind. Sam could not keep working in the house, clearly, and the price that a slave of such wretched appearance might bring in Montgomery would never cover the cost of an adequate replacement. Sending Sam to the fields would amount to the same loss.

Mosely recalled hearing of another young surgeon in Montgomery:

Marion Sims. Rumor claimed that Sims had saved the life of an overseer suffering from a growth in his gut and had cured the face of a horribly deformed woman from Hayneville. It was said that plantation owners were bringing their slaves to town with their cotton harvest so that Sims could operate on them for a variety of ailments. Perhaps Sims could convince Sam to undergo a procedure.

Sam was twenty-six years old when he first visited Sims's Negro Hospital in April 1845. It was a ramshackle structure behind Sims's office on Perry Street, little better than a slave cabin, with eight cots on one side of the room and, on the other side, a barber's chair and an examination table partitioned off by a sheet hanging from the ceiling.

Sims had arranged to be alone in the clinic when Sam arrived. He invited the slave to sit in the barber's chair and performed a tender examination. The whole undersurface of Sam's lower jaw was hard and bony, whereas everything inside his mouth, from the third molar forward on either side, had been replaced by a growth that oozed bloody pus.

The gentle examination was a ruse. Mosely had written to Sims of Sam's reluctance to be cut—but perhaps it was an opportunity. In Charleston, Wagner had profited from the public performance of a capital surgery of the jaw, and McClellan had done the same in Philadelphia. Sims himself had recently followed suit with another slave who had been only too willing to be cut. But what of slaves who refused to submit to any procedure that would be more painful than whatever punishment they might receive for refusing it? The problem was not only mechanical. Some surgeons lacked the wherewithal to perform extensive surgeries without consent. Sam's case demonstrated that medical fortitude was exactly what savvy plantation owners might require—and pay handsomely for. Sims could earn a nice fee, publicly demonstrate his skill, publish the case, and, as a bonus, put his name to a piece of medical hardware that would prove the practicability of capital surgery regardless of whether a patient was willing.

Sims patted Sam on the shoulder. He told him not to fear and to return in two weeks' time.

Several months before, Dr. Thomason, of Lowndes County, had sent Sims an eighteen-year-old slave named George. Like many plantation owners, Thomason had just enough medical training for the title, but he

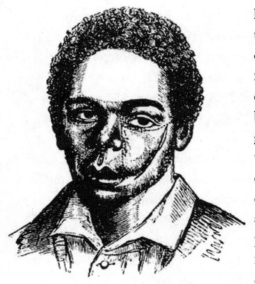

lacked the skills to undertake anything beyond the simplest of procedures. He'd removed a growth
from George's upper left gum several times, but when the boy's cheek
began to bulge, he sent him to Montgomery. Sims found George's gums
to be purple; they bled at the slightest touch. The cause was a tumor, of
course, as large as an orange, with
a tense, elastic feel. One-third of it
projected outward from the slave's
face. The rest was lodged under his
cheek and eye.

Sims spent several days removing George's decayed teeth in preparation, and the boy was given brandy and water, as needed, during the
operation. His cheek was opened with the cut recommended by France's
famous Dr. Velpeau, a curving incision that stretched from the edge of
his left eye to the corner of his mouth. To make a flap that could be lifted
away, Sims cut the wing of the left nostril and the connective tissue of the
inner upper lip. Thrusts of a bone knife separated the palate from the jaw
and the sphenoid bone. Then he attacked the mass itself, cutting through
mucous membrane and snipping the bones of the roof of the mouth with
Liston's bone forceps. During the most difficult portion of a thirty-five-
minute procedure, George's exposed eye and its appendages had to be
supported by an assistant using the bent handle of a silver spoon, like a
ladle. When at last the mass came loose, it left its curved impression in
the boy's face.

After the operation, Sims was left with two regrets. He wished he had
hired a sketch artist to render a likeness before the procedure—though
the extensive scarring would not matter, as George was a field hand—and
he regretted not taking more bone away with the tumor. How could he?
George was a willing patient to a point, but no man could have controlled
him if they had begun sawing bone along with the mass. By the time R. R.
Mosely's slave Sam appeared to offer the chance of correcting both mis-

takes, Sims had heard that George's
tumor had returned and was even
larger than before.

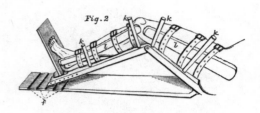

He set about elaborate preparations for Sam. In 1838, Josiah Nott,
who had now made good on his
plans to move to Mobile, published in the *American Journal of the Medical Sciences* an account of the duel he had attended at Lightwood Knot
Springs in South Carolina. He articulated in detail his innovation of the
double inclined planes to immobilize the injured student's pelvis. Sims's
device was similar. He drew up plans and took them to a carpenter, and
then wrote to Mosely for consent to attempt a vigorous operation.

Sam returned to the Negro Hospital on May 15, 1845. He was surprised to find that Dr. Sims was not alone this time. More than twenty-
five men were gathered inside, sitting quietly as though waiting for a
frolic to begin. Dr. Sims instructed Sam to stand still as one of the men
began to sketch his face, and then Sims steered him to the barber's chair.
This time, a flat plane board—as long as a coffin, outfitted with many straps
and buckles—was suspended between the edge of the chair and a stool
several feet away.

Sit, Sam, sit, Dr. Sims said.

Sam hesitated, then straddled the plane board to ease himself into the
barber's chair. The moment he was settled, Sims's assistants seized Sam's
arms and legs. There was a struggle, but the men—fifteen were Sims's
Montgomery colleagues, ten were students—fought with Sam from every
quarter. Sims's plane board proved itself be of the proper length, even
though he had only guessed at Sam's height. Straps of the sort used for
horses immobilized the young man's knees, ankles, and thighs. Additional
straps were passed around his abdomen, chest, and shoulders and made
movement all but impossible. Cuffs secured his wrists, and his elbows
were pinioned to his sides. Last, a strap was wrapped around his head
and fastened at the rear, permitting movement of the neck to any desired
position by pulling a length of leather along the course of the spine.

Sims was barely able to deliver the sixty drops of laudanum that
were intended to ease the pain of the procedure. Sam was so alarmed the

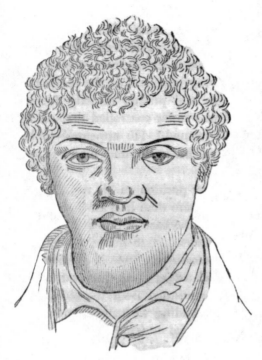

drug seemed to have no effect on him. At the first cut, the boy made a last furious effort to free himself. Sims noted to the others that his precautions had been warranted, and that his device was proving itself adequate to an obstacle that less manly physicians regarded as insurmountable.

A cut around the base of Sam's chin enabled the dissection of flaps both upward and downward to expose the tumor and the diseased jawbone. Ligatures secured facial arteries and immobilized the tongue. An additional fang was removed to make room for a narrow saw, but the saw quickly proved inappropriate to the job. Liston's bone tool was equally ineffective.

Sims next tried a handheld chain saw that was meant for dividing a woman's pubic bone in difficult births. He'd never used it before. So far, he'd been successful in avoiding conditions of the female pelvis, and cases he heard about from Lowndes County had only cemented his decision to avoid the female sphere. There was a woman who had been bled of sixty-two ounces during childbirth—her doctor had held camphor to her nose, believing it would help. Another pregnant woman had been given opiates, and her belly was blistered before she delivered a putrid child. The uterus of still another woman had descended and fallen out of her body, the mass gangrenous with a whitish, leaden color, giving off a fetid, cadaverous odor. Such medicine might be remunerative, Sims thought, but it was wholly distasteful.

The chain saw worked perfectly, passing through each side of Sam's jawbone in a few seconds. The wound was left open until the bleeding abated, and it was only now that the laudanum seemed to take effect. A student sat up with Sam that night, and over the next few days it became apparent that apart from a scar on his jaw the only outward evidence of the slave's former growth was a tendency for his chin to sag or collapse into his face when he reclined. His value as a house servant had been preserved.

Sims was so pleased with the result that he wrote to Lowndes County to have George sent back to Montgomery. Sam was still recovering when Sims operated on George for a second time. The boy looked a horror. The skin of his cheek was threatening to rupture from the pressure of the returned growth, and his eye was now bulging from its socket—he could neither close it nor move it. The operation lasted ninety minutes, as long and tedious a procedure as anyone present could remember. Sims's proddings dug down nearly to the base of the boy's brain. This time, Sims erred in plugging the cavity with a sponge to control the hemorrhaging. Rather than staunch the bleeding, the sponge invited it. George collapsed into nausea and vomiting and nearly died. He recovered from immediate danger, but the mass had begun to reappear even before he returned to his plantation. The growth destroyed his eye and filled his mouth and throat, and in a few months' time the young slave died of the disease's advance on his brain.

* * *

Seven years earlier, Sims had nearly left medicine completely. One of his brothers had died in Mississippi after entering into a partnership with a man named George Browne, who had secured $100,000 of funding for a Vicksburg clothing business. The news of the death and the opportunity—Sims could assume his brother's stake, no investment required—arrived shortly after he and Theresa had settled in Mount Meigs.

Co-partnership Notice.

THE firm of Brown and Sims was dissolved on the ﾠ ultimo by the death of Mr. C. W Sims.
GEORGE Y. BROWNE.
oct. 1

THE Subscribers have entered into co partnership under the firm of Browne and Sims.
GEORGE Y. BROWNE.
.'. MARION SIMS.
oct. 1—3t

Theresa had given birth to a girl, and another child was on the way. As a doctor, Sims was scraping together $3,000 per year. The work was uninspiring, and it was unclear how his career might advance from there. In 1837, exuberant bank lending practices triggered a collapse in cotton prices, and the resulting panic quashed the possibility of transforming the meager profits that one might realize from country medicine into true wealth, as Dr. Lucas and Theresa's father had done.

Browne's clothing venture launched in 1838, when it appeared the recession would be short-lived. Sims and Theresa sold their home and packed a wagon for Mississippi. Then a letter arrived. The crisis had not been averted, the funding had been lost, the deal was off.

By then, Theresa's mother and her brother Rush had followed the newlyweds to Alabama. They settled in Lowndes County, and Sims's father and sisters also ventured west and looked farther south, to Butler County. Resolved to remain in Alabama, Sims and Theresa purchased a new home in the settlement of Cubahatchee, in Macon County, closer to Sims's practice among the plantation slaves of the Abercrombie family and Tom Zimmerman. Sims spent an idle year on horseback, hunting game with his pointer dog as he rode his rounds, shuttling from plantation to plantation, charging a dollar for tooth extractions, two dollars for enemas, three dollars per mile for calls in rain and snow, and a flat rate of five dollars if he was woken at any time between 10:00 p.m. and dawn. The work was easy, but it came with hitches. He'd once been forced to take legal action for a fee of $14.18¾. He won, but his attorney took $4, the judge $2, and serving the writ cost an additional $1.

Surgery would have to be his salvation. He took note when word came from South Carolina that a doctor named Toland was making many thousands per year performing the German physician Johann Dieffenbach's surgery for crossed eyes, and a separate procedure for clubfoot. Sims ordered medical journals from Europe, taught himself the new surgery on slaves, and within a year he had cemented his reputation with the knife by curing every case of crossed eyes and clubfoot in or near Montgomery.

More significantly from a medical perspective, he stumbled on a new method for extracting foreign objects lodged in the ear. One day, Rush called him to Lowndes County to attend to a five-year-old slave boy with a small fake gem stuck deep in his ear canal. They pinned the boy down on a staircase, and Sims was flushing blood from behind the object with a syringe when the pressure of the water caused the bit of glass to come suddenly shooting out of the ear. A few months later, his captain from the Creek campaign, Dr. Hugh Henry, sent him a four-year-old girl with a bit of chinaberry stuck in her ear. The following year, he treated a man who'd had a cherry pit lodged in his ear for twenty years. The syringe worked admirably each time. A survey of his growing library of medical texts revealed that the simple procedure had not previously been attempted— not by Kentucky's Gross, nor France's Velpeau, nor Philadelphia's Gibson. A surgeon's reputation could hardly be built on syringing the ear, but it was Sims's first chance to align his name with the greats of medical history in a paper for publication.

In 1840, prompted by another bout with malaria and a church community in Cubahatchee corrupted by drink, Sims and Theresa moved into Montgomery. The town was perched at the end of a horseshoe bend of the Alabama River, where paddle-wheel boats impossibly stacked with bales of cotton paused on their journey south to Mobile. The wealthy white population was mostly situated on a hill above town, in handsome homes whose spaciousness embodied the hospitality that was the right and due of the South. Tradesfolk and the black population were spread through a downtown dominated by a new hotel called Montgomery Hall, and by the Rialto Theatre.

Sims acquired property on Perry Street, not a hundred yards from the hotel. He sold his gun and gave away his dog, and bought a buggy like the one Theresa's father had used. Heedless of the histrionic Kappa Lambda men, whose ethics crusade had been gaining momentum despite the fact that its leaders had been publicly exposed, Sims placed an advertisement in the newspaper. He boasted of ortho- 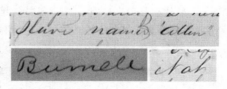 pedic instruments he had ordered from New York for the cure of wry neck and crooked legs, the deformities of muscular retraction. Soon, he counted prominent white citizens among his patients: the Crommelins and Goldthwaites and Pollards of Montgomery, the Duncans and Fairs of Autauga County, and Dr. Nathan Harris, the wealthy lawyer and widower who had moved to Alabama from Georgia despite a rumored fondness for the slave children he had fathered before his wife died. Still, a good portion of Sims's practice was among Montgomery's Jewish population, the frazzled Irish, and the blacks for whom he constructed a small hospital in his backyard. He continued to perfect procedures on slaves, and then advertise his skills for the better classes of society. Sims had more slaves of his own now: Abigail and her three children, Amanda, Martha, and Minerva; Harriet with her Emma and George; Burnett and Nat and Allen. When Sims went on rounds in his buggy, it was young George who rode alongside him as errand boy and messenger.

Theresa's mother offered financial support, and on holidays they visited her in Lowndes County, where there were barbecues and squirrel hunts, the occasional violin concert, and scandals when traveling gamblers attempted to woo local girls. They socialized well at fetes and frolics in Lowndes and Autauga both, with Pratts, Hilliards, and the famous preacher-turned-author William Henry Milburn. Prominent citizens like Senator William Rufus King gathered to celebrate and discuss growing anxieties over the slavery question and the ongoing banking crisis. In 1840, Sims attended a ball at the Rialto for Senator Henry Clay, who years before had helped Adams rob Jackson of the presidency. Now Clay was running for president himself. It was here that Sims at last met Josiah Nott's colleague from Mobile Henry LeVert, a humble man who had married up. Indeed, he was overshadowed by his flamboyant wife, Octavia, a prominent socialite. They were somehow related to Senator Clay.

When Sims's first son was born, in 1841, he debated between his mentors McClellan and Pattison in choosing a name for the boy. In the years since Sims graduated from Jefferson, McClellan had achieved further renown with another capital jaw surgery, the removal of a tumor in the upper maxilla. The procedure required him to dig deep under his patient's eye and stuff the resulting cavity with lint. But McClellan had also been mysteriously disgraced, ejected from the medical school he had founded. Sims settled on Granville Sharp Sims for his boy, to honor the rogue grave robber Pattison, whose more masculine approach to responding to criticism had paid off. It was a trait Sims resolved never to forget.

* * *

The following year, opportunity appeared in the form of a young woman named Margaret who wandered into Sims's Perry Street office with a blue veil over her face, folded double to obscure everything below her eyes.

Margaret explained that she was twenty-one years old, from North Carolina, a resident of Lowndes County for two months now. She had heard of Sims's achievements as soon as she arrived. Could he help her?

She lifted her veil to reveal a horrific double harelip. Parallel open fissures stretched from her mouth to both nostrils, and between them a bony protrusion grew out from her face like the snout of an animal, covered with a gristly, shriveled segment of lip. Margaret could neither speak nor drink without effort, and she had lived her life hiding her face from all who knew her.

Sims promised a cure within a month. He invited doctors to observe and assist in the procedure, secured a dentist to make teeth for her, and hired a sketch artist to draw an approximation of the woman's face for publication. He performed two operations, first dissecting the remains of the lip from the bony protrusion and sawing the snout away, and next closing the fissures by connecting them to the remainder of the lip. The result wasn't perfect, and Margaret refused to submit to any additional cutting, but the work was good enough for Sims to make a point of demonstrating the results to a famous dentist who visited Montgomery a short time later. The dentist helped him secure publication in a prominent journal. Sims's article on syringing the ear soon followed in the *American Journal of the Medical Sciences*. These were promising developments, and the move to Montgomery to focus on surgery appeared to be paying off.

In early June 1845—days after Sam and George left the Negro Hospital—Hugh Henry arrived in a rush, with an appeal to Sims's vanity. A young slave on the Westcott plantation had been in labor for several days, he explained, but the baby would not come. Sims groaned. He insisted, as he had often done with Henry and others, that such medicine was not in his line. Henry would not relent. He had been in attendance when Sims used the chain saw on Sam's jaw, and he was convinced that Sims's skill with instruments offered the only hope for the mother and child. Henry also knew that Sims was not as financially established as many physicians in Montgomery. He noted that he had already negotiated substantial fees for cesarean section and instrument delivery. It did not matter whether either the mother or the child survived.

Sims packed up the chain saw he had used on Sam, along with his little-used obstetric forceps, and together they rode a few miles outside of town to the Westcott plantation. The girl was perhaps seventeen, small of stature, barely conscious. Henry's bleeding of her had only made things worse. How could she push the baby out when she was depleted of blood as well as exhausted? Checking for a fetal heartbeat would have been a waste of time. Sims quickly opted for the forceps over the chain saw. He knew the forceps might cause injury, but the girl was delirious beyond pain, and a slave besides. With leverage and muscle, the baby came away easily enough, and Sims passed it off to the plantation granny—he had no idea whether it was successfully revived.

As they were preparing to leave, Sims heard Mrs. Westcott say the slave girl's name—Anarcky. His ears perked at the sound of it—it was so close to the name of the girl who had nursed him through his first bout with malaria, already nine years ago. That girl would now be about this girl's age. Sims did not look back. He pocketed his fee and fully expected never to see Anarcha again.

Henry returned to his office within the week. The young slave had rallied from her ordeal, he said, but she had experienced a great sloughing inside, a breaking away of dead tissue, and now both urine and feces were flowing freely from her vagina. Sims shuddered—he had no choice. The look in Henry's eye revealed that he too understood that Anarcha's injury might have been the result of Sims's forceful application of the forceps. In any event, the slave girl was still his patient, for a fee that had already been paid.

They made their way back to the Westcott plantation. The girl held his eye for a knowing moment before she averted her gaze. Sims couldn't be sure—it might have been the same Anarcha. Nine years earlier, he'd been the delirious one. How many young slaves had he examined since then?

They put Anarcha into the position they had used for the delivery. Already the effect of freely flowing feces and urine was apparent on her labia and thighs; the whole area was irritated and raw. Her vagina had mostly returned to its usual size, which made viewing the condition extremely difficult. Working together, Sims and Henry managed to glimpse the source of the mischief: there was one great hole opened along the front wall of Anarcha's vagina, creating a gap of communication with her bladder, and there was another hole along the back wall, opening a fissure into her rectum. Even as they watched, urine seeped in pulses from Anarcha's vagina, out onto the mattress that was stained with her birth blood.

Yet the forceps, Sims discovered, may not have been the culprit. At home, he dug into his books and determined that the condition was fistula. Most often the accident was limited to a single hole into the bladder, vesico-vaginal fistula, and generally it was not a tear or a cut, as from an instrument, but a rift that opened several days after birth, when necrotic tissue killed by the unrelenting press of the baby's head fell away. Fistula was enticingly mysterious; the condition had baffled the world's leading medical minds for centuries. Central to the problem was that the wound was simply difficult to reach. How could you hope to stitch closed a hole that you could barely see, in tissue that was both delicate and often moist with mucous secreted by the cervix? By all accounts, the condition was horrific—never directly fatal but making a misery of life. There had been occasional cures. A doctor named Gosset in England had closed a fistula using silver wire for suture material. Another doctor named Mettauer had succeeded more recently with lead wire in Virginia. There were others as well, but no one knew why a few had triumphed where so many had failed. There was no accepted procedure, and no doctor had attached his name to a device that enabled a cure.

The sources all said that fistula was relatively common, but Anarcha's was the first case that Sims had ever seen. That was hardly a surprise. His disinclination toward medicine of the female pelvis was widely known, but the truth was even worse—he hated it. Clearly, honor awaited the man who could cure fistula once and for all. But Sims quickly set aside the possibility. Even if he overcame his loathing for that particular precinct of therapeutic investigation, the consistency of failure in the record made the possibility of success remote at best.

He returned to the Westcott plantation and informed Anarcha's young owner, William Westcott, that her value as a slave was ruined. She would soon be unable to work, and though fistulous women could give birth, the offensiveness of her presence would likely make a slave marriage impossible.

* * *

Far more promising was the mysterious deaths of slave babies from lockjaw—tetanus.

Sims first saw a lockjaw case not long after he arrived in Alabama. He was called to attend to an infant suffering from periodic spasms. He found it in the middle of just such an agonized clench, head tipped back in a mournful wail and face caught in a sardonic grin, like that of a cackling old woman. Sims dreaded a reprisal of his initial medical failures in South Carolina. Again, the education he had received and his books were of little help apart from describing the infant's inability to nurse. After nine days, it died in the midst of harrowing throes.

By 1839, Alabama physicians were taking note of an unusually high incidence of babies with anxious stares and restless hands just before the spasms began. Invariably, they died. Sims was as baffled as ever when his own daughter began to exhibit similar symptoms, and Theresa discovered that she could alleviate the spasms by turning the girl on her side.

The medical community agreed on one thing: infant lockjaw was limited to slovenly pauper communities. Among cultivated and refined intellects, it was unknown.

In July 1845, Sims was called to the Stickney plantation, west of Autauga, for another infant fallen to lockjaw. It was shortly after he received a visit from the wealthy Dr. Harris, in regard to a slave named Betsey. Like the girl Anarcha, Betsey had begun leaking urine from her vagina after a difficult birth. Sims performed an examination of Betsey and confirmed that it was another hopeless case of fistula. He sent Dr. Harris away.

The call to the Stickney plantation came just a few days later. The unfortunate child, one of a set of twins born to a slave named Patsey, was just as hopeless. Sims agreed to an examination—perhaps he could pull a paper out of the experience.

He took a colleague along with him. As he was demonstrating the rigidity of the baby's body during the spasms—first lifting it up by its legs, stiff as if with rigor mortis, and then by its neck—Sims felt something odd on the back of the infant's head. One of the bones of the skull was protruding slightly. Rather than growing together to a smooth curvature, the skull plates seemed to have become mechanically stuck in an overlapping position.

A theory formed at once. What if the cause of infant lockjaw wasn't slaves' slovenliness at all? What if it was the position that babies were kept in, causing their skulls to grow abnormally? The bones would cause pressure among the veins, perhaps bleeding in the brain, and the blood in turn would pressure the spine, which would result in seizures. That would explain why Theresa had been able to alleviate their daughter's symptoms by turning her on her side. A quick glance at the wedge-shaped crib in which the Stickney slave baby was kept confirmed it. The cradle seemed practically designed to cause the deformity.

The baby died in four days' time. Sims arranged to have the corpse brought to Montgomery for an autopsy, and he invited half a dozen medical men to observe. As he suspected, he found the bones overlapping. The marrow of the spine was pressured by a coagulation of thick black blood.

The case was certainly a discovery, and from there it wasn't hard to imagine cures: reposition infants whose skulls had not yet become fixed and, for those sunk deeper into the course of the disease, employ a knife to pry up the skull plates to cause them to snap into proper position. It was an intriguing possibility, and Sims set about gathering case reports from his colleagues to write a paper. He now had a number of students who had been attracted by his surgical successes, and he sent several of his young apprentices into the countryside to hunt for additional doomed babies.

A short time later, Tom Zimmerman, Sims's old employer from Macon County, paid a visit to Montgomery.

Remarkably, Zimmerman too had a fistula case for Sims. A young slave girl, Lucy, had given birth at about the same time as Anarcha and Dr. Harris's girl Betsey. She couldn't hold her water. It was truly odd. Sims had never even heard of fistula before that year, and now he had encountered three cases in two months' time. He diagnosed Lucy on Zimmerman's description and declared it hopeless. Zimmerman protested. He'd been angry when Sims moved into Montgomery, and now he argued that a real doctor would never refuse to see a case simply because he had run off to the city seeking fame. Like it or not, Zimmerman would send Lucy to Montgomery by the next train.

The girl arrived the following afternoon. Sims examined her, and it was just as he expected. Her fistula was not as severe as Anarcha's, but the excoriation of her labia and thighs was more advanced. The flesh had begun to rot. The stench was unbearable. Even though the fistula was simple, Sims could barely see it. He gave Lucy some instructions to care for her damaged skin and told her she could sleep in his Negro Hospital for the night. She would return home by train the following afternoon.

* * *

In the morning, Sims packed his buggy and was about to set out for his daily rounds when his little slave George ran excitedly up to the office. Mrs. Merrill, a respectable seamstress married to a gambling scoundrel, had fallen from her horse. It was unknown whether she had fractured a limb or broken her skull. A doctor was needed at once.

He hurried up the hill to the white districts of Montgomery. He found Mrs. Merrill prostrate in bed. She was a large woman, more than two hundred pounds, and she explained that her pony, startled by a hog, had thrown her. She landed precisely on her rump, all her weight compressing at a single point. She had no broken bones, but there was a great pain in her back and a miserable feeling of needing to void—and of something still further down, pressing inside.

Sims choked back a sigh. He suspected the cause, and confirmed it with a digital examination beneath Mrs. Merrill's clothes. The woman had retroverted her uterus. Rather than an injury that truly called on the skills of a surgeon, she had precisely the type of condition that he had been passing off to Hugh Henry and his students for years now.

Still, it was an emergency. After a moment of panic, Sims found himself recalling the procedure for impacted uterus that Dr. Prioleau had awkwardly described in his South Carolina classroom: a finger each in the rectum and vagina, and a simultaneous action of pushing and pulling. Sims couldn't bring himself to do it. Just the other day, he'd been obliged to insert a finger in a man's rectum, and the ungrateful fellow had whined so miserably Sims had resolved never to attempt it again.

But he had to do something. He guided Mrs. Merrill into Prioleau's knee-chest position, nates raised high in the air and chest pressed onto the mattress, and almost at once the difficult position gave Mrs. Merrill pain from the sheer difficulty of sustaining it. He instructed her to lift her skirts, threw a sheet over her, and then reached to insert a finger into her vagina. He found the dislocated organ easily enough, but his finger was too short to nudge it back into place. He tried again with both his index and middle fingers, and for a time he attempted all sorts of maneuvers and positions, pumping vigorously with palm up and palm down. He shoved with greater and greater might, and the seamstress was soon awash in sweat from pain and the awkward pose.

Then—all at once—her womb seemed to vanish! He had felt it clearly at one instant, and in the next it was gone. Even the walls of her vagina seemed to disappear. Sims's fingers were left flopping around an empty nothingness, like the insides of a hat. He had no idea what he'd done to the poor woman.

Why, doctor, Mrs. Merrill said, I am relieved!

Sims knew better than to show any outward sign of surprise. You may lie down, Mrs. Merrill, he said.

The woman flopped onto her side, and the moment her body settled onto the mattress, a powerful shot of air came surging from her vagina, like an escape of gas from the bowel. Mrs. Merrill was mortified. Sims comforted her, and again he disguised his true reaction—a thrill of inspiration. The bolt of air explained what had happened. The knee-chest position, which shifted all her organs forward in the trunk of her body, and the placement and action of Sims's hand, had resulted in an inrush of air that inflated her vagina like a balloon. As with the syringing of the ear, it was pressure—of air, rather than water—that did the work of shoving Mrs. Merrill's uterus back into place. When she lay down, the air came bursting back out of her again.

As Sims packed his bag and left, his mind raced home to the slave girl Lucy, waiting for a train. What if the knee-chest position and the inflating action of the vagina could be replicated? Wouldn't that enable a surgeon to see a fistula clearly and thereby effect a cure? It was possible, but there were additional complications. Even if sutures were possible, how could one prevent tension from causing the silk to cut through the delicate membrane of the vaginal wall? And how to stem the flow of urine that would cause the line of union to rot before it healed? Even more fundamentally, how could one compel slaves to submit to a series of experimental surgeries? Sawing off a jaw was one thing, but you couldn't very well tie a woman down and prevent her from flexing the deep-seated muscles that would confound any attempt at vaginal surgery. Fortunately for purposes of this last concern, the condition was so horrific that surgeons who had attempted procedures in the past had reported no difficulty in finding women who were willing to undergo almost anything in pursuit of a cure.

Sims stopped at Hall, Mores & Roberts on the way home. He needed a tool to better activate the inflating action of the vagina. He thought back on the bent handle of the silver spoon that had been used to hold up the eye of the slave George as Sims had worked to free the adhesions of his tumor. A table spoon would be too small, but Sims found a large pewter spoon with a gently curved handle. The possibilities churned as he hurried home. The honor he pursued could not be doubted—the body of the fairer sex was a frontier, and doctors all over the world had raced to link their names to anatomy and procedures: the Fallopian tubes, the pouch of Douglas, the glands of Montgomery. There was a rush of exploration underway. Even better, the extensive literature on vesico-vaginal fistula from Europe was proof that the condition did not afflict the poor nearly so much as infant lockjaw. If Sims could contrive a cure for fistula on a slave, the gains that could be realized were immeasurable—and not only in Alabama. It was both providential and convenient that three fistula cases had found their way to him. Everything would work in his favor. The women would be willing because they were desperate, and their masters would leap at the chance of salvaging their investment.

Arrived home, Sims called on two of his students. They found Lucy in the Negro Hospital, stinking of urine and preparing to leave for the train. They instructed her to disrobe and climb up onto the examination table. The students pressed Lucy's head down and positioned her knees, and then each took hold of one of her nates and pulled up and away. Lucy's vagina began to dilate even before Sims touched her. There was a soft puffing sound as air began to rush in. Sims sat down behind her and positioned his mirror to direct the sun's light onto her vulva. He bent the handle of the pewter spoon ninety degrees and then turned it around to insert it and pry up on the girl's perineum. Her vagina opened just as Mrs. Merrill's had done, and Sims looked inside.

The fistula was there—as clear as a tear in a piece of paper, as tantalizing as a bit of treasure glinting on an ocean floor. Sims felt the thrill of a mariner at the first glimpse of an undiscovered land. He could see the hole, he could see Lucy's cervix, he could see all the way to the cul-de-sac of her vagina. He could see everything, as no man had ever seen before.

Eight

ON MARCH 11, 1843, LIEUTENANT MATTHEW FONTAINE MAURY, RECENTLY selected as superintendent of the US Naval Observatory, pointed the department's small telescopes at a strange light that had appeared of late in the noonday sky, leading many to believe that it was a daytime comet like the one historians spoke of from 44 BC, or the comet spied by Tycho Brahe just before sunset on November 13, 1577, as he was returning home with a catch of fish.

The construction of the observatory's huge dome would not be completed until the following year, so Maury and his assistants relied on smaller instruments that reminded the superintendent of a telescope nicknamed "the Squirt"—it resembled a doctor's syringe—that he and a cousin had used to examine the skies from an Irving Place rooftop in Manhattan. Maury and his staff were hoping to glimpse the nebula of the comet, but they were forced to settle for a view of its curved train, fading over several hours into the haze of the west.

Maury was a grandson of Reverend James Maury, tutor of a young Thomas Jefferson. Reverend Maury was the patriarch of a large family that would go on to become influential in politics and cotton. Children and cousins spread out from Charlottesville, first to Fredericksburg and Richmond and Washington City, and from there to Mobile, New York, London, and Liverpool. Matthew Fontaine Maury's family first settled on a plantation called Topping Castle in Virginia, fifteen miles southwest of the Bowling Green, a famous home in Caroline County that had once been a stopping point for George Washington. When Maury's father fell on hard times, the family decamped for Tennessee.

It was Maury's older brother who pulled him toward the navy. John Maury enlisted and returned home full of tales of wild shipwreck and child-eating cannibals. Not even his brother's subsequent mid-voyage death of yellow fever would dissuade Matthew Maury from dreams of life as a midshipman. Defying his parents' wishes, he enlisted.

His first cruise was aboard the USS *Brandywine*, ordered to escort Lafayette home after his yearlong tour of America. On this first voyage, Maury learned the basics of navigation using the stars and planets. He became preoccupied by the vision of the Magellanic Clouds, luminous bodies high overhead, like tandem ghosts linked by an invisible string.

The *Brandywine* dropped Lafayette in Europe, then sailed for Rio de Janeiro. Over the next several years, Maury visited Macao, Manila, Cape Town, the forbidden city of Canton, and the Sandwich Islands. At home in 1830, he continued his education in navigation, got engaged in Virginia, and visited another cousin in Caroline County, a navy recruit like himself named William L. Maury.

On a return voyage to Rio, Maury began to jot down notes for a book that would improve on the navy's existing navigation guides, reducing the more difficult math and astronomy problems to core practical skills. In school, Maury intimidated his teachers; at sea, his drive for knowledge annoyed his shipmates. In 1834, he married and he wrote his practical guide.

"The spirit of literary improvement has been awakened among the officers of our gallant navy," read a glowing review from the prolific editor of the *Southern Literary Messenger*, Edgar Allan Poe.

In 1837, frustrated by bureaucratic entanglements, Maury managed a gold mine and conducted harbor surveys in North Carolina and Mississippi. He was promoted to lieutenant. In 1839, on a journey to meet his ship for another harbor expedition, he was thrown from an overloaded carriage. He fractured his thigh; it was unclear whether he would ever be fit for sea duty again. During his recovery, he penned a number of anonymous articles highly critical of graft and fraud in the navy. The *Southern Literary Messenger* now championed the whistleblower Maury as a refreshing candidate for secretary of the navy. Maury wished only to go to sea. He was denied a berth aboard the frigate *United States*, either because of his crippled leg or because he had ruffled the feathers of superiors now bent on stalling his career.

In 1842, the family of his naval cousin William L. Maury bought the famous Bowling Green plantation in Caroline County, Virginia. The home itself was now called Old Mansion, to distinguish it from the town that had adopted its name. Old Mansion became a stopping point for Maurys traveling north and south.

Later that same year, Maury was named superintendent of the US Naval Observatory. Seven months after that, he aimed the depot's small telescopes at the great sun-grazing comet headed for the farthest reaches of space.

The observatory had a number of missions, including the maintenance of a soggy library of logbooks assigned to every navy ship captain. This, Maury realized, was an untapped trove of information. Untold lives, time, and money could be saved by mining the logbooks for what they revealed of the currents of the seas, flowing as strong as rivers within them. The observatory coordinated its astronomical work with a new telescope at Harvard and another in Alabama. In April 1845, Maury gave a personal tour of the newly completed observatory to former president John Quincy Adams, now a congressman. The young superintendent and the elderly politician peered together through the new refractor at a cloudy nebula in the constellation Orion, appearing like an engraved filigree on the blade of the huntsman's sword.

On November 26, 1845, Biela's Comet, known since 1772 for its six-year orbit, was spotted in Italy. On January 13, 1846, Maury found the comet with the observatory's main telescope. Immediately, he noticed something odd. There was another object below it. It was reddish in color, a fraction of Biela's intensity. Subsequent observations proved the two objects were linked. The second blazed with whitish light as Biela's dimmed behind it. A few days later, Biela's reemerged. It was clear—they were in orbit about each other.

There was no mistaking the larger suggestion: Biela's Comet was undergoing physical disembodiment. Lieutenant Matthew Fontaine Maury was the first to glimpse the breaking apart of a celestial body. The comet was shattering from within. The ongoing disintegration was evident from glowing trains that curved away from each body like flowing veils. Together these tails formed an arched way in the heavens, framing stars shining from the deep abyss of space.

* * *

Constantly in pain, incontinent of urine or feces, bearing a heavy burden of sadness in discovering their child stillborn, ashamed of a rank personal offensiveness, abandoned therefore by their husbands, outcasts of society, unemployable except in the fields, they live, they exist, without friends and without hope.

—Dr. Reginald Hamlin,
cofounder, with Dr. Catherine Hamlin,
of the Addis Ababa Fistula Hospital, 1966

Now, Anarcha was the monster in the woods.

The rule on the Westcott plantation was: after birth, no work for five days, and it was five days after the baby that was not her baby was pulled from her womb by the fire tongs that were not fire tongs of Dr. Marion Sims that Anarcha's mind stitched itself back together again. She got up, and at once she was aware of something inside of her bursting and splitting—not painfully but as though a tight string had snapped or a knot had been snipped loose with scissors—and she hid what came sliding out of her, small chunks or strips that looked less like flesh than like the star jelly that had rained from the skies on November 13, 1833, the night the stars fell. Not long after, a noxious shower began streaming out of Anarcha and spilling down her thighs, as though her womb had been cursed by an angry god or split by the blade of a knife.

The Westcott slaves had underthings made from old sacks or bags, so there was no staunching what came from her, and there was no hiding the smell at all. A slave told an overseer, or an overseer passed her by and noticed the rancid odor of rot and shit, or William Westcott came to see if she was ready to work and to take stock of how quickly she might be able to become pregnant again, and it was her master who noticed the odor and Dr. Henry was sent for at once. Dr. Henry laid her back and spread her legs wide, and it was worse now because her mind was not clouded by the pains and Pheriba's teas and the ax underneath the bed, and Dr. Henry held a kerchief to his mouth as he looked inside and didn't say anything at all to Anarcha, and then Dr. Henry stood up, and as he left he told the missus that he would return shortly with Dr. Sims.

Dr. Sims arrived, and Anarcha looked him straight in the eye. Letters from many years later hint at Anarcha's boldness in refusing work, but even now, when she was young and vulnerable, she would have wanted Sims to recognize her, and to remember when she cared for him, when he was the one close to dying. She'd be careful, of course, not to stare too long or too hard because it risked a whipping to look at a white man like that. They laid her down again. Both men squatted on stools between her legs, and there was quiet discussion between them, and then they rose and left and did not return. The following day, Anarcha heard that Dr. Sims returned to the plantation to speak to William Westcott, but she didn't see him, and the next time William Westcott looked at her she knew what had been said because his look revealed that she was now worthless, no-account, like a husk that had held an ear of corn but now wasn't good for anything.

Or even worse—because slaves used husks for lots of things, for ticking and mats and medicines. But now, even the slaves treated Anarcha like a corrupted thing. Not all of them—not Pheriba, not her brothers—but most avoided her for the sores on her legs, like the sores of smallpox, and for the smell of gas and waste that came from her, because they believed that it was not gas and waste that was coming from her but flying ants, or snakes, or frogs, or turtles, or thousand-leg worms, or ground puppies, or spiders. Slaves were sometimes terrible to each other, and perhaps there had been a slave who was jealous or angry that Anarcha did not work in the fields when she was pregnant, and the slave went to a hoodoo doctor, or a root worker, or a free issue, or a two-headed slave, or a charm doctor like that which was called *traiteur* in Louisiana, and the charm doctor had taken a bowlful of spiders or thousand-leg worms and put them to dry and beat them to dust and then put the dust onto the white people's food—hoodoo didn't work on white people because they took the oil out of their straight hair, while slaves put oil into their kinky hair—and when Anarcha ate the white people's food when she was pregnant the dust went inside her like eggs and the eggs hatched and the critters crawled around and ate at her insides, and that's why her birth did not take its natural course and not even the white doctors knew what to do about it. Now she was afflicted with foul-smelling frogs or snakes that kept on eating at her as they slithered out of her body.

Others believed that Anarcha had given birth to a baby with a caul draped over its face and the white doctors didn't know the proper thing to do with the veil of tissue, which was to peel it away and wrap it in paper and put it in a trunk until it disappeared. So Anarcha was cursed, and it was like when witches bewitched the cows and you couldn't get the butter to come no matter how much you churned it, and the curse could be lifted by reading the Bible three times backward, but how could you read the Bible backward three times when you couldn't read it forward even once?

Not even Pheriba knew what medicine to try. She told Anarcha about a Georgian woman named Aunt Darkas who was blind and 128 years old, and she had a well, and she would listen to your complaint and lift water from the well and pass her hand over it, and you drank it to get better. There was a conjure doctor in Kentucky named Linda Woods who had bottles filled with a rainbow of colors, and you shook the bottle until it was all one color and then rubbed it on yourself and bathed in a bath of life-everlasting weed, and there was a slave named Dr. Jones in Texas who wore a long black coat like a preacher and sideburns for whiskers, and he walked the streets like he was in a deep study, and he would curse you just as soon as he would cure you. And there was a Shawnee in Indiana who claimed to be able to take lizards out of your body by soaking your feet in a tub of boiled poke roots, but what the Indian really did was hire a child to get some lizards and then he slipped them into the poke-root bath when you weren't looking so that you would think you were cured.

Inside of two weeks, as the skin of her thighs and between her legs began to rot, Anarcha became like a chicken in the yard with a knot on the side of its head. Eventually, it would sink to drooping around, and then it would die, and everyone would know not to eat that chicken because it was poison.

* * *

She went to the woods for two months. If she was closer to the river she could clean herself more easily, and she wasn't a runaway because no one was hunting her.

Pheriba gave her matches and a pocketknife and hog-jowl grease for the wounds on her skin, and she told Anarcha how to find the cave that the slave man had turned into a home for his slave wife, where they'd had free babies. Anarcha found it on the second day, after a night on which she slept in a tree and heard for herself the woman-screaming panthers in the woods, but up close you could tell it wasn't a woman because at the end of the squall there was a low, throaty growl, and no woman, slave or white, could make a sound like that. The cave had been hidden by pine limbs and torn-off brambles that had died, and other brambles had grown over them so that you could walk by it and think you were passing an ugly tree or a sick bush, and that's what Anarcha did, once, twice, and noticed it only the third time, and she spent the afternoon clearing out the entryway.

The ceiling of the cave was reinforced with pine logs, and there were pine-log beds against the wall and a pine-log table and two chairs. There was a twig broom for sweeping the dirt floor, and there was an old grinder for grinding snails and worms for food, and the stove that Pheriba had said was there was still there, and it worked after Anarcha cleared the top of the pipe and everything that had got inside of it burned away.

She cooked only at night and used oak bark for fires to make little smoke. Even though she wasn't a runaway, she had to be careful because Creeks stole slaves and hunted runaways for bounties, and also because there were many runaways in the woods, slaves who would rather go to the land of sweet dreams than submit to another whipping, and if she saw them in the daytime and they weren't afraid of her—word spread of a cursed girl in the woods—then she shared what food she had, but at night she had to be sure that her scent did not get mixed up with the runaways whose feet she could hear pounding through the woods like deer.

Surely, Anarcha's brothers Ben and Joe brought her food, snapping the neck of a chicken on the walk to the cave or stealing a loaf of light bread that had been put out to cool and was still warm inside when Anarcha broke it open and ate it. Her own time was spent gathering wild blackberries, and she once saw a bear stealing corn just the way she did it, climbing the fence and putting the ears of corn into the crook of its paw one by one, and then climbing the fence again just like a person. She ran out of hog-jowl grease for her wounds and began using soot instead, and she used sand from the riverbank as soap for her clothes and beat them with tree branches, and when she ripped her clothes she made thread to fix them with wool that she picked off a sheep she found dead and half-eaten in the woods. There were many dead things in the woods. In two months, she ate skunk and crow and hawk, just like Raw Head and Bloody Bones who ate all the meat he could find or steal, and despite what Pheriba had told her, Anarcha too began to suspect that she had been cursed, and now she was like the wildmen of the woods. There was nothing meaner or lower than a shunned slave.

After two months, Joe came running up to the mouth of the cave calling her name, and he said the master wanted to see her, William Westcott. Dr. Marion Sims had returned to the plantation and asked for her. She had been called for. Anarcha felt a cold slither run up her spine, as though her body really was filled with thousand-leg worms. Even in the woods, news had come to her, through Joe or Ben or runaways who stopped for bits of bread and scavenged turkey, of experiments that Dr. Sims had performed before and since he pulled the baby out of her. Like another hungry monster, Dr. Sims had not contented himself with operations on slaves' feet and eyes. He had tricked them into coming to his Negro Hospital in Montgomery, it was said, and he had tied them down and cut into their faces just to show other white doctors that it could be done.

Anarcha first washed in the river. Then she and Joe walked two miles to the Westcott plantation, slowly and painfully for all the sores between her legs and the misery that had begun to gather in one of her feet, and when she arrived she was confused because she expected to be loaded at once into a wagon and taken for experiments, and maybe that was for the best and maybe it would be even better if she died because what more could she have than a life alone in the woods with a load of slow-growing miseries, always eating and slowly dying? But she wasn't put into any wagon, and instead she was asked to sit down at the table in the Westcott house, which she hadn't done since she was a young girl and went to Sunday dinners so the missus could take stock of her health. Dr. Sims looked her in the eye and invited her to look back. He told her that she wasn't alone in her suffering. There were others who had come after her, and still more had been found in the areas around Montgomery, ten in all, women leaking urine, and at least one other leaking feces as well.

It was a terrible condition, a curse, Dr. Sims said, but he sounded excited as he said it. Women had suffered from it for hundreds of years, he said, slave women and white women alike, from the Old World and the New World, and it was incurable, there had never been a cure, but Dr. Sims had an idea for a surgery, he said, and he believed that he could cure her, he could stop the leaks. Anarcha could see that he was earnest. Dr. Sims was less like the Shawnee who slipped lizards into your poke-root bath than he was like an old woman who believed that passing her hand over well water gave it the power to heal. Yet Anarcha did not understand why he was asking her. Why did he need her to approve? When had anyone ever asked her permission for anything? She could tell that William Westcott had already approved, had agreed to turn her over to Dr. Sims, who was now telling her that the surgeries would hurt, of course they would hurt, but there was a very good chance for a cure because Dr. Sims had seen something that no other white doctor had seen. But why did he need her consent? Couldn't he just tie her down and do what he wished? And did he really believe it would be a choice? Or did his eagerness suggest, just as with the slaves he'd tied down to impress white doctors, that what he truly sought was not a cure for her, but one for himself? Anarcha did not have time to decide, and it did not matter in the end, because to be placed between misery and hope, between pain and promise, is to be given a choice that is so false it is indistinguishable from a command issued with the threat of a whip behind it.

* * *

The cursed women began caring for one another right away, but they didn't begin assisting in the surgeries until several years had passed.

Anarcha met Betsey and Lucy first, and the others arrived over the next few months after Dr. Sims's men Burnett and Nat and Allen added a second level to the Negro Hospital behind his office in Montgomery. When they were finished there were twelve beds upstairs, four down-stairs, and the women cooked for themselves and ate together outside and they got water from a fountain to one side of Montgomery Hall, a hotel a hundred yards away, the tallest building in town. The hotel leased slaves as servants, and also as nurses for wealthy guests who checked in because they were sick and there was nowhere else for them to go. Dr. Sims leased Anarcha to Montgomery Hall as soon as he saw her caring for the other women in the Negro Hospital. She leaned over a new arrival, a girl who could barely walk and hadn't eaten in some time, and Dr. Sims looked at Anarcha, and looked away, and he looked back again, and that was when Anarcha knew that Dr. Sims had recognized that she was the girl who saved him.

With plentiful water the women could wash often, and Dr. Sims gave them a supply of proper underthings that they hand scrubbed frequently, and there was always a houseful of linen and drawers hung to dry beside the Negro Hospital, fluttering in the breeze. Their rooms wouldn't ever be fully free of miasmas, but as the women arrived they shared remedies for the stench of urine and gas. A salve made from chitlings, lard, and camphor that had an odor to it. The Indian turnip that runaways used to fool dogs. Or soaking your clothes overnight in wild rose or cape jasmine or sweet bazil or magnolia leaves, and letting them dry with the perfume still in it.

For their wounds they used the medicines that Dr. Sims gave them in small bottles, syrups and powders. When he wasn't looking, they used tur-pentine and okra blossoms on open sores, sugar and cobwebs if they were bleeding, or they smoked the wounds with burnt wool, and then dripped soft rosin onto the charred fabric and bound it to the injured spots.

Dr. Sims was having instruments made and performing the duties of his practice, and Anarcha and Lucy and Betsey and the other cursed women worked in Dr. Sims's office, or they worked for Dr. Sims's wife and helped care for her children and wet-nursed Dr. Sims's baby son who was born on December 25, 1845, and was named Merry Christmas Sims, though that baby was never healthy. Or they were leased to Montgomery Hall or to families nearby who needed servants. The free black population in Montgomery was not permitted to wander at night or gather in groups, but the cursed women, some of whom had come from plantations more remote than the Westcott or Lucas plantations, eased into the city life of Montgomery. There were cockfights in the streets, and once there was an attempt at a bullfight but the bull wouldn't charge, and the city was being made the capital of Alabama, so construction began not far away on a great stone building, and sometimes the militia paraded through town in white pants and blue tops, three rows of fifteen white soldiers with rifles on their shoulders and drummers leading the way, and women in hoopskirts stopped to watch and stray dogs ran alongside the men as they marched up the runneled street. Weekly, Anarcha passed the slave market where excited criers implored prospective owners to examine slaves' fingers and toes to prove to themselves that the men and women for sale were good cotton-picking slaves, each worth ten bales just as surely as a respectable man is worth a julep at eleven o'clock.

Anarcha had never set foot in the plantation homes of Rose Hill or Bright Spot, and Montgomery Hall put the Westcott plantation house to shame. She never entered through the front of the hotel. There were drawing rooms near the front of the building, though no one drew anything in them, and instead men talked and drank and smoked there. There were public bedrooms across from the drawing rooms, and behind the bedrooms there was a dining room with two walls of huge windows, the glass stretching taller than a house. Beyond the dining room an immense porch reached out to the ballroom, which was open and tall inside like a church, and off the ballroom a promenade gallery gave dancers a place to sneak away to, to escape the eyes of chaperones. Prominent families, the Youngs and Abercrombies, kept private apartments behind the drawing rooms, and Montgomery Hall was frequented by many more prominent citizens, Bibbs and Holts and Taliaferros and Goldthwaites and Merriweathers. The hotel was run by the wives of the men who owned it, and Anarcha's skill as a nurse was soon recognized, and when she was not caring for the cursed women at the Negro Hospital, she worked at the Hall and cared for important people who needed tending.

There were servant quarters at Montgomery Hall as well, outside in back, near the icehouse where cooks made ice cream and boiled custard, and Anarcha did not stay in these quarters but sometimes she stopped there on the short walk back to the Negro Hospital, and the cursed women could holler to her from there if they needed to. They called to Anarcha on the day they found the plank board that Dr. Sims had used to tie down the slave George. The rumors about Dr. Sims were true. Some of the women were horrified and fearful of the pain they would be forced to endure under Dr. Sims's knife, and others were fearful but also hopeful that they might be able to return to their children and their husbands. Some feared only remaining uncured and being sold to sugar plantations in Louisiana where they would be worked until they died.

After Christmas and after the New Year, Dr. Sims was ready to begin the experiments. He gathered all the cursed women in the Negro Hospital, which had no other patients now, just the women living together, and he demonstrated his procedure on a piece of burlap with a rip in the middle of it. When he spoke, it wasn't like he was talking to the women or Anarcha at all. Rather, the speech itself was an experiment, practice for some future audience of white people and white doctors.

The burlap was like their insides, Dr. Sims said. He briefly rolled the piece of burlap into a cylinder to illustrate this. But a rip in a piece of fabric was not exactly like what had happened to them, he explained. It was more like a piece of them had rotted like fruit and died and fallen out, and so the hole inside them was more like a worn-down hole in a shirt at the elbow, and the only way to darn it was to snip away the frayed parts and sew together the fresh bits of cloth. The shirt wouldn't fit like new, but at least there wouldn't be a hole in it.

Also, Dr. Sims said, the inside of a woman was not tough like burlap. It was delicate, like the lace that fine ladies wore, and it was moist mucous membrane. Closing a hole inside a woman was like sewing closed a hole in a wet piece of tissue paper.

There were three problems that needed to be solved, Dr. Sims said. The first was the position of the experiment.

He told Lucy to undress, and Lucy took off her clothes and climbed onto the examination table in front of all the cursed women and she got onto her hands and knees as she had already demonstrated for them one night, with her clothes on, when they got to talking about what was going to happen to them. Lucy sank her chest down onto the table so that her buttocks shot up into the air. Dr. Sims explained how he had first looked inside Lucy with the bent handle of a pewter spoon, and he showed them that very spoon and the tool that had been fashioned to replace it. It was a long piece of metal and it looked like something you might use to force open a locked door, or if you squinted right it looked like a snake rearing up to bite you.

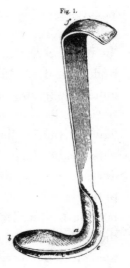

Fig. 1.

He would perform experiments in the morning, Dr. Sims said, when he could use mirrors to direct sunlight so that he could see, and he told Anarcha and Betsey to stand alongside of Lucy and lay hold of her and lift, and they did so tenderly at first, touching Lucy's rump and easing each side upward and forward. Next, Dr. Sims slid his new implement into Lucy's vagina sideways and turned it upright and lifted it toward her lower back, and he seemed contented that the action of the tool was the same as that of the spoon. All the cursed women saw how Lucy's vagina inflated with air, and with a ray of light shining from the mirror they could see the hole inside her just as clear as the rip in the piece of burlap.

When Lucy climbed down from the table the air came out of her again with a sound—she had warned the cursed women about this as well. Dr. Sims ignored it.

The second problem was the stitches, he said. Just as stitches could come loose when you sewed a hole in a damaged piece of cloth, so might the silk thread pull on the tissue and tear the stitches out before the body healed itself. Dr. Sims had solved this problem, he said. He held up between his thumb and index finger a small bar, a piece of metal shorter and thinner than a match, with holes bored through it, and using the piece of burlap he showed the cursed women how he would position two such bars on either side of the holes inside them, and the bars would be stitched into the tissue with the silk thread connecting them, and when the bars were cinched together by pulling and tying the thread, the tension of the thread would be on the metal and not on the flesh. With a few quick flourishes, Dr. Sims cinched closed the hole in the piece of burlap.

The last problem, Dr. Sims said, was urine. Unchecked, urine would flow over the stitches, and the tissue would rot and the stitches would cut out even if there was no tension on them, and urine was the reason that doctors for centuries had failed to cure the holes inside of women. To remedy this, Dr. Sims would insert a long thin sponge made from slippery elm bark. The middle part of the sponge would be covered with a thin skin of ox intestine, and the top of the sponge would remain inside the cursed women to catch the urine before it rotted the line of stitched-together flesh, and the urine would be sucked through the middle of the sponge and it would come out the portion of the sponge that would dangle outside of the women as nature took its healing course. Then Dr. Sims would remove the sponge and the stitches and the metal bars, and the women would stop leaking.

Everything depended, Dr. Sims said, on the cursed women remaining completely motionless, during the experiments and for a long time after that. That's why Dr. Sims had seemed to ask for their permission, Anarcha thought. The only hope for a cure required a slave who wanted to be cured.

After the experiment, Dr. Sims said, for five days, or nine days, or however many days it took for nature to heal the stitched flesh, the cursed women would care for one another, using a large squirt to clean one another's skin and genitals, warm or cool water, as preferred, at least twice a day and more if possible, and they must take care to throw the water onto the dirtied parts with enough force to dislodge even invisible buildups of urine. After the experiments, the women who had been experimented on could lie on their backs or on their sides, but under no circumstances could they stand up. They would be given a drug that would empty their bowels before the experiment, and their bowels must not move for at least a fortnight in bed. They could eat only crackers and tea and perhaps a little coffee in that time. They could have no meat, fruit, or cornmeal, even water should be kept to a minimum. To ensure that their bowels remained frozen, Dr. Sims would supply them with opium, which was a great expense but he would endure it. The opium should be given at least twice per day, in as great a quantity as could be borne. Opium would help with pain and ease hunger and seize the bowels, Dr. Sims said, and also it would create hope. Instead of foreboding and suffering, the cursed women would spend their fortnight of recovery in pleasant dreams and delightful sensations.

Dr. Sims made ready to leave. He was confident, he said, that he could cure them all in six months' time. They all had good masters, he told them, who wanted them to be cured, and the experiments were a great expense, he repeated, but Dr. Sims was hopeful. He was hopeful that the cursed women would assist in whatever ways became necessary. This was essential, he said. He paused and looked out the open door toward his office. The cursed women could be cured, Dr. Sims said, but if they were not cured, he was not sure what would happen to them. They might never return to their plantations. They might never see their families again. They might remain cursed forever.

Nine

Second pregnancy—Nathan Harris—First experiment—
1848 epidemic—Third pregnancy—Dr. Jarvis—
William Rufus King—Autauga County—Washington

ANARCHA LEARNED SHE HAD BEEN SOLD ONLY AFTER SHE GOT PREGNANT
and began to show and it became a question of where her second baby
would go. Dr. Sims had told the cursed women that it was possible for
them to have babies, and in fact after the first experiments he didn't dis-
courage them from having babies so long as they didn't all have babies at
the same time, because what the experiments were supposed to prove was
that a cursed woman could become a cured woman who returned to her
plantation to have more babies for herself and her master. Dr. Sims's first
experiments did not succeed, and sometimes they went horribly wrong,
but sometimes he came close to a cure, and when he did, it was a chance
to see what happened when a partially cured woman gave birth, whether
her hole would open up again. Mostly it did, and there were more experiments.

Anarcha met one of the servants at Montgomery Hall, Lotley or Alfred
or Frederick or Bill, or she grew friendly with Dr. Sims's Burnett or Allen,
and it was then that she learned what it meant for a man to be with a
woman. They stole moments. They stole moments the way that slaves stole
waffles and chickens, and now she knew what it was like to hold a man,
because it was the first time her hands were not bound. Lotley or Burnett
did not find Anarcha to be loathsome. City men were less likely than plantation slaves to believe the cursed women were filled with lizards.

fifteen Dollars for two of Sot Boy Bill

Lofley, Alfred - Frederick

Dr. Sims experimented on Anarcha three times before she got pregnant, and when she began to show she learned that her baby would not
be taken to the Westcott plantation because William Westcott was not her
master anymore. Dr. Sims told her that she needn't worry about the details,
it was complicated, but William Westcott had decided
after Anarcha's first experiment failed that she was not

Anacha

going to be cured and so now she was owned by
Dr. Nathan Harris, Betsey's master. Dr. Sims said

Anacha ,,

that Dr. Harris was a very good master and very
good to his slaves, and Betsey said that Dr. Harris was an older man who
had come from Georgia and had recently married a young Alabama
woman, and the slaves he bought in Alabama had been told by the slaves
he'd brought from Georgia that Dr. Harris had liked his female slaves in
Georgia very much, and several children had resulted from all that liking.
Dr. Harris owned a plantation and slaves in Lowndes County, he owned
property and more slaves in Autauga County, and he owned property and
slaves in Montgomery too, and because he had medical training like Dr.
Sims he took pity on the cursed women whose masters didn't want them
anymore, so he bought them all even though they were worthless, and
that was why Anarcha's baby would go to Lowndes County or Autauga
County, and when the time came and Anarcha's baby arrived—this time
the baby was a large boy, but nature took a true course—she was permitted to let the baby boy suck for five days and then the nameless baby was
sent to Autauga County to be raised by slaves that belonged to the young
woman who was now Dr. Harris's wife.

Lucy had been first for an experiment. At the appointed time, the white
doctors that Dr. Sims had invited to observe the experiment arrived, and
they waited and smoked in the examination room and waved their hands
in front of their faces to push away the smell of the Negro Hospital, which

had persisted even though Dr. Sims had ordered the cursed women to scrub clean the examination room and to clean themselves as well and put out flowers to mask the sickly sweet odor the cursed women had grown accustomed to. The doctors asked the cursed women questions about their holes, and they examined Dr. Sims's new instruments, and they looked over the notes that he had left out for that purpose, and then Dr. Sims arrived, and the cursed women were sent upstairs, and Lucy nervously watched them file past the hanging sheet that made a wall between the examination room and the rest of the Negro Hospital.

The cursed women sat upstairs in a circle. They heard Dr. Sims again deliver his speech about the three problems he had solved with science and inspiration, and if the experiments succeeded, he told the doctors, it would be a leap forward for medicine and for all American doctors, not just himself. There was commotion as the doctors moved the barber chair outside and positioned the examination table so that they could gather around as Dr. Sims worked, and there was some disagreement as Dr. Sims's young medical students struggled to lift the flesh of Lucy's buttocks. Dr. Sims instructed them to do it as Anarcha and Betsey had done it, but for a time there was confusion about what exactly they had done. Then there was quiet, though sometimes there was a sharp whimper from Lucy that she attempted to stifle, and sometimes Dr. Sims talked aloud about what he was doing, about how every previous doctor had failed, and you could hear the white doctors shuffling about, taking turns to look inside, and instead of the twenty minutes that Dr. Sims had said the experiment would take, Lucy stayed in that pose for nearly an hour, and at last there was a great shuffling of feet and furniture downstairs, and Dr. Sims called for the cursed women to come down and help turn Lucy onto her side and carry her to a cot. Lucy was wet with sweat and she was woozy and delirious from the first dose of opium she'd been given, and if she was having dreams, they didn't at all seem like they were pleasant or delightful dreams, as Dr. Sims had said they would be.

Nor did her dreams become delightful over the next few days, as Anarcha and the cursed women threw water onto her with the large squirt and cleaned the places and sores between her legs firmly but gently as though she was a baby, and gave her crackers and more doses of opium as Dr. Sims instructed. Within several days a fever came over her, and the beating of her heart grew very fast, and at night she barely slept, and the women took turns sitting up with her. One morning, Anarcha sent one of those less afflicted with miseries in her feet out to the woods for life-everlasting weed and horsemint and some scrapings of red oak bark, and they gave these to Lucy as teas, but her fever was not eased, and her suffering did not abate in any way. Dr. Sims came twice per day, and he said something about poison in her blood but he did not say who might have poisoned her, and he hoped she would improve with rest and opium but she did not.

They changed the ticking on her cot and gave her new blankets when she sweated through them, and her skin got so hot it was as though a fire was baking her from the inside out. On the fifth night, she woke the cursed women with cries, and they sent for little George who rode with Dr. Sims on his buggy, and George fetched Dr. Sims, who came to the Negro Hospital in his nightshirt with a lantern. He was puzzled because the experiment had gone well, he said, he had closed the hole, and the cursed women agreed that Lucy was not leaking and that urine was coming from the sponge that dangled from her and collected in a small tin that they emptied regularly, so they knew the urine was not rotting the tissue around the stitches. As they stood over her, Lucy's breathing sped up like the panting of a dog, and for a moment she shook all over like the slaves that got happy at church in the quarters on the Lucas plantation, but she was not happy and she gave out a long, throbbing sob that echoed into the streets of Montgomery. It was then that Dr. Sims decided that the experiment must have failed. They needed to pull everything out of her to save her life.

They had to wait for morning light. Little George stood outside with a mirror, directing it inside to another mirror, and Lucy continued to fade into the dawn, and it seemed that the last bits of life were draining from her when the cursed women gathered around to hoist her onto the examination table and hold her upright. Anarcha and Betsey lifted her flesh, and this time Dr. Sims had Anarcha hold in place his tool that looked like a snake, because there was no student to assist him. He talked to himself as he peered inside and worked. The hole was still closed, or mostly closed. He removed the stitches and the bars, and discovered what was wrong only when he attempted to remove the urine sponge: it was stuck. Even touching it caused Lucy to writhe as the women held her. Dr. Sims attempted pulling at various angles with gentle force, but no angle seemed better than any other. Finally, he laid hold of the string that ran through the sponge and he gave it one great vicious tug and Lucy screamed as though she had been stabbed and she fainted. There was a gush of blood and piss, and Dr. Sims staunched the bleeding with felt, and it was not for some time that they were sure that Lucy would survive, but she did.

* * *

When Dr. Sims's assistants grabbed your flesh and lifted, it was like they were touching something dead. The cursed women held one another with firm tenderness, more cupping than clenching, but the assistants squeezed you into their fists and they moved you as a butcher moved meat. The white doctors crowded in around Dr. Sims during the experiments, and amid the fear and the painful tugging you could feel the warm tickle of their breath on the backs of your thighs, and sometimes a stray finger grazed you there as well. Some experiments were more painful than others. The cursed women who had been whipped said that a painful experiment was like being whipped while giving birth, but there was no whipcrack and there was no overseer counting the lashes, and whereas an overseer wanted you to scream from the pain so that all the slaves could hear it, if you flinched at the pain of Dr. Sims's experiments you might be punished for that too.

Dr. Sims attempted another experiment with his sponge, on Betsey, but he gave it up on the second day of her fever instead of the fifth, and Dr. Sims's students helped this time when he pulled the sponge out, and Betsey bled but not as much as Lucy bled. A week passed with no experiments, and Dr. Sims gathered the cursed women around Lucy and Betsey on their cots and showed them what had happened to Lucy's hole on the swatch of burlap. What had started as a two-inch hole had begun to heal, and now only three small holes remained. That's how Lucy would have stayed had the healing been allowed to continue.

Three small holes was no great improvement, Dr. Sims allowed. A cup of urine would trickle through a small hole just as surely as it streamed through a large hole. But even the first failed experiment had demonstrated that a cure was possible. Now he had a device to replace the urine sponge. It was a stick of gum elastic with a wire running through it, and by pulling the wire you made one end of the stick open up like a flower, and Dr. Sims showed the cursed women how to insert the stick into the bladder, open it, and then close it again to remove it so that it would not get stuck inside like the sponge. The urine would flow through the stick, and several times per day the cursed women would remove it and clean it.

Anarcha was the next to be experimented on. The stick did not give her fever, and she remained in bed and was given opium for nine days, and then Dr. Sims gathered the white doctors to remove the stitches and demonstrate a great success and triumph. But it was not a success. Like Lucy, Anarcha was left with two small holes where one of her large holes had been. Nevertheless, the flesh had healed as flesh heals, and Dr. Sims was praised by the white doctors, but it was not a cure, and he was not satisfied because there were still holes and Anarcha was still leaking, and when Anarcha gave birth after two more experiments and nine months of pregnancy, her partially closed hole opened up again completely.

All of the women were experimented on, but there were no triumphs, and when six months passed and none of the cursed women became cured women, Dr. Sims said nothing at all about it. He kept on experimenting, though over time, fewer and fewer white doctors came to watch. He kept the women supplied with food and clothes and opium, but he was wrong about the opium because it was never pleasant or delightful, and one of the things the cursed women learned early on was how to care for one another when their stitches were removed and the opium was stopped. Some of the women didn't want it to stop. At night, they talked. A few of the cursed women had come to think that the experiments were torture, and they wished to return to their plantations, hole or no hole, and some thought life in the city was better even with the experiments because the stink of the city covered up the stink of their holes, and because they had found men here who knew they didn't have any turtles inside of them. Others preferred the experiments to picking cotton, because in addition to picking cotton their overseers and masters gave them unwanted attentions and forced them to bear yellow babies. And some of the cursed women wished to stay at the Negro Hospital, and they even hoped for more experiments, but not because they wished to become a cured woman. Rather, they were now doubly cursed by their holes and by the opium.

Anarcha had two holes, so she could be experimented on twice as often as the others. After she gave birth to the baby who was sent away name-less, she was operated on several times more, on both of her holes. She lost count of how many times, though it was more than the others, and Dr. Sims gave her the devil's share and even liked operating on her because some of the women screamed in agony at the experiments, despite the possibility of being punished for it, but Anarcha never moved or made a sound, though the pain was fierce and cut down into her soul. In January 1848, when both of Anarcha's holes had been reduced to smaller holes, Lotley once again made her pregnant, or perhaps Lotley was gone now and it was Alfred who made her pregnant this time, and Dr. Sims examined her because he wished to see her holes after her time with Alfred, but he did not tell her what he saw inside. As time went by, Dr. Sims told the cursed women less and less about what he was doing and why he was doing it, and by then he had replaced the sticks of gum elastic with short, bent tubes of silver for the urine. He attempted to hide it, but the cursed women could tell that he was now worried there would never be a cure.

In 1848, diseases passed through Montgomery like runaway ghosts. Many doctors got sick, and a doctor from far away, in the North, traveled to Mobile, and he fell sick like many did in Mobile. He rode a riverboat north to Montgomery and came under Dr. Sims's care. The sick doctor's name was Jarvis, and he believed he had ship fever. Dr. Sims resisted the diagnosis at first, but eventually admitted the man had typhus. He put Dr. Jarvis into the largest room in Montgomery Hall, and he arranged for Anarcha to be the nurse that looked after him, and the closest Dr. Sims ever came to acknowledging that Anarcha had once saved his life was when she visited Dr. Jarvis for the first time. The man was very ill, but Dr. Sims told him that he could feel easy about his recovery because Anarcha was caring for him. Even Dr. Jarvis could tell that there was more than hope in Dr. Sims's words—there was knowledge. Dr. Jarvis looked at Anarcha differently after that. He looked at her differently because he was a Yankee, and the cursed women and all the slaves knew that there were Yankees who wanted slavery times to come to an *"kindest and best nurse"* end. That's why runaways ran away north. But there were other rumors about Yankees too, such as that Yankee men called all slave women Dinah even if Dinah wasn't their name, and that Yankees weren't even truly people but something else, and certainly not gentlefolks, and that what a Yankee wanted most was to skin a slave alive. Dr. Jarvis was not a Yankee who wanted slavery to end, nor did he hope to skin anyone alive, and Anarcha cared for him as he bled from his bowels, as his tongue turned white, and he muttered on about how Anarcha was the kindest and best nurse anywhere to be found, and she gave him opium for a pain in his hip until at last he was able to sit up and drink porter beer and crack the bones of boiled birds. In March, he returned home to Yankeedom.

Anarcha tended to another man who immediately replaced Dr. Jarvis in the large room in Montgomery Hall. He was a famous man, a politician who had named the town of Selma, Alabama, refusing to name it for himself even though others had suggested that he do so. His name was William Rufus King, but everyone called him Mr. King because he was powerful, and he owned plantations in Selma and Lowndes County and elsewhere, but mostly he lived in Washington City because he had been a senator in the Congress of the United States. He had also been a diplomat in France, and he had lived with another powerful senator, Mr. James Buchanan, and even the slaves heard that they had been called Miss Nancy and Aunt Fancy, and it was true that Mr. King sometimes seemed more like a missus than a master.

Mr. King had fallen ill just when he was supposed to go back to Washington City to be a senator once again. He came down with a terrible cough, and when he wasn't coughing he told Anarcha that if he was dying, that was just fine because Earth is not our true abiding place. The sons and daughters of men, he said, must be prepared for the awful change that awaits us all. Anarcha gave him lobelia tea and peach brandy, and when Mr. King was woozy but his cough let up, he told her about the balls he had thrown in France, how he had advocated for an expansion of a dozen war steamers to the United States Navy, and how he had almost died in a shipwreck on the way home. When he was woozier still, he spoke with longing of Mr. Buchanan, who had been considered for the Supreme Court. Mr. King was most anxious to see Mr. Buchanan. Mr. King admitted that Mr. Buchanan's letters caused him both pleasure and pain, particularly when they spoke of wooing boys and of a young man named Jemmy who would remember Mr. Buchanan as long as he remembered hickory oil. Sometimes, Mr. Buchanan instructed Mr. King to burn his letters after he read them.

Mr. King had often acted as a nurse for Mr. Buchanan in Washington City, so Mr. King shared with Anarcha the cures that his family had used for a variety of ailments. For camp itch, soak a copper coin in vinegar for twenty-four hours. Boiled rice and rhubarb for diarrhea. Boiled rhubarb and sugar for infant cholera. Salt, sage, and bay rum for your hair, and add rusty nails for color. Salt, tartar, and lemon to clean the blood. In morose moods, Mr. King complained that he had held on to his cotton too long this year, confounded by his own cupidity. For this reason, he would soon write his will, but he had no idea what he would do with his slaves because he had so many of them. A few he planned to leave money so that they could go to Liberia, or Washington City, or any free state they wished.

Mr. King wasn't fully healthy when he returned to Washington City. Anarcha heard news of him years later, long after the cursed women had become Dr. Sims's assistants. By then, they'd seen the surgery done so many times they likely could have done it themselves, and sometimes they were tempted to do so. Anarcha gave birth again, her third child, a large girl who was taken away after five days. She never did see that girl again. And then she was cured, in 1849, when Dr. Sims closed at least one of her two holes, and almost immediately all of the cursed women were experimented on again, and some of them were cured and some of them weren't, but all of them were sent away from the Negro Hospital, some to their plantations, some sold by Dr. Harris. Several years later, on the Duncan plantation in Autauga County—Betsey and Lucy were also sent to Autauga—Anarcha learned that Mr. King was no longer a senator. He had become vice president of the United States of America! However, he had never gotten well. It was tuberculosis, Dr. Sims told her. Doctors in Washington City had advised him to go to Cuba for the warmth and the air, and he became vice president there. But almost at once, the tuberculosis grew worse. He set out for home. Everyone in Alabama heard that the vice president of the United States had arrived at his plantation in Selma. He died a few days later. He had been vice president for a month.

In Autauga, Anarcha became the plantation's doctor woman and midwife. She wasn't well, she still had holes, and a small cabin was constructed for her away from the rest of the slave cabins. She cared for the sick with what she'd learned from Pheriba, and she caught babies with what she'd learned in Dr. Sims's Negro Hospital. She did not see Dr. Sims again for several years, but in Autauga she met her son, her second baby, the one who had sucked from the breast of another slave mother.

His name was Washington.

Ten

AT FIRST, IT WAS SIMPLY AN OPPORTUNITY TO AFFIX HIS NAME TO PROCE-
dures and devices. It *had* to be devices—just as J. F. G. Mittag and medical
school had taught him. The full scope of the opportunity, however, did
not become apparent for some time.

After Sims and Theresa and their children moved into Montgomery
in 1840, it was clear—if medicine was to provide a sense of honor and the
lifestyle that his wife expected and deserved—that the idle years tending
to plantation slaves in Mount Meigs and Cubahatchee had been a waste of
time. In Montgomery, Sims was pleased to discover that doctors weren't
nearly so combative as the cliques he had glimpsed in the north. They fos-
tered one another's careers, shared expertise, and assisted in procedures
and experiments. Woefully, some of them were aligned with the Kappa
Lambda men, but even if Montgomery medicine was out of date—and
even if its physicians lacked the ambition that was a common trait to all
true men—Sims's Alabama colleagues each distinguished themselves in
one form or another.

On the one hand, there were the old medical workhorses like Hugh
Henry and Dr. Silas Ames, who had once been in practice with poor
James Lucas's preceptor, Charles Lucas, and who was now doing work on
meningitis. And there was Dr. Samuel Holt, who was a great theorist of
medicine, when he wasn't tinkering with vacuum-tube inventions. Holt

had once likened the work of physicians to that of a mariner who sails without a compass, trusting in his knowledge of the movements of the stars and planets.

On the other hand, there was the new generation, young physicians with modern educations who, by dint of inherited wealth and social advantage, were outperforming Sims. Dr. James Berney had also attended medical school in South Carolina, but he'd then gone on to the University of Pennsylvania and followed up with additional study in Paris, like Josiah Nott and so many others. He established a successful practice in Charleston, moving to Alabama a full two years after Sims did. Dr. Carnot Bellinger had distinguished himself with an important paper about hernias that reapplied a *Macbeth* quote about assassination to surgery: "If it were done when 'tis done, then 'twere well it were done quickly." Dr. Alexander McWhorter was young but had inherited a plantation from his father—Sims could expect no such bequest—and Dr. William Baldwin was also Sims's junior but he was already rich with slaves. Baldwin had luckily inherited his practice when his former partner was tried for attempting to kill a circus performer who had attempted to steal his wife. Now, Baldwin was moving into banking. Dr. Hardy Wooten, in Lowndes County, attended Jefferson in Philadelphia after Sims and fancied himself a writer; he circulated essays called "On Literature in General" and "Procrastination Is the Thief of Time." He was an amateur astronomer as well; in 1843, Wooten kept his fellow physicians apprised of the passing of the Great Comet, the subject of much discussion in Washington City and abroad. Its tail stretched from the horizon to the meridian, Wooten reported, and at the same time a star of considerable magnitude was mysteriously darting all about the heavens. A few years later, when Sims sent invitation cards for his first fistula experiment to all his colleagues from Montgomery and Autauga County and Lowndes County, it was Wooten who wryly noted, before the procedure began, that it was appropriate that Sims was attempting to cure a case of a woman's inner break and crumbling precisely at the moment—only days earlier—when the superintendent of the nation's new naval observatory, the precocious Lieutenant Matthew Fontaine Maury, had become the first person in the world to observe the breaking apart of a celestial body.

The first experiment was a disaster. Sims's medical students had found it almost impossible to replicate the ease with which the slaves Anarcha and Betsey had elevated Lucy's nates to expose her fistula. Sims talked as he worked, pointing out to his colleagues the rising and falling of Lucy's cervix as she breathed. This proved, of course, that no such operation could be performed on a white woman unless her tight-fitting garments were loosened. He laid out each of the steps of the procedure for which he should receive sole credit as innovator: the position, his speculum, the clamp suture, and the bladder sponge that would draw urine away by capillary action. Everyone present understood that the clamps were a variation on the quill suture long in use, but the device and the procedure as a whole were novel enough that Sims could attach his name to every part of it.

If Lucy had died when the encrusted sponge had to be yanked out of her, the fistula experiments would have come to an end right there. He hadn't anticipated urinary salts turning the sponge into a stone. He tried and failed with the sponge once again, then attempted a gum elastic device. From there, he began experimenting with the amount of tissue he would remove in freshening the edges of the fistula. He worked with a jeweler to commission specula of various sizes, clamps of different lengths, with more or fewer sutures, and eventually he altered the distance of the clamp from the edge of the fissure. Success always seemed imminent, but nothing worked.

It was in the earliest days, not long after his slaves completed the second floor of the Negro Hospital and the fistulous women that his students had found hidden in the areas around Montgomery began to arrive—some having leaked urine for years, some dangerously emaciated—that Sims confirmed his suspicion about the girl Anarcha. Although the condition was taking a toll on her appearance, she was not as old as some of the others. Nevertheless, she was emerging as a leader among them, and it was something she did—the way she touched the brow of a feverish slave with a wet cloth, or insisted that another drink a tea that was likely infused with one of their slave cures—that cinched it. Anarcha was the same girl who had watched over him as he veered precipitously between malarial chills and sweats. There was a kindness in her, and a knowledge;

someone had taught her something of medicine. Sims never let on that he recognized her, just as he never let on that her two fistulae might have been the result of his clumsy forceps delivery of her baby. Immediately on recognizing her skills, he leased her to Montgomery Hall as a nurse to help defray the costs of keeping the slave women in his backyard.

He owned a dozen slaves now, or near a dozen; it was hard to tell as the tax collector counted the women in the hospital as his, even though the deal he'd made with their owners was that he was merely keeping them for the period of the experiments. Furthermore, a number of Sims's own slaves weren't technically his. After the financial crisis, there had been a wave of plantation owners dying insolvent, leaving their wives destitute. There was discussion of legislation that would permit women to own property—held in trust by a man, of course—and in the interim, men were transferring assets to their wives. In 1841, Sims transferred slaves to Theresa. A boilerplate contract specified that Abigail and her Amanda, Martha, and Minerva, and Harriet and her George and Emma, belonged to Theresa but would remain in Sims's possession and under his control.

Possession and control aside, how could Sims take pride in owning any slaves at all—how could he feel that they signaled his prosperity—when he was forced to use the slaves he did own to cover his debts? In 1847, Burnett acted as collateral for a debt of $726.30 that had been accruing since 1845. The funds were due January 1, 1849, or the boy would be seized. Sims paid off that obligation, but six months later, he used eight-year-old Bill to cover a debt of $184.24. In 1850, Sims's slave Allen stood against

a loan of $500 to be paid back in four months' time,

and in 1851, Henry Lucas agreed to cover Sims's debts in the amount of $1,306.78, with Harriet, George, Emma, and Nat listed as securities. None of this was secret. How could any of it remain so with the unscrupulous R. G. Dun credit investigators skulking around for rumors and slander, cursing Sims as a man of high standing but little means? All Montgomery knew he was poor. And soon, all his colleagues recognized that the fistula experiments were failing.

* * *

After it became clear that closing a fistula wasn't going to be as easy as he'd hoped, infant lockjaw appeared once again to be the quickest route to status outside the congenial but insular world of Montgomery medicine.

The case on the Stickney plantation had revealed that lockjaw was likely a function of the position in which babies were kept. Now, Sims made a study of what had been written about lockjaw in Moreau's *A Practical Treatise on Midwifery*, and he consulted Quain and Wilson's definitive set of lithography plates on anatomy, and he read a number of recent articles on the subject in the *New Orleans Medical Journal*. Eberle had claimed a lockjaw cure, but it seemed obvious to Sims that Eberle's baby had gotten well simply because one wouldn't lay an infant on its back after blistering it there—his cure was an accident. Similarly, a tale of a woman curing an infant with a concoction of oil was a case of having luckily placed the baby in the proper position.

He grew more and more convinced of his sudden insight: the condition was mechanical, and it could be cured by mechanical means. He examined the heads of dozens of slave babies, healthy and not, and when not he made every effort to perform an autopsy and procure the infant's spine for examination as well. He achieved a success in August 1845, prescribing no physic at all, and in September his brother-in-law Rush confirmed Sims's theory of overlapping bones with some clever use of his pocketknife. A few days after Theresa gave birth to a son on Christmas Day, 1845, Sims received word from another doctor who had come across a case too late to be saved. The timid physician felt that an autopsy would have been inappropriate, but he was confident of the presence of the true culprit, Sims's crowded skull plates.

In March 1846, in the dramatic aftermath of his first fistula failures, Sims saved two babies with changes of position. That was all that needed to be done if you caught the problem in time. For more advanced cases, he began a new set of experiments, manually manipulating slave babies' heads. Pressing hard to push the infants' unfused skull bones against their brains, he found that he could alternately create and diminish the symptoms of lockjaw, to the point where he could unlock a baby's lips and then fasten them again around its mother's breast.

Later the same month, Sims was invited to the autopsy of a lockjaw infant owned by Montgomery circuit court judge George Goldthwaite. Sims had made Goldthwaite's acquaintance through Betsey's owner, Dr. Harris.

It was William Baldwin who invited Sims to the autopsy. That was suspicious from the start—Baldwin had openly disagreed with Sims's first lockjaw paper. Not only did Baldwin think the facts of lockjaw failed to comport with Sims's mechanical theory, he'd accused Sims of seeking out cases to support his thesis. Baldwin argued that infant lockjaw was associated with a wound of some kind, most likely at the site of the severed umbilical cord, which was so poorly cared for by slave midwives.

Baldwin's confederate Dr. William Boling, another of the new generation of Montgomery physicians, was also present at the autopsy. Like Wooten, Boling had attended Jefferson after Sims, but that hadn't stopped him from beating Sims to Montgomery to establish a thriving practice and publish on pneumonia, opium eating, and the dangers of the tartar emetic. Now, Baldwin and Boling were partners and coconspirators in the planning of a statewide medical association, one to be formed in concert with the formation of the American Medical Association, whose first meeting was to be held in New York in a little more than a month's time. Sims wasn't hostile to any of this. He had even assisted Baldwin and Boling in experiments on dogs to demonstrate that quinine was being overprescribed. However, he suspected both men knew that he believed work on dogs to be a waste of time when there were better subjects for experimentation all around them.

The autopsy was of a six-day-old male infant. Seven hours after death, its fingers and toes were still tightly clenched, and what remained of the umbilical cord was enlarged and hardened. Baldwin explained that, despite Sims's theory, the mother had insisted the baby had not been kept on its back. The men took turns feeling the tiny corpse's head. As soon as he touched the skull, Sims realized it was a trap. He tried to insist that the bones were *slightly* overlapping, but his colleagues united against him. Baldwin claimed the skull was typical of an infant of its age, and Boling said that if the skull was remarkable in any way it was for its regularity and uniformity.

Worse than embarrassing Sims in front of a local colleague, Baldwin went on to publish about the Goldthwaite slave baby case. Just months after the publication of Sims's own lockjaw piece, Baldwin showered him with false praise, and then insisted that his theory of infant lockjaw was wholly in error.

Sims refused to budge. Perhaps the cause of the spasms was more situated in the brain than the spine—he might allow that much—but he did not waver from an insistence that the condition's cause and cure were best suited to doctors equipped with the will and the skill to employ a knife to effect. What he needed was a case that would enable him to demonstrate that surgical intervention could change the fate of a lockjaw baby even when the disease was far advanced. As though on cue, two such cases arrived in quick succession.

* * *

In January 1847, a slave named Ann belonging to Mrs. Somerville gave birth to a baby with a remarkable head—flattened in the front and mashed backward, elongated toward the cranial vertex at the crown of the skull. Lockjaw set in a few days after birth, and Sims was called in when the disease was only partly advanced. The history of the case was remarkable in that it seemed to demonstrate that even a mother who held her baby in the hard crook of her arm could cause the skull plates to grow overtop one another. Sims immediately found the baby's head to be amenable to the digital pressure that alternately created and relaxed the symptoms of the disease.

Mrs. Somerville assented at once when Sims asked to bring the child home for observation overnight. He fully intended to puncture the infant's scalp that evening with a short, strong blade. He would pry up the misplaced bones. He refrained from doing so, however, resolving to wait until the case was nearly hopeless—when his cure could be attributed to nothing else. Several days later, he punched into the living infant's skull and pried up the parietal bone, an action that produced a frightful display of muscular spasm. In keeping with his revised theory of the spine, he arranged for the child to be kept upright at all times. The position alone seemed to help. He repeated the puncturings at regular intervals, and soon the dramatic contractions of the baby's face and hands began to relax.

The success was short-lived. The following month, Sims encountered yet another case in which the pressure of the mother's arm was the source of the mischief. The baby of a slave named Frances had begun to fret five days after a normal birth. Sims first saw the infant in the disease's early stages. Once again, he would wait to puncture the child. The following day, he was called deep into the country on a case. He returned home late that evening to find a snide note from Boling waiting for him. Frances's baby had taken a sharp turn for the worse. When Sims couldn't be found, Boling had been called in. He had sat with the infant all day long.

The baby would likely die very soon, Boling wryly wrote, but Sims needn't worry, as care would be taken to ensure that it was placed into the proper position first.

Sims rushed out the door, purchasing on the way a crooked awl meant for woodworkers and cobblers. The tool would be even better suited to the puncturing work than his knife. He arrived in a rush and laid the spasming infant, deluged in perspiration, facedown across its mother's legs. Before he could press into the head, a spasmodic quiver thrilled across the baby's entire frame. It went silent and limp. The mother, the mistress, Boling—all believed the child dead.

Sims took the infant up in his arms and began shaking. He threw water into its face to excite the respiratory act. It wasn't until he'd given up and was wiping the baby's face dry that another whole-body quiver came. At once, Sims turned the baby over and carved the point of the awl into the back of the head to pry up first one parietal bone, then the other. The infant spasmed and took a gasping breath, and its eyes flew open like the eyes of a corpse in an anatomy class, falsely woken with electric shock. For the next twelve hours, Sims kept the baby alive with further punctures and prizings. It died at dawn the following day—not as most lockjaw babies died, in violent throes, but with its life slowly flickering away.

Sims took the baby's body with him when he left, but already he had decided to give up on infant lockjaw.

He published two more papers about it. He was able to salvage this much, at least. But how could the work bring him renown when not even his colleagues were aligned with his theory? The future would judge him, he decided, and surely the surgical cure of infant lockjaw would be regarded as the first major discovery of Dr. J. Marion Sims. Until then, he would need more for his career. Medicine for slaves, in the form of either clever cures for lockjaw or the plank he'd devised for Sam that made possible procedures that were otherwise too painful to be practicable— innovations such as these could nurse his surgical reputation, but that was all. He needed a cure that promised a profit, an ailment that did not distinguish between rich and poor.

Everything depended on the slave women in his backyard.

* * *

In June 1847, Sims and Theresa, who was pregnant again, attended the Autauga County wedding of Dr. Nathan Harris. Harris was marrying Margaret Duncan, who was several decades his junior and the sister of Harris's law partner, John Duncan. Sims had known the Duncan family since his earliest days in Mount Meigs. Along with Margaret and John, there was a sister, Catherine, and their parents, whose romance had begun at the 1825 fete for Lafayette at Henry Lucas's Rose Hill plantation. The Harris wedding was held at the Duncan plantation, Violet Hill, which had hosted some of the grandest soirees in the history of Alabama. Violet Hill was known for its private racetrack, for rows of marble stepping-stones that snaked through the property, and for hothouses with chimneys at both ends that grew pineapples, rare flowers, and tropical plants from Africa.

Nathan Harris was one of the best lawyers in the state. He was so well regarded that people forgave him strange rumors—not only that he'd fathered slaves in Georgia but that he'd written them into his will. There were concerns that he treated his Alabama slaves a little too well, and there were whispers when he accepted a fifty-dollar fee to defend a slave accused of manslaughter. Harris's legal practice was successful nonetheless. He worked on everything from wills and trusts and business partnerships to defending plantation owners against accusations of cruelty to their servants. His training as a physician was limited, but it prepared him well for medical litigation. He could recite from memory from both Theodric Beck's *Elements of Medical Jurisprudence* and Joseph Chitty's more recent book, *A Practical Treatise on Medical Jurisprudence*. Sims had once retained him in a matter, and Harris had represented Baldwin and Charles Lucas and Abercrombie and the Westcotts and Senator William Rufus King and Rush Jones, who had begun to move into the dry goods business, as his father once had, and who now supplied Harris's plantations with sherry and brandy and balls of lampwick and yeast powder and castor oil. Rush signed as an official witness for the newlyweds' marriage license.

Sims and Theresa rented a carriage for the twelve-mile journey to Autauga County, passing along the way some of Alabama's grandest estates: Ellerslie, Thornfield, the Mill, the Elms. Sims was surprised, approaching Violet Hill, when he glimpsed Anarcha, Betsey, Lucy, and a number of the slave women from his own Negro Hospital. They were caring for children outside the Violet Hill slave quarters.

Nathan Harris now owned all the slaves Sims was experimenting on. Sims had told the slaves' masters the same thing he'd told the women: he expected them to be cured in six months' time. When they weren't, it hardly mattered that Sims had resolved to permit some of the women to become pregnant so they could send slave babies back to their plantations to be reared or sold. The masters didn't want them; it was as though they too thought the women were cursed. Several were returned to their plantations, most likely to be sold for whatever could be got for them, and Nathan Harris bought the rest, informally and almost for nothing. Sims had told Harris of Anarcha's value as a nurse. That's why she and the others had been brought to Violet Hill for the wedding, he realized—it released other slaves that didn't smell of urine for house service.

Just before his marriage was solemnized, Harris, as many others had done before him, arranged for a significant portion of his property to be signed over to his young betrothed.

Anarcha appeared on a list of slaves now owned by Margaret Harris, née Duncan, though Margaret's property was held in trust by Judge Goldthwaite, the same Goldthwaite who had owned the lockjaw baby that William Baldwin used to fool Sims. Goldthwaite attended the Harris wedding as well, mixing with the Pratts of Mobile, who had cousins nearby, and E. Y. Fair and his wife, who were practically Nathan Harris's neighbors. Sims and Theresa greeted Goldthwaite and exchanged pleasantries. They never knew him well, but it was clear that he was destined for higher office. In 1852, Goldthwaite was named to the Alabama Supreme Court, and in 1856, he became the court's chief justice, though he mysteriously resigned his position after only thirteen days. After the Civil War, Anarcha's onetime trustee owner ran for the US Senate from the state of Alabama. Goldthwaite won, served a single unremarkable term, and died three years later.

* * *

A great deal changed in the months after Sims's final lockjaw case. He wasn't sure if Baldwin and Boling were behind it, but a rumor spread that his fistula experiments were now growing desperate. There were quiet, secretive whisperings: the use of slaves as experimental fodder without any imminent hope of success was not in keeping with the spirit of the code of ethics that had been passed when the American Medical Association was officially formed at its second meeting, in Philadelphia in May 1847.

The Kappa Lambda men had won. It was said they'd played an out-sized role in drafting ethical prohibitions that seemed to Sims to have been designed to ensure that a doctor who came from modest means would never be able to advance his station. Physicians should avoid gloomy prognostications that magnified the necessity of their services, the code asserted. It was derogatory to the dignity of the profession to publicly advertise cures for particular diseases. No physician should hold a patent on a surgical device. How could any doctor, Sims wondered, expect to make a living under such strictures? Worse, the Medical Association of Montgomery—Sims dutifully paid the five-dollar initiation and one-dollar quarterly fees—adopted the entirety of the AMA's ethical code and added a few constraints of its own. Some of these clearly targeted Sims's work: Doctors should not exhibit or explain instruments employed in operations particular to females. Cures for such procedures should not be publicly boasted of. No doctor whose practice was based on a singular dogma, or who rejected the accumulated experience of the profession, could be considered one of its regular practitioners.

At any rate, the truth was bleak. The fistula experiments *were* growing desperate. The problem was simple: it was essential to Sims's career that the clamp suture provide the cure, but it wasn't working.

Sims studied again and again the accounts of the doctors who had succeeded with fistula before him—Gosset in England, Mettauer in Virginia, Hayward in Boston. He borrowed from each of them. After the sponge almost killed Lucy, the gum elastic catheter Sims used was based on the implement Gosset described. It worked for a year. Then he abandoned it in favor of the silver tube used by Mettauer and Hayward, though Sims bent it into an "S" shape so that it would lodge behind the pubic bone. More recently, Sims had had his jeweler fashion a length of lead wire for suture material, as Mettauer had done, but when he attempted experiments with it he found it virtually impossible to twist the wire into a knot. Either the wire snapped because the metal was too soft or the knot remained too loose to hold the edges of the wound together.

What gave him hope was that none of the doctors who had cured fistula had invented a device to enable their procedure. Furthermore, although their accounts appeared in reputable journals, they were short and poorly presented. There were no woodcut illustrations of tools, anatomy, or process. The physicians had made no true effort to profit from their good result.

Ironically, the first glimmer of hope came at the moment when the experiments seemed like an utterly foolhardy quest. Sims sent out invitation cards for yet another fistula experiment. No one arrived at the appointed time; even the students who were supposed to assist in the surgery failed to attend. On a whim, recalling the ease with which Anarcha and Betsey had lifted Lucy's nates, Sims called on the slaves to assist in the procedure.

It wasn't only Anarcha's skill as a nurse that had caught Sims's attention. When she thought he wasn't watching, Anarcha quietly offered instruction to the others, and without Sims either intending or fostering it the slave women had become a corps of skilled attendants. They were more adept than himself at extracting and cleaning and reinserting the catheters. They were patient companions to the convulsions of the lingering aftereffects of opium. And the fastidiousness with which they kept the hospital tidy, masking the smell of urine as much as possible and attending to one another's most intimate needs, was almost enough to make one reconsider the race's well-established reputation for grime and slovenliness.

Anarcha and Betsey hesitated when Sims instructed them to assist in the procedure. It was as though they feared he was luring them into a transgression for which they would be punished. He repeated the instructions more firmly, ordering them to take positions alongside a girl who had been one of the more difficult subjects. She tended to cry out at the pain, and when Sims or one his assistants warned of punishment, the tremors of her sobbing made the work all the more difficult.

The difference with the slaves assisting him was apparent at once. Anarcha and Betsey lifted the girl's nates in a way that offered him a clearer field of vision, and they held the girl's hand and spoke gently to her as Sims worked. She winced once and cried some, but she was far steadier throughout the ordeal. Nevertheless, Sims saw at once that this experiment too would fail. The clearer field of vision revealed that he hadn't yet mastered the problem of how to fix the clamps in place. Either they remained too loose or they buried themselves too deeply into the membrane of the vaginal wall. As well, the sheer number of experiments he had already performed—dozens in Anarcha's case, probably half as many for the others—was a problem. Each failure resulted in additional scar tissue, and now, at best, he was hoping that cicatrix would fuse to cicatrix. Either that, or he was snipping away additional dead tissue and creating even larger holes that, once clamped, would be subjected to even greater tension than in earlier failed experiments. What he needed most was fresh experimental subjects. Regardless, with Anarcha and Betsey assisting him, Sims recognized something new. All along, the problem had been his inability to reach deep enough inside to properly secure the clamps.

Sims closed the girl's fistula as best he could. As predicted, the clamps cut out in a few days' time. Still, the experiment was a success. After years of work, he at last understood the problem.

* * *

In 1848, the whole world got sick. An epidemic of scarlet fever in Mobile killed more than a hundred, and a meningitis attack in Montgomery afflicted dozens, chills leading to a comatose state that left victims with swollen, ashy white tongues protruding from between their teeth. Sims and his colleagues discovered reddish pulp and lobes of pus in the brains of those who died of it, and others recovered after speculative treatments of mercury, valerinate of zinc, and liquor potassae. This last was a cure suggested by a Connecticut physician named Jarvis who believed he had contracted ship fever on a journey to New Orleans.

Jarvis and Sims became friends, and Sims arranged for Anarcha to attend to him at Montgomery Hall. One morning, when Jarvis's fate was still in doubt and Anarcha was not present, Sims told Jarvis that he needn't worry because the young slave caring for him had once seen Sims himself through a bout of malaria. Jarvis survived, and he was immediately followed at the Hall by Senator William Rufus King, who had brought a case of consumption home with him from France. Sims was not his physician, but given the rampant chatter about King and his political roommate in Washington City, Sims wondered whether there would soon be news that

*Mr. King (at the Hall) has been
sick and Anarca, our Anarca, is missing
him, so you may feel easy about her recovery—*

President Polk's secretary of state, James Buchanan, had also contracted tuberculosis.

Worst of all, Sims's youngest son—the boy Theresa had named Merry Christmas for the holiday on which he'd been born, in 1845—fell ill with the same disease that had foiled Sims's earliest medical efforts in Lancaster. It was now fifteen years since Sims had begun medical school, and neither he nor anyone else was closer to understanding how to cure chronic diarrhea. The boy died in October 1848. Over time, the woe of the death proved to be a nudge added to Sims's ambitions and Theresa's longing for experience of the broader world. All seemed to point to a fate beyond the confines of Montgomery.

For that, Sims still needed to make his fortune. It was from this perspective that he failed to understand his Montgomery colleagues' preoccupation with infectious diseases. He knew now that his colleagues resented his longing for acclaim; he could sense it as his papers on Sam and George were published, and as he began to correspond with physicians in the North. He had begun to be shunned, even when his goals were for the honor of American physicians, southerners in particular. Likely, they sensed that his enthusiasm flagged whenever the medical community was called upon to attend to epidemics. It was dangerous: the treatment of disease was imprecise and hardly scientific, and how could one make a name or a living curing conditions that did not require the tools or procedures that would ensure one's entrance into the annals of medical history? Josiah Nott, in Mobile, was an excellent example. He was thriving, and he was now more famous as a racial theorist than he was as a doctor. At the end of 1848, he gave a series of popular lectures at the Louisiana University entitled "On the Connection Between the Biblical and Physical History of Man." Nott argued that just as our growing knowledge of astronomy, the movements of stars and planets, had challenged our religious assumptions about the heavens, so had the science of race demonstrated that the biblical story of creation had been in some way adulterated. In light of science, who could now continue to hold that blacks and whites were of a common origin? Or that Germany was not the parent stock of modern civilization? Nott had established himself as the leading voice espousing scientists as the revealers of facts and laws that, more than scripture, shed light on the will of the Creator.

So why did Nott also preoccupy himself with foolish theories of disease? He had offered the preposterous claim that yellow fever traveled not by miasma but by mosquitoes that carried the affliction from host to host. Worse, Nott had enthusiastically signed on to Mobile's Can't Get Away Club, doctors and nurses who banded together and refused to flee whenever the city was struck with outbreaks of vernal fevers, bilious colic, and dysenteries. In 1853, there was a great exodus as yellow fever gripped Mobile. Stories reached Montgomery of streets powdered with lime like snow, huge burning tar fires, carts filled with coffins as high as cotton bales, and church bells tolling for the dead throughout the day and night. Of the three thousand who remained in the city, five hundred perished, members of the Can't Get Away Club among them. Dangers to one's own person and family aside, Sims thought, it made no sense that physicians who knew they were God's most perfect instrument would subject themselves to dangers that might wipe them from the face of the earth.

It was in the midst of the meningitis outbreak in Montgomery that Sims's brother-in-law Rush arrived at Sims's office one day to confront him over the fistula experiments. Days before, Sims had been forced to put up another slave as collateral for a loan to keep the experiments going. He suspected that Theresa had let news of the arrangement slip to her brother. Rush was agitated. He'd recently lost a patient to the epidemic—neither blistering over the upper dorsal vertebra nor extracts of nightshade had done anything to prevent the boy from sinking into unconsciousness. Frightening convulsions soon killed him.

Rush asked his brother to have a serious word. He closed Sims's office door behind him.

The fistula mission was foolhardy, Rush said. The cost was too great.

Sims was putting his family in financial jeopardy, and his honor as a physician was being tarnished by rumors that he was using slaves as fodder and medical assistants. Who else could be helping him when the doctors of Montgomery had grown concerned with the propriety of his work and now refused to even attend his procedures?

Rush spoke with the tone not of a man expressing a private opinion but of one empowered as an ambassador. Perhaps this was not Theresa's doing—perhaps it was his Montgomery colleagues. Rush claimed that Sims was overworked. That much was true. First, there were the duties of his usual practice, and of late he had performed another radical jaw surgery on an elderly slave whose mouth was so unnaturally large that Sims was able to demonstrate that a tumor and the bulk of a patient's jaw could be removed without external mutilation. Additionally, there was the responsibility that all Montgomery physicians had to combat epidemics as they traveled north from the swamps and bayous. Last, there were the fistula patients, the experiments that absorbed his imagination at every idle moment and secretly offered him hope. More than most, Rush knew that Sims's fancy and ambition were already looking beyond the shallow horizons of Alabama.

Nevertheless, Rush offered his brother-in-law an opportunity. He and William Baldwin were considering a joint venture, a dispensary to be located just steps from Sims's office. Perhaps Sims could buy into the business and secure a future for his family and children? Sims agreed, but his resolve to see the experiments through only hardened at his brother's words. Every manly impulse in him fired in protest at the suggestion that he should accept the life of a simple country doctor, or become a peddler of pills.

A few months later, on November 13, 1848—exactly fifteen years since the night of the falling stars and his first day in medical school—Sims experienced an odd state of mind, late at night, lying in bed next to Theresa. It was a few weeks after Merry died. The passing was merciful, after so much suffering for both the boy and his mother. But the grief had not yet fully transformed into the message that Sims should seek a safer home, one that did not frown on his hubris. He awoke in the darkness, or he did not fully wake, as he remained sunk in a groggy state of semi-awareness. In later years, when he recalled the trance of this evening, it seemed that he had traveled somehow to a timeless place where past, present, and future were stitched together, a mass sutured and healed by the first intention of memory. He imagined the reverie to be not so different from deliriums produced by chloroform and ether, the agents that doctors, by 1848, had begun experimenting with and that were said to eliminate pain entirely. The drugs were promising to transform the world of medicine, to end the reign of the kind of surgeons that Sims had idolized and emulated—those known for speed and courage with a blade, and for hands so nimble they seemed to have wits of their own.

The whole world was changing. Just as the secrets of the stars had given themselves up to the telescope, so was the microscope promising to solve long-standing medical mysteries, to overturn deeply rooted assumptions. The changes were political as well. The misguided emphasis on ethics among physicians had been echoed by a rising chorus of abolitionists absurdly calling for a sudden end to slavery. Nott and others had responded wisely. Only the truly ignorant could believe that slaves were able to care for themselves. It would be wholly cruel to impose freedom on those who were unfit for it. At the Democratic convention in early 1848, Sims thrilled at the passage of resolutions threatening Alabama's secession. The following year, Montgomery's new capitol building caught fire, even before its clock was installed. The entire populace stepped out onto Market Street to watch the flames licking out from the stone edifice. The blaze seemed like an omen, a precursor of a larger conflagration that everyone could feel coming. This was staved off by the passage of the Compromise of 1850. California was admitted to the union in exchange for revisions to the Fugitive Slave Act. Southerners could reclaim runaways that crossed over to free states. The compromise satisfied no one. Soon, abolitionist pamphlets could be found left in train cars between Montgomery and Columbus, Georgia. In 1852, word came from Mobile. Nott and LeVert had crisscrossed the city to interrupt sales of *Uncle Tom's Cabin*, a blasphemous novel that had grown popular in the North.

Montgomery now had a theater and an opera, and a new artesian well was being dug on Court Square. But the city had never stopped being a wild place, frequented by roughs and bandits. In 1851, a doctor was stabbed through the lung by the very man he was treating. There were wild shootings in Greensborough and Tuscaloosa. By 1853, a number of Sims's friends had died of dengue fever and smallpox, and for all the attempts that had been made to control quack medicine in Montgomery, newspapers were awash with advertisements for galvanic cures for nervous ailments, for the use of an oiled flatiron to kill ringworm as dead as Julius Caesar, for gunpowder to staunch bleeding, for a fur vest as protection against pulmonary diseases, and for Dr. Brown's bitters recipe of poplar bark, goldenseal, bayberry, and columbo root.

And there were still runaways—slaves stuffed into Montgomery's jails, not dissuaded by any law, and easily caught because it was always known in which direction they fled. Perhaps it was the thought of runaways that sent Sims—suspended in his trance—back to the fears of his youth, to the runaway slaves and the monsters in the woods. But he was not frightened, and his mind drifted to his experiments as it always did, poring over its intractable puzzle like absent fingers worrying a stone. He lilted further back to a memory of the woods, fishing as a young boy, using a knife to split a bit of lead shot, which he then pinched onto the end of his line as a weight.

Sims never doubted that his efforts were the will of a divine mind working through him. But he never felt more like that mind's implement than when the old split shot emerged from the deepest recess of his memory and revealed how it might finally solve the mystery of his experiments. Running a bit of shot up the length of the sutures and cinching it tight with forceps would enable a deeper, more secure knot and keep the clamps in place. The solution rang perfect in his mind. By an act of will, he ascended from his sleepy daze—the vision, thank God, climbed with him to wakefulness—and he roused Theresa to share the joy of his discovery.

Poor Theresa! She was deathly sad at the loss of her son, but with her husband mostly gone in the day on calls, she hardly had time to grieve. There were still five living children and their home to care for. Theresa groggily tried to follow along as Sims attempted to demonstrate his innovation in a handful of sheets hastily shaped into an anatomical model. Theresa didn't understand the medicine, but she understood Sims's inspiration.

It was more than a cure, it was the gift that was being offered to them in response for the loss of their child, and it was proof that the experiments had not been a waste of time, as her brother had suggested.

It mattered little that the next experiment, conducted in two days' time, was a complete failure. Sims had practiced the maneuver of slipping on the shots and pinching them tight, but he'd never thought of what they would do to the silk over time. No matter. The solution came at once. Using the shot, he could return to wire—not Mettauer's too-pliable lead, but Gosset's stiffer silver. Perhaps Henry LeVert had been right all along. Silver might work.

It was Anarcha's turn to be experimented on. In the months since he had come to rely on them as assistants, the slave women had become only more and more adept at their jobs. Once or twice, Sims noticed Anarcha leaning back to look in at his work, studying the swift movements of his fingers as he placed the clamps, and concentrating with a greater intensity than any of the students or colleagues who accepted his invitations solely for the prurient novelty of witnessing surgeries performed on women. They had been only too happy to see him fail, Sims realized. But Anarcha watched with the fervor of one who hoped for success, for herself and the others.

It took his machinist a week to fashion the silver wire, and the demands of his practice caused months of further delays, but at last he gathered the slave women together, and he saw that they could sense his excitement. The procedure worked perfectly. Anarcha hardly made a sound, though she broke into a sweat. The shot rode down the silver wire, the clamps nestled in alongside the more severe of her two fistulae, and they tugged together to as neat a line as any skilled seamstress could produce. It was an excruciating week as she healed—Sims barely had time to visit Anarcha as they awaited the result. No one had counted how many times she'd been experimented on. But all of them knew she'd suffered the most. At last, the day came. Anarcha climbed onto the table again, Betsey and Lucy lifted her nates, and Sims slid the cold tongue of his speculum inside of her. The line of union appeared pink and healthy; the clamps were not buried into her tissue. He snipped them free, and the line of union held.

He had cured a fistula.

BOOK
TWO

Eleven

IN GEORGIA, A SLAVE WOMAN DROPPED A TRAY OF FOOD, AND HER MISSUS chopped her in the head with a butcher knife. Another missus sneaked into her slave's room one night and cut off the head of the slave's baby because the baby was the master's—the master beat the missus, and he kept going with that slave after that, and she had more babies.

In Arkansas, a master put his slave's head in the screw that was used for packing cotton and ran the mules around until the slave's head was mashed. A slave man was sold away after his missus killed his wife by hitting her in the small of the back with a ten-inch-wide battling stick that was used for laundry. The battling stick broke at the blow, and the master was afraid to go on owning the slave husband after that. A large, burly slave named Green was told to pick up an eight-hundred-pound hogshead of molasses and carry it a piece. Afterward, a ball of blood the size of a goose egg came out of Green's mouth, and he died the next day.

In Texas, a slave cook brought potatoes to the table that weren't done all the way through. The missus grabbed a fork and stuck it in the cook's eye and put it out. A slave named Brown was chained to a woodpile and covered with oil and set alight, and after the fire smoldered down, white women and children collected Brown's ashes for souvenirs. A slave woman ran away and got caught. She was dragged home behind a horse, and the next morning they cut off her breasts and rammed a hot iron down her throat and killed her. A group of slaves were driven through the winter, and when one slave woman couldn't go any farther the driver shot her, kicked her, and left her for dead. A slave woman refused to admit to stealing money from her master—the master tied a rope around her neck, attached it to a rock, and threw her in a creek.

Slaves that were fished out of rivers after being murdered and dumped were found so covered with shrimps eating on them that you could barely see their flesh. Those that saw it never wanted to eat shrimps again.

In Kentucky, speculators wanted to buy a slave girl, but not her baby. Her baby was beaten to death in front of her, and then she was sold. A slave man was lashed five hundred times and left to die, and the whippers let the bloodhounds on him so that they would know the smell of slave blood, and the next morning the whippers found the dogs licking at the dead slave's back.

In Indiana, dogs were loosed on a slave who had been whipped, and the dogs tore him to pieces and ate some of what they pulled off of him. The slave lived for a time, and they doused him in alcohol before he died.

In Mississippi, a master disfigured all of his slave babies, putting a pin into their eyes so that he could recognize them should they ever run away when they grew up.

In Virginia, a slave woman praised God when her baby died because it was one her master couldn't sell, and a thirteen-year-old girl was whipped so hard that ever thereafter she suffered spells. A slave girl ran her finger around inside a chimney to black her eyebrows the way her missus did. Her missus took a log from the fire and hit the slave on the head and cursed her for mocking her betters, and later the missus said that she thought the girl's thick skull and wool cap would protect her better than it did. The slave girl was sold.

In Alabama, a slave was whipped nearly to death for throwing the child of an overseer into a pot of boiling lye, and a slave woman and her two children were sold off because she grabbed two overseer men by the privates and ripped their privates out at the roots, because that was a slow death. In Chambers County, a pregnant slave was tied to a hackberry tree and whipped until she died, and afterward if you got close to that hackberry tree you could hear her baby crying.

* * *

Anarcha met her son Washington again when he was two years old and she got to hold him and nurse him, but he called another slave mother and he was carried around the quarters by other children, and Anarcha watched him from a distance for signs that he was her son and she saw some. In 1851, Washington was sold with a number of other slaves to E. Y. Fair, who was a man like William Rufus King in that he was very wealthy and spent a lot of time in Europe but still owned plantations in Alabama. In August of that year, E. Y. Fair bought a number of slaves from Dr. Harris, including George, Yellow George, Carson, Mariah, Daphny, Wind, Leak, Charity, Minny, and Washington. They all went to a plantation in Lowndes County, and Anarcha never saw Washington again.

She had another baby in 1850. It wasn't long after she arrived at Violet Hill, in Autauga County, that a small cabin was built for her, and slave men began to visit her at night. There was no discussion of marriage or jumping over any brooms, the men just came to her and didn't say anything at all, and Anarcha didn't know if they came because they wanted to or because the new master, John Duncan, who wasn't her owner but who was in possession and control of her, sent them to her. There was a slave named Jerry, like her father who might not have been her father, and Jerry was older than her, and there was Sumter who was much younger than her, and there was Barney, and Abram, and Israel, and Anarcha went with them nightly, though it wasn't like Montgomery, where it had been easier to keep clean and she had come to understand a bit of what pleasure was. More likely, this was another plantation chore, and the men arrived and did their work, and soon Anarcha was pregnant again. When she gave birth, the master, John Duncan, named the girl Venia, but Anarcha decided the girl's name was not Venia but Delia, and she swore an oath to keep Delia close and never let her get whipped or sold or taken away from her by some other slave mother.

It had been four years since Anarcha lived on a plantation. She had been much younger then, and now she was a woman and she heard the horrible stories of what happened on plantations both near and far, stories that slaves didn't tell to children. Nor did the stories make their way into the city, though slaves who ran away were sometimes caught and brought to town and jailed, and there was an opportunity for stories to travel, but not on what on plantation slaves called the grapevine, though Anarcha had no idea what stories had to do with grapevines because the only grapevines slaves knew were the ones that grew grapes. Later, these grapevines got used as ropes stretched across roads at night to upend patrollers who rode too fast in the pursuit of runaways, and they didn't see the grapevines stretched across their paths. They hit the vines and fell and broke their bones, and sometimes they died from falling.

Violet Hill was the fanciest plantation Anarcha had been on yet, and because she was now the plantation nurse or doctor woman—Dr. Harris told John Duncan of her value, just as Dr. Sims told Dr. Harris and Dr. Jarvis—she could visit the house, particularly in the early months, before she gave birth again and her holes opened up once more. Or at least one of them did, and anyone could tell which from the smell. Violet Hill had acres of flower gardens and rare plants from Africa, including one that had cost $500, as much as many slaves were worth. In front of the house's piazza there was an evergreen hedge heart bed for more flowers, and children played games around the heart bed, and the young Duncan women, including Margaret—who was Dr. Harris's wife and who was now technically Anarcha's owner—and her sister Catherine, who was a great beauty and belle, sat on the piazza and the porches on the sides of the house and sang love songs with a guitar on moonlit nights. Inside the house, Anarcha ran her finger along the silver candlesticks and claret decanters and toilet tables and butter coolers and custard cups and Violet Hill's fourteen calico window curtains. And because she was the nurse she could access the medical chest that Dr. Harris, who visited Violet Hill often, kept well stocked with trusses and syringes and lancets and syrup squills and lunar caustic and Number Six and ipecac and Seidlitz Powder and Tilden's Extracts and blue lick water and gold foil for teeth and Davis's Pain Killer and Reynold's Specific and Morse's Invigorating Cordial.

Some of these medicines worked and some of them didn't. When they didn't, Anarcha relied on what she had learned from Pheriba, who had died while Anarcha was in Montgomery. The misery in Anarcha's foot had grown worse in four years' time, and Dr. Sims's cure did nothing at all for her leg, and now she walked with the help of a cane or walking stick, and she enlisted several of the young slaves—Mary who was twelve, Martin who was six, and Judge who was three, and Charlotte's children Alice and Winston—to go to the woods to gather all the things for Pheriba's cures. She described for them the spiked purple star flowers of pennyroyal, the sparkling green suns of goose grass, the blue twinkling moons of feverweed, the pale constellations of snakeroot in bloom, and the white-sprangled stalks and yellow bouquets of life-everlasting weed. Just as Pheriba had done, she kept all these in jars and boxes in her cabin and tended to the slaves as was necessary, and apart from that she caught babies, even though she was very young compared to the grannies that usually caught babies, but she had learned how to catch babies because of her time in Montgomery, and because her own pregnancies had taught her more than she ever wanted to know about when nature was taking its course and when it wasn't.

Stories came too of other slaves who worked as nurses or herb doctors or did hoodoo work. There was Penny Brashiers in Oklahoma, who worked with plant medicine but sometimes bled you like a white doctor by making a cut over your misery. There was Cain Bobertson, who was a hoodoo doctor with a curing hand for spells and fits, and Cain used horns to extract blood filled with wiggle tails. In Florida, there was a doctoring slave named Charlotte who was famous for the white doctors who sought her out for the cures she made when she wasn't making quilts, and in Georgia, white doctors went to a slave named Nancy for cures made from pepper and tansy tea. Big Sarah, in Mississippi, was seven feet tall and weighed 390 pounds, and she made cures from red shank and prickly ash and the roots of bamboo and black haw. In Perry County, Alabama, Aunt Tildy worked as a midwife but was also a doctor woman and she advised matches in the hair for headache and a dime with a hole in it around your ankle to avoid getting poisoned. And in Greene County, there was a plantation that had been founded with the help of two slave women, both named Peggy: Short Peggy and Long Peggy. Between them, the two Peggys raised three hundred children, and Long Peggy was freed after she gave birth to twenty-five babies.

Anarcha wondered whether her own story had traveled by grapevine or by some other means to places that didn't already know about her. Sometimes at night at Violet Hill, alone in her cabin, nursing Delia or mixing medicines or making a sweet-smelling salve that covered the room's stench, her stench, she wondered whether what she had endured in Montgomery, and the success that Dr. Marion Sims had claimed on her, had become a tale told by others.

* * *

William L. Maury—known as Lewis—first heard the story of Anarcha indirectly, through his cousin Matthew Fontaine Maury.

After he witnessed the breakup of Biela's Comet in 1846, Matthew Fontaine Maury's interests expanded beyond using data from old captains' logbooks to shave weeks off the voyage from New York to San Francisco. There was the effort to lay telegraph cables across the Atlantic Ocean. He played a role in the formation of an international meteorological body. And there was the ongoing effort to build railroads that would increase the facility of intercourse across the empire of wilderness that stretched from Missouri to the Pacific Ocean. In the service of this last vision, Maury attended the Memphis Railroad Convention of 1848 and served on a committee with a peculiar South Carolinian named J. F. G. Mittag. Mittag told Maury of his former student Dr. J. Marion Sims, who even then was performing trailblazing medical experiments in Alabama, and who was on the brink of a great discovery for the health of women. On a visit to Virginia, Maury told his cousin Lewis of Sims's medical experiments and of their young kinsman Richard Maury of Memphis, who at fourteen was already planning a life as a physician, much like the medically adventurous Dr. Sims.

Lewis had followed his more famous cousin into the navy. He had embarked on his career long before his father, anxious to try his hand as a farmer, purchased the Bowling Green plantation in Caroline County, along with its impressive home, Old Mansion. In 1838, Lewis was assigned as lieutenant on the USS *Vincennes* under Commander Charles Wilkes during the much-vaunted Exploring Expedition of the South Pacific, which lasted until 1842. In the Samoas, Lewis passed several weeks on the island of Sapapele, where for some reason the women were more gracefully formed than on the surrounding islands. In the Fee Jees, Lewis commanded one of three raiding parties in an attack on the town of Sualib. Lewis's party was the first to approach the village, fortified with a mud-and-water moat and an exterior wall fashioned from cocoa-nut trunks. The defenses posed little challenge to the raiding parties' muskets and rockets. In a pitched battle of arrows and balls, Lewis witnessed one of the Fee Jee warriors attempt to dislodge a rocket fired into the thatched roof of one of the town's structures. The rocket exploded, and the native disappeared in a cloud of blood and fire.

Later, on the west coast of North America, Commander Wilkes christened Maury Island, in the Puget Sound, for his loyal lieutenant.

Back home, emulating his cousin, Lewis tried his hand at essay writing to chronicle an adventure from a still earlier expedition. Lewis and several shipmates had attempted an ascent of Corcovado when their sloop of war stopped for several days at Rio de Janeiro. The story was ripe for telling, with descriptions of the great aqueduct that supplied the city with the precious element, and the cobras and reptiles that hassled their climb. Yet Lewis lacked his cousin's gift for words; he abandoned the effort. Between voyages, he married Mary Hill Beckham, and it was the difficult labor of his young wife's second birth—their second daughter, Mary—that caused Lewis's interest to pique when his cousin told him the story of the female experiments of Dr. J. Marion Sims.

Members of the Maury family could lodge with relatives on either side of the Mason-Dixon line, from Mobile to Tennessee to Virginia to New York City. Lewis and Mary lived in Washington City for a time, where Lewis's older brother had been an alderman for years. In 1852, John Walker Maury was elected mayor. Just then, Mary became pregnant again, and Lewis received orders to report to the USS *Saratoga*, one of a squadron of vessels that would set out in support of Commodore Perry's expedition to Japan, with orders to exert vigor if necessary to open trade routes. Mary would retire to Old Mansion.

Lewis wrote to his father from Manila. The windows of Philippine homes were made from ground oyster shells instead of glass, and chain gangs worked on the city's cobbled streets. Cockfighting pits were ubiquitous, and the population of 150,000 was a beguiling mixture of creoles, mestizos, negroes, malays, and Chinese. Several months later, Lewis described for Mary the pirates he'd chased in the fall, and the hurricane that had shredded the *Saratoga*'s sails. On the other side of the world, Lewis wrote, all things are capsized. He asked Mary to remind a friend who had traveled west with the rush of forty-niners to save him a bag of the precious dust.

He received mail rarely at sea. In 1853, he was given command of a barque, the USS *Caprice*, and received orders to sail to Shanghai with forty souls. They would ferry anthracite and coal between China and the Loo Chau Islands, to keep Perry's Japan vessels well stocked. In August, one of Lewis's crew spotted a hole in the daytime sky. At night, it appeared large and faint, like a grainy star cluster in the forward paw of Ursa Major, the Great Bear. Over several weeks, the comet grew in magnitude and moved with intent toward Hydra, the longest star pattern in the sky. Shortly thereafter, when the *Caprice* dropped anchor in Shanghai to collect a translator for Perry, Lewis received a batch of mail that included a dire letter from home. As with the birth of baby June, Mary's labor had been long and difficult. This time, she had perished. She had given birth to a son, but he had died not long after. Lewis's daughters would await his return at Old Mansion.

Despite the news, Lewis carried out his orders. He received word that Perry himself had noted his pleasure with the mark of Lewis's consideration.

The Perry Expedition ended in 1854. Lewis's first orders on returning home were wholly uncomfortable. He was to travel to New York for special duty—administrative work on the Navy Retiring Board, what would come to be called the "plucking board."

In the years Lewis had been gone, Matthew Fontaine Maury had become even more famous with the publication of *The Physical Geography of the Sea*, a popular version of the book Poe had once praised. Now, finally, the navy was taking seriously the anonymous suggestions that Maury had once made about eliminating graft and waste in the service. Ironically, this took the form of a bureaucratic body designed to snip away dead weight: officers incapable of carrying out the duties associated with their rank. Owing to his lame leg—and a measure of spite from those he had irked—Maury wound up on a list he had inadvertently proposed. And now his cousin was among those who would decide whether his career would end.

After traveling to Liverpool to promote his book, Maury returned to the States to lie low while his fate was decided. He visited his family in Fredericksburg, taking carriages fifteen miles south to relatives at Old Mansion and Bowling Green, and diverting from there to Richmond, where Robert H. Maury had a home just blocks from the Virginia State Capitol. Maury could reside here while beginning to dabble in secret experiments. He wondered whether the explosives that were sometimes used in whaling could be turned into tools of war—something like a torpedo or mine. Maury performed preliminary tests in a large iron bathtub on his cousin's third floor.

The laboratory in the basement of Richmond's famed Egyptian Building—just two blocks from his cousin's home—was made available to him for supplies. Before he visited, he was warned of what he might find: a visiting doctor of uncertain reputation was conducting experiments on animals in the basement. It was said the stench was remarkable, and there were disturbing rumors of what exactly was happening there.

One afternoon in 1855, Maury walked to the Egyptian Building. He caught a scent of scat as he approached the cellar door, on the side of the structure. Inside, he encountered a slave woman who had been tasked with assisting the mysterious physician's experiments. She was tending to the animals' cages.

Perhaps it was her lame leg. With a hobble of his own, and a cane like the slave's—he thought she looked older than she was—Maury felt compelled to strike up a conversation, a shared dose of misery among like sufferers. He had complicated feelings about slavery. He owned but few slaves himself, and his time in Brazil had made him wonder whether Brazil or someplace like it could become a repository for Virginia's slave population—not freeing them of course, that was impractical, but at least cleansing Virginia of the scar and the stain of an abominable practice.

The girl's voice, with an accent of the Deep South, confirmed it. She was much younger than she appeared. Maury suspected that her affliction, whatever it was, was aging her prematurely. He questioned her. She was from Alabama. She was here to be operated on by Dr. Charles Bell Gibson, who was not the doctor performing the animal experiments. Gibson was a Maury family friend. As the girl provided additional details—she'd had woman problems, problems of birth, she said, and she'd been experimented on many times in Alabama, and now they were giving her something to breathe that put her to sleep, to experiment on her some more—it dawned on Maury that he'd heard the story before. That queer chap on the railroad committee in Memphis, Mittag, had told him the story of Dr. J. Marion Sims.

Maury said the name Sims aloud, and the slave girl's eyes lifted to his. She looked at him with a brave, uncommon intensity—a risk for any negro, free or slave, in the city of Richmond.

Maury's thoughts snapped to his cousin, who had recently suffered the loss of his wife to problems like that which the girl described. As he rushed home to write to Lewis of the encounter, he realized he'd forgotten to ask the girl's name.

As it happened, Lewis had learned more of Dr. J. Marion Sims in New York City. Shortly after Lewis had made his way to the city, notices appeared in the papers of a lecture Dr. Sims would deliver to propose a new hospital dedicated to the conditions of women. Lewis did not attend the lecture, but accounts the following day revealed that Sims had

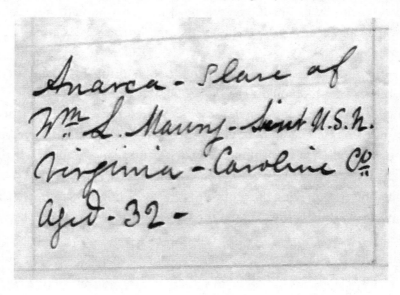

described the extended period of experimentation in Alabama and the group of extraordinary young slave women who were both his subjects and his assistants. Sims was quickly gaining notoriety in the new field of "gynecology," and not only was Lewis's young cousin, the would-be doctor, planning to follow in Dr. Sims's footsteps, another family friend, Thomas Addis Emmet—the Emmets, the Jeffersons, and the Maurys were among the old society families of Charlottesville—had become Sims's assistant at the hospital that opened less than a year after Sims proposed it.

The message from Lewis's famous cousin in Richmond couldn't have been clearer. Many in the Maury family knew that his period of grief over Mary had ended. He was now courting Anne Fontaine, who had recently come of age. Anne and Lewis's daughters got along well, they had all traveled once to Niagara, and the only hurdle now was convincing older Maury relatives that it wouldn't amount to much if cousin married cousin. The famous Lieutenant Maury in Richmond seemed to approve. His silent suggestion made sense. Lewis had lost one wife to childbirth. What better gift could he offer his young, would-be bride than a celebrated servant who had been part of a series of experiments about dangerous births? A girl who seemed capable, who wasn't likely to run away for her debility, and who was clever enough to be assisting yet another doctor in a series of experiments. In anticipation of his offer of marriage, William L. Maury sent word to Richmond. Buy the girl, and send her to Old Mansion in Caroline County, Virginia.

* * *

In 1851, in Autauga County, Alabama, Anarcha gave birth yet again. The baby was a large girl, very large, the largest baby anyone had ever seen. There was a doctor present because Anarcha had had difficult births in the past, but it was not Dr. Sims. It was either Dr. J. D. Nixon, who charged three dollars per visit, five dollars for a vaginal exam, and ten dollars to deliver a placenta, or it was Dr. E. H. Robinson, who charged only two dollars per visit and had seen Mariah before she was sold away.

the largest child she ever saw

The breech baby was a girl, and though Anarcha was in labor for less than a day the baby girl died and she never had a name.

Not long after, one of the Duncan children, eleven-year-old Maria Caroline, fell ill. Dr. Nixon was called, and his cures didn't work. Dr. Robinson was called, and his cures didn't work, either. Maria Caroline's mother carried her to Anarcha's cabin and asked her to try. Anarcha brewed Pheriba's devil's shoestring cure for fever, her belladonna cure for cleansing the blood, her life-everlasting cure for colds, and her poke-root cure for smallpox even though it was clear the girl didn't have smallpox. Nothing worked. Young Maria Caroline died. The Duncan family didn't trust Anarcha as a doctor woman after that.

In 1853, Dr. Harris took her away from Violet Hill. He told her that he was going on a long trip to see the North, Yankeedom—he wanted Anarcha to come along as nurse to his children. Like Dr. Sims, he presented the journey as an option, but Anarcha knew it wasn't an option. She made it clear that her baby Delia would come too. She was surprised that Dr. Harris didn't object.

Anarcha had seen small trains, and she had ridden them when they were pulled along the tracks by horses or oxen, and she knew that there were now trains that moved very quickly without anything pulling them at all. Like grapevines, horseless trains brought stories from great distances, packed in baggage and mail cars. It was said that trains brought babies too, perched atop the cow catcher or left behind like the baby Moses, dressed in nice baby clothes and set on the tracks rather than hidden in the bulrushes. If the stories a train brought were good, the train gave three quick whistles as it arrived. If the stories were bad, it gave three long, mournful wails instead. One of the stories the trains brought was that trains had not been the idea of white people at all—rather, a blacksmith slave man had looked at a pot of boiling coffee one morning, and he had the idea of putting wheels on it and using the steam to make it roll without horses. That's why horseless trains all looked like they had a giant wash pot on top of them, for boiling water.

The travelers were Nathan Harris and his young wife, Margaret—they told Anarcha that Margaret was her true missus, it was written down on official papers in Montgomery—and Margaret's sister Catherine, who had always wanted to go north to meet a husband, and then the missus's children, Richard, Catherine, and Charles. Both Richard and Catherine had been born before Anarcha had come to Violet Hill, but Charles had not yet been born, and when he came Anarcha caught him, with the missus's sister Catherine there to help, and of course the traveling party also included Anarcha and Delia, who was now barely more than three years old but already knew how to keep quiet and play with rag dolls full of flower petals, just as Anarcha had done when she was a girl. The party rode one of the old horse-pulled trains from near Montgomery to Columbus, Georgia, and from there they switched to a horseless train that was the biggest and loudest thing Anarcha had ever seen, but beyond that first glimpse of it when they climbed inside she didn't see much, and she held Delia between her knees to protect her. Delia hollered when the train began to move because it was so fast, the fastest thing that ever went through the country, and Delia became sick from the swinging and swaying of the train, too sick to eat the ginger cakes that Anarcha brought for her.

From inside the car, it looked like the woods were leaving them all behind.

There were different trains and different cities in the weeks to come, and they passed through Washington City and Baltimore and Philadelphia and then New York. Anarcha saw about as much of the cities as she saw of the trains. On the trains, she sat with the children in a car near the front, and her missus and Catherine Duncan sat in a car near the back of the train, and sometimes Nathan Harris came through the train and stopped with the children, but then he walked forward to the smoking car, where men gathered to smoke cigars and talk. When they stopped for water and wood, Anarcha made the children a stomach tea from the bark of oak trees she found near the tracks. Soon, the swaying of the train lulled them all to sleep, even Delia. As they dozed on the benches, Anarcha looked out at people who gathered to watch the horseless marvel roll past, white people and black people both, slaves below the Mason-Dixon line, and then free black people north of it. These were the first truly free black people Anarcha had ever seen. You could tell they were free from their clothes, and even from a blurry glimpse you could see how they stood and held their heads high, and what Anarcha thought in seeing them was what any enslaved person would have thought on first witnessing the effects of freedom: this was what runaway slaves had been running away to, not a line, not a law, but the little measure of dignity that was afforded by a piece of paper that said you were not a thing. Once they got off the train, Anarcha and the children were hurried into carriages and then into hotels that were not so different from Montgomery Hall in Alabama, and Anarcha stayed with the three children of her missus and Delia stayed with her, and Anarcha let Delia and Charles suck and she fed and cared for the others while her missus and Nathan Harris and Catherine Duncan left the hotel to see the White House in Washington City and Independence Hall in Philadelphia, and City Hall, the Stock Exchange, and Green-Wood Cemetery in New York City. When they were gone, Anarcha lay on the bed, but only briefly when the children were asleep, and at night the missus's children slept on the bed and Anarcha and Delia slept on the floor beside them, and Anarcha's experience of the cities was mostly the rotten smells that came in strong gusts through the windows.

* * *

On May 6, 1853, they boarded a train at Canal Street in New York. It was the largest train they had been on yet, more than two hundred people wandering up and down the long row of cars between the smoking car at the front and the passenger cars toward the rear, and the train stopped at Twenty-seventh Street to add another passenger car, and then they left the city, rolling north toward Boston. This train went even faster than the trains that had brought them north and east, and Nathan Harris was sitting up front with Anarcha and the children, and there were several doctors in the car with them, men like Dr. Sims, talking loudly about a meeting of doctors they had just attended in New York. There was a white bishop in the car dressed in bright colors and joking, and everyone was very jovial, all of them marveling that they must be traveling as fast as forty miles per hour—just think of it! In the slow, crawling distances farther south, Anarcha had come to understand the system of flags and balls that the railroaders used to send messages, like the horns and whistles masters used to give orders to slaves. White flags signaled track changes near depots, and a large red ball—large enough to be seen from a distance, so that a speeding train could screech to a stop—signaled when wooden bridges spanning draws were open. If the ball was raised on a pole it meant all was well, the train could proceed as it pleased, and if it was lowered it meant stop right now.

The train stopped at Stamford to wood and water, and then sped on toward the bridge that crossed the river draw at Norwalk.

Later, Anarcha would recollect the vision of the ship, the *Pacific*, an oceangoing side-wheel steamer, looming above the treetops, with its masts and its giant paddle wheel in the middle of the ship, not on the end like smaller steamboats on the rivers of Alabama. It quickly replaced the train in her mind as the largest man-made thing she'd ever seen, and still later Anarcha would hear stories of how the *Pacific* vanished at sea after setting a record for crossing the Atlantic, 45 passengers and 141 crew lost with only a message in a bottle to hint at the iceberg that sank it. Anarcha and everyone on the train saw the ship. There were many exclamations because it was so large, like a slowly drifting mountain. The ship had just come up the Norwalk River, and seen from the perspective of the train, it looked as though it was sailing through the land itself. The vision of the ship perhaps explains why the engineer did not heed the lowered ball indicating that the drawbridge at Norwalk had been raised, so that the *Pacific* could sail through. The bridge was not yet closed. The train continued churning toward the draw at full speed. After registering the marvelous ship, one of the passengers, a man who had been chatting amiably with Dr. Nathan Harris, glanced out the window to look ahead at where the track curved, just before the bridge. He announced no small concern that the train might be thrown on the curve—they were moving so swiftly and running so heavy. In the time it took for his words to pass from mouth to mouth through the car—just seconds—the train came to the bend, and now they could all see that even if the train made the turn, and it did, its wheels screaming as though in anticipation of what came next, the drawbridge over the Norwalk River was still raised.

Oh, God—we are gone, said the kind man speaking to Nathan Harris, and he was right. In the next moment, it seemed that the car and the benches fell away from beneath them and there was a terrible moment of pause that was followed by otherworldly sounds: a thousand timbers splintered by a thousand strokes of lightning, and a single scream shrieked in unison by every voice on the train. Witnesses from the shore watched the engine, the baggage car, the mail car, the smoking car, and the first two passenger cars sail sixty feet across the draw. The train slammed into the bank on the opposite side, and some of the cars were stove to atoms, and the others hit the water and began to sink, creating great eddies and whirlpools.

above the water; and dashing through the window he drew out in succession Mr. Nathan Harris, of Montgomery, Alabama, his three children and their nurse, together with others, and put in with them for the shore. On landing, Mr. Harris endeavored to

In Anarcha's car, all the windows shattered at once. Passengers were tossed through the air like chaff, and in an instant everything was a mass of ruin and there was water, water everywhere. Anarcha had been holding Delia, and when she found herself afloat she was still holding Delia, and they were the lucky ones near the surface. Nathan Harris was still near them, and the Harris children were nearby, and it was less than a minute before bystanders managed to climb on top of the submerged cars and begin to hack through the roof with axes. But it was a minute filled with wailings and howlings of despair, and Anarcha watched the bleeding, ghastly face of a man break the surface of the still-rising waters, only to be grasped from below by an arm wrapped in soggy lace, a submerged woman blindly seeking purchase. The woman pulled the man under again, and neither reemerged. Nathan Harris was the first to climb through the hole that was made in the roof, and Anarcha shoved his children up one after the other, and then Anarcha pushed Delia up through the hole, and if that had been all the saving that was possible, it would have been enough. Anarcha was grabbed from above and yanked through all the same. Harris and his children and Anarcha and Delia were shuttled ashore on a small boat, where they were reunited with Anarcha's missus and Catherine Duncan, and Nathan Harris tried to give a purse full of money to the man who saved them, but the man refused, and nothing at all was said about whether Anarcha had saved Dr. Harris's children. They watched, shivering, as others were saved and bodies were brought to shore, the faces of the living and the dead like a collection of nightmare phantoms. There was a drowned woman clutching her drowned child, and there was a beautiful sixteen-year-old girl with the back of her head caved in, and some among the living struggled in vain to return life to those who had been brought ashore lifeless. For four hours, the women of Norwalk spread quilts from their homes over the faces of those irrevocably lost. There were a number of doctors among the dead.

They returned to New York. They took adjacent rooms at a hotel, and through the wall Anarcha heard Nathan Harris and her missus and Catherine Duncan talk and plan about what they should do now. The trip to Yankeedom was over. Catherine Duncan wished to remain in the North, perhaps visit a water cure. Sometimes their voices rose and sometimes they fell because they knew that the wall was thin, and sometimes instead of saying words out loud they spelled them instead, in case Anarcha was listening. Anarcha and Delia were discussed at length. A slave could not remain in New York, Nathan Harris said. But why should they pay to transport a worthless cripple all the way back to Autauga County, where they would be taxed sixty cents for her, work or no? Perhaps they should manumit her—release her into the city and take the baby girl rightly called Venia home with them. No, Margaret Harris said. Anarcha was her property. Despite the stench, Anarcha was capable of increase. One should never discard property for nothing.

By May 21, 1853, all but Catherine Duncan had returned to Alabama.

Twelve

Emmet—Emigrant Refuge Hospital—A winter journey—The
baths at Florence—Sims in New York—Proposal—Emmet meets
Anarcha—An enslaved man, stabbed—Silver wire

LIKE ANARCHA, DR. THOMAS ADDIS EMMET WAS A YOUNG CHILD ON THE
night of November 13, 1833, the night the stars fell. His parents woke him
to view the spectacle from a continuation of the piazza on the north side
of the family home in Charlottesville, Virginia. Many years later, Emmet
would recall the sky filled with glowing forms of many colors, bursting in
every direction. The family's servants were particularly struck, shouting
proclamations of conversion and singing hymns until sunrise.

The Emmets socialized with many prominent Charlottesville families, including the Jeffersons, Carters, Walkers, Pages, and Maurys. Maurys in particular had been close with Emmets in New York for decades,
with memorable games played among friends at the racquet courts near
Broome Street. Both families boasted of officers in the United States
Navy. Of these, Emmet would hold great admiration for the talents and
attainments of Lieutenant Matthew Fontaine Maury, who when Emmet
graduated from medical school was one of the best-known men in the
American scientific community for his work on the seas and the stars.

Emmet's father had practiced medicine in Charleston for only a short
time before Thomas Jefferson named him to the medical faculty of the
newly minted University of Virginia. Emmet followed fitfully in his
father's footsteps, studying medicine first in Flushing, New York, before

being expelled and at last graduating from Jefferson Medical School in Philadelphia, where he spent a full four years.

Before he began to practice, Emmet, along with his mother and sister and a throng of three thousand New Yorkers, attended the first American performance of Jenny Lind at Castle Garden in Battery Park. The event was as notable for the voice of the "Swedish nightingale" as it was for her manager, P. T. Barnum, who exploited the occasion to gratuitously extoll his other acts: the Italian plate spinner, and the negro that Barnum had schemed to present to the world as a white man in blackface. There was a rumor that Barnum had hired Lind without ever having heard her voice. Reputation was more reliable than personal opinion, Barnum said. For weeks before her arrival, quadrilles and polkas and poems were composed in her honor, and by the time her ship made port there were offered for sale Jenny Lind gloves, Jenny Lind bonnets, and Jenny Lind riding hats, shawls, mantillas, robes, chairs, sofas, and pianos.

It was a wholly different class of immigrant that Emmet was called upon to attend to after the concert, when he was appointed resident physician at the Emigrant Refuge Hospital, on Ward's Island in the East River. In the following three years, Emmet worked ceaselessly to treat as many as 11,000 patients, with 1,900 cases of typhoid among them. Obstetrics was a large part of the work; up to ten babies per day were delivered at the hospital.

During the terrible blizzard that struck New York in the winter of 1853, Emmet took it upon himself, as the youngest man among the hospital residents, to trek from his home, on Fourth Avenue near Twelfth Street, to Ward's Island. On the morning of the storm's third day, a steam snowplow at last cleared the railroad tracks. The three-mile journey from Canal Street to 110th Street took two hours. It was another three hours on foot from the train station to the ferry house, slogging through drifts of snow that were sometimes taller than Emmet himself. No ferryman would agree to brave the frozen river piling up with huge cakes of ice. The reverse current of the tide drove thick floes up on top of one another. Emmet secured oars into the grommets of a flat-bottomed skiff and rowed himself across, sometimes dragging the boat across the ice. He managed to visit patients who hadn't seen a physician in more than four days. He barely made it home, and came down with a case of rheumatic fever for his trouble, suffering heart palpitations and fainting spells.

He was long overdue for a rest. He was advised to travel south and sailed with his mother and sister to Bermuda. He attended a military ball, witnessed an hour-long battle between two colossal whales in the harbor, and was impressed by the story of a twenty-seven-foot shark that had been caught and killed. The desiccated leg bones of a man, still clad in a high cowhide boot, were found in its stomach.

One afternoon on the voyage home, Emmet was handed a copy of the *New York Herald*. Tragedy had struck. Shortly after the sixth annual meeting of the American Medical Association in New York, seven New England doctors, on their way home, were killed with their wives when a train of the New Haven Railroad line ignored an open drawbridge and vaulted into the muddy bed of the Norwalk River. Remarkably, just a short time later, when Emmet took his mother for a course of exercise, diet, and sleep at the noted water cure establishment at Florence, Massachusetts, Emmet met one of the survivors of the disaster. The first person he encountered in Florence was Catherine Duncan, of Alabama. She told him the tale of the accident, and before long they were spending significant time together.

Catherine returned to New York at the same time Emmet and his mother did. The couple's courtship continued into the fall. One afternoon, they went for a walk, venturing north from Twelfth Street, passing the homes near Twenty-second Street that marked the edge of the city and venturing into the quaintly rural area between country and town. Here, apart from a tavern or two, it was all immigrant shacks and grazing land for goats. Bellevue Hospital loomed to the east, and to the west you could see all the way to the Hudson River, where ships coursed slowly along the horizon. Above, they spied the nick of a comet that in recent days had appeared like a hole in the sky, causing a sensation in the papers. It was now leaving a short, curving trail, like a scalpel tracing a fine incision.

They approached a lone house standing queerly on the east side of Madison Avenue, between Twenty-eighth and Twenty-ninth Streets. Emmet recognized the sign outside as that of a physician. He remarked to Catherine how odd it was for a doctor to have hung his shingle so far from anything like a neighborhood, away from paying patients. Catherine responded with a remarkable coincidence. She knew the name printed there—Dr. J. Marion Sims.

Emmet knew Sims too. He was a recent arrival in the city. A year before, he had caused a stir with a long and elaborate publication in the *American Journal of the Medical Sciences*—including twenty-two woodcut illustrations—which claimed to once and for all provide a simple surgical solution for vesico-vaginal fistula, the age-old condition that had bested almost every surgeon who had undertaken to master it. Though he had not presented his paper publicly, Sims had attended the previous year's meeting of the AMA in Richmond. He had been active in convincing others to attempt his procedure. Now, Sims was endeavoring to procure a fistula case in New York, to demonstrate his skills to the city's medical community. He was capitalizing on his breakthrough, of course, and it was said that he hoped not only to establish a profitable practice but to propose—as others had proposed in recent years, albeit unsuccessfully—a hospital devoted to the maladies of women.

Catherine had known Sims for as long as she'd been alive, she explained. Not only that, but the surgical experiments that had already brought Sims more than the typical doctor's share of renown had been performed on a number of servants in Montgomery. They had been loaned to Sims by their masters, and one of them had belonged to her brother-in-law, a lay physician himself. Out of pity for the servants, the brother-in-law, Dr. Nathan Harris, had purchased all of the women when the experiments proved more difficult than first anticipated. The slave who had been Sims's first cure after years of effort now belonged to Catherine's sister, Margaret. This very girl had traveled north with them. She and her child had been on the train that sailed into the Norwalk River.

Unannounced, the young couple rang Sims's bell. To them, he appeared as a tiny, frail man, womanish of appearance. He was overjoyed when he recognized Catherine and exclaimed to Emmet as he shook his hand that he had known the girl's parents for ages, and Catherine since she was a very young girl. There was no hiding the fact that Sims was not well. He was exceedingly thin, his pallor was bad, and his cheeks were caved with the stresses, perhaps, of working to sustain this large, lonely house and to provide for the many children that could be glimpsed cavorting about inside, behind him. If Sims greeted them with all the conviviality he was able to muster in his weakened state, then it all drained from him the moment Catherine told the story of the train wreck. Sims, however, appeared less distressed by the deaths of the seven doctors than by the news that the young slave he had portentously cured was among those who had been tossed into the waters of the Norwalk.

Anarcha? Sims said. Is she—well?

Anaka, yes, Catherine said. We all survived.

Sims stared a moment, as though Catherine's reply did not give him the information he desired, but he was unable or unwilling to press for more. He appeared relieved to hear that the slave girl had returned to the South. He begged leave of the young couple and offered Emmet a wink and a word of advice. Alabama girls were the very best girls in the world.

Catherine returned to the South to care for her sister—she had been ill ever since the accident—but not before she accepted Emmet's proposal of marriage. February 14, 1854, was tentatively chosen as the date for their wedding, but the letter confirming the date was delayed by a heavy storm that washed out roads. Emmet did not receive final notice of his imminent betrothal until six o'clock in the evening on February 10. He hurried to his Fulton Street tailor for the two hours it took to be fitted for a suit and then, luckily, he made every connection successfully over three days, arriving in Autauga County on the evening of February 13. As Emmet was not Catholic, like Catherine, the wedding was held at the home of Dr. Nathan Harris. It was after the ceremony that the new Mrs. Thomas Addis Emmet pointed out the servant girl Anarcha tidying an unoccupied room. Did Emmet recall the Dr. Sims they had so briefly encountered in New York City?

Emmet did. In the interim, he'd heard additional rumors about Sims, confirming the romantic tale Catherine had told him about the Alabama experiments. The man had persisted gallantly for years, the story went, causing great strain to both his purse and his health. In New York, Sims had at last found a fistula case upon which to demonstrate his technique. Some were already heralding Sims as a hero of American medicine, proof that doctors of the New World could succeed where those of the Old World had failed. Others voiced reservations about his methods and ethics. Even if Sims was highly skilled, the argument went, the profession should be wary of blindly sanctioning his procedure. What if less expert hands found it more difficult to perform? What if a patient was left worse off as a result? Already, some were asserting that Sims's method was not as easy to execute as he had claimed.

Emmet sensed a far graver problem during his wedding reception. He approached Anarcha to make the acquaintance of the young servant who had unwittingly played a role in what many were calling a dramatic leap forward in the practice of surgery. The girl had kept her distance from the festivities. She glanced up as Emmet drew near. A mysterious expression of shame and resolve flashed across her face. Emmet understood why only when he pierced the atmosphere that surrounded her—when her air hit him. It was a sweetly rank odor of urine and feces, inadequately masked by unseen flowers and herbs. He knew in an instant what it meant. The girl who was the first cure of an incurable condition had not been cured at all.

Anarcha impressed him as he asked for her personal history, and for details of the experiments. He was surprised to learn that they were approximately the same age—she looked much older—and were she his patient, he would have immediately advised bed rest for her limp, likely foot drop. Anarcha described Sims's technique and the demands of surgical aftercare with an expertise that would have impressed Emmet in a medical school student, let alone a slave nurse.

Before leaving on his honeymoon—a tour of the South—Emmet remained several days in Alabama. He seized the opportunity to write a letter to Dr. Sims. Surely the girl had been genuinely cured, Emmet wrote, but somehow her cure had been undone, likely by subsequent pregnancies. Now that Sims and Emmet were connected both professionally and through the bonds of marriage and friendship, he wrote, duty compelled him to inform his colleague that the slave girl the New York medical community was already calling a pivotal success was leaking quite as if she had never been cured at all. If Sims wished the girl's condition to be addressed in any way, Emmet was at his service.

On the afternoon they were to depart on their nuptial journey, Sims's reply arrived by frantic telegraph message: Anarcha to Virginia. Charles Bell Gibson. Egyptian Building, Richmond.

* * *

In April 1853, Sims hadn't seen Anarcha for several years. He wasn't sure where she was.

News arrived of the death of the vice president and Anarcha's onetime patient William Rufus King. Cuba had failed to cure King's tuberculosis. Already, there was talk of raising a monument to him there. Immediately following the news of King's death, Sims was forced to use his slaves Amanda and her children Edward and Haile as collateral on a loan for

$1,000, from a man named McQueen. Neither the end of the fistula experiments nor the drugstore partnership with Rush and Baldwin had solved his financial difficulties. He was as close to ruin as he'd ever been. Immediately after that, however, a young slave was mortally stabbed, offering the promise of completely changing Sims's fortunes.

He was called to the case, and he never asked whether the boy had been a victim in a brawl among his fellow unfortunates or the recipient of a particularly severe punishment from his master. The latter was more likely, as it would have been unusual for a slave to be in possession of a cutting implement of the size that had inflicted the young field hand's wounds.

There was a puncture to the boy's left side, between the sixth and seventh ribs, and two deep gouges in the abdomen. The sack of the peritoneum had been sliced open as well, as evidenced by large knobs of lacerated intestine wriggling out of the wounds. The thoracic penetration had passed downward from above, piercing the diaphragm muscle and rupturing the stomach, the contents of which had seeped into the pleural cavity. Sims recalled his father-in-law's reputation for disemboweling slaves and putting them back together again. Sheer fantasy: the boy wouldn't live another day. But the case was perfect, in its way, and if Sims worked quickly he could use 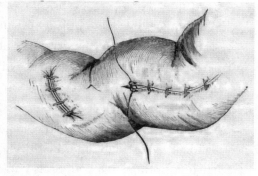 the young slave to prove something essential about abdominal surgery.

As he had done with his first successful fistula experiment, Sims employed interrupted silver sutures to close transverse and diagonal lacerations on the slave's intestines. The whole of the bowel was then stuffed back into the peritoneum. There was no need to close the exterior wounds. As anticipated, the boy died twenty-four hours later. Sims brought the body back to Montgomery. Rush and another colleague attended a post-mortem.

Sims bisected the peritoneum—the procedure had been a success. For an inch around the sutures in the bowel, plastic lymph had begun to glue the wounded parts to the peritoneal coat. There was no inflammation. The boy had lived long enough to begin to heal without infection, without slipping into the peritonitis that made abdominal surgery a death sentence. It proved that the frontier of abdominal surgery could be explored—with silver wire.

After the success with Anarcha, Sims performed clamp suture procedures on the remainder of the fistulous slaves. With silver wire, it worked about half the time. Quietly, he let his Montgomery colleagues know that he had achieved a success, but to publish he would need to perfect the method. This meant additional operations on women whose vaginal walls were not already toughened with scar tissue. He sent Anarcha, Lucy, Betsey, and the others away. At the same time, he took on an assistant, Nathan Bozeman, the protégé of the famed Dr. Samuel Gross of Kentucky. Bozeman was ambitious like Sims, but they were opposites in every other way. Bozeman was a large, mustached bear of a man, yet of a much milder demeanor than Sims. It wasn't hard to find more fistula sufferers: after word spread of a cure, even white women began to present themselves at Sims's office. Bozeman quickly learned the clamp suture procedure, and Sims was freed from the drudgery of the simpler cases, enabling him to perform the sorts of experiments with silver wire that Henry LeVert had never had the courage to attempt.

He employed silver sutures in a wide range of surgeries. In May 1850, he used silver on a gentleman who had lost the left wing of his nose to an accident. A fortnight after he'd healed, the man reappeared with a peculiar bump under his scar. Sims had failed to remove the entirety of the suture, but even after weeks with a bit of silver embedded in the man's face, there was no trace of infection. In 1852, Sims used silver to close a wound on the face of a young boy. The cure was so perfect that removing the suture was like lifting an earring from an earlobe long used to wearing it. In the same year, Sims used silver in another invasive case of osteosarcoma, removing the principal portion of the lower jaw of a fifty-year-old slave woman. The ten-inch incision was closed with eighteen sutures that remained in place three times as long as any doctor would have dared with silk. Between 1849 and 1852, Sims performed three operations to remove diseased breasts and three amputations of the leg, all requiring between eight and seventeen silver sutures. Used in conjunction with plaster treated with isinglass fish jelly, Sims achieved union by first intention in every case.

There were a few failures. He reasoned that if he was now able to cure a fistula, he should be able to create one to remove bladder stones more easily. He performed two such procedures on young slave girls, but both failed, even with silver. Similarly, he used silver to strangulate warty growths on the face of an old woman and for a difficult hemorrhoid patient. In each case, the growths healed around the wire and persisted.

Despite the setbacks, even these latter cases offered promise. What if silver could be used to tie off the thin stalks that attached cancerous growths and polyps to the inner walls of the uterus? If one used silk, the stalks would rot, causing mischief. Silver could be the solution to cancer surgery. It was a promising theory, but it was academic without addressing the other dangers of uterine and abdominal surgery.

Then came success with the doomed slave's intestines. With this, a host of surgeries now performed only in the direst of circumstances began to look to Sims's imagination not only possible but routine. For some time, he had been thinking that the fistula work would be his salvation, in the form of a clinic that would make his name. Now, his vision began to grow, and for the scope of the idea and the audacity required to implement it, Sims would consult a powerful visionary whom he would later be proud to call a friend: P. T. Barnum.

Thirteen

P. T. Barnum—Joice Heth—Baldwin's speech—Summers in
New York—Jenny Lind—Horatio Storer—Caroline Thompson—
Planning a hospital—AMA meeting—New York colleagues—
Comet of 1853—Henri Stuart

DOCTORS KNEW WELL THE STORY OF THE SLAVE JOICE HETH, BORN IN
Madagascar in 1674. In 1835, she was purchased by P. T. Barnum. Heth was
161 years old. She had been the nurse of the young George Washington.

Barnum was a former grocer from Connecticut, a failure in the mer-
cantile and newspaper businesses but a success in running lotteries. When
the Connecticut lottery was outlawed, he moved to New York. He soon
learned of a woman of impossibly aged appearance on display in Philadelphia, said to have an intimate connection to the father of the country.

Barnum traveled to see her and found her wholly satisfactory. She
was a thousand years old if a day. She sat reclined in a seat but couldn't
move. She was blind, and her eyes had sunk so deep into their sockets
they appeared to have disappeared completely. The nails of her hands
were four-inch claws, and her mouth showed a single, elongated fang. She
didn't have enough flesh to entice a Jersey mosquito, but she would chat
happily with whoever wished to converse with her, singing bits of ancient
hymns and offering recollections of "dear little George."

She had few visitors in Philadelphia. Barnum was sure that he could
do better in New York. He sold a portion of a Connecticut grocery interest to purchase Heth for $1,000, having talked her owner down from an
initial asking price of $3,000. The condition of the sale stipulated that he

would own her for only a single year. Surely, he thought, the slave would be dead by then.

Barnum arranged to have her displayed at Niblo's Garden, an open-air saloon on Broadway that for more than a decade had been impressing paying customers with hundreds of colored-glass lanterns in the evenings. Profits and traffic had increased greatly in the last year with the addition of a theater. Blurbs and snippets about Joice Heth's arrival in the city began to appear in newspapers even before Barnum invited editors to Niblo's for a private showing. When editors refused to attend, he bribed them for coverage. Breathless articles subsequently appeared in the *New-York Sun*, the *New-York Evening Star*, the *New-York Daily Advertiser*, the *New-York Courier and Enquirer*, and the *New-York Spirit of the Times*. Attendance was twenty-five cents. Showing Heth first in New York and then elsewhere, Barnum was soon making $1,500 per week.

New York doctors were among the first to publicly doubt the authenticity of Heth's age. Some argued in print that she wasn't a person at all but an automaton. Barnum knew the trick: when your spectacle is revealed to be a fraud, turn the fraud into a spectacle. As anticipated, Heth died on February 19, 1836. The same newspapers that had once trumpeted the reality of Joice Heth now clamored with a second round of free advertising—calls for a public autopsy. (Public dissection of bodies would not be outlawed in New York until 1854.)

Most prominent among the doubters was the professor of surgery at the New York College of Physicians and Surgeons, Dr. David L. Rogers. Rogers was known for having invented a device for excising enflamed tonsils, and for having performed one of the first successful ovariotomies in the country. He had a flair for spectacle. He had conducted a public autopsy of the famous pirate Charles Gibbs, executed in 1831 for the murders of four hundred people. Rogers kept Gibbs's penis, said to be of notable size. He arranged for a facsimile of the organ to be donated to New York's Grand Anatomical Museum.

Rogers had already seen Heth at Niblo's. He announced prior to the autopsy that it was unlikely Heth had the same ossification of the arteries he had once seen in a 115-year-old woman in Italy. Barnum arranged for

Rogers to examine Heth's body at the City Saloon, near Broadway and Fulton, directly across from St. Paul's chapel and churchyard. More than a thousand spectators, many doctors and medical students among them, paid fifty cents to attend. Rogers declared Heth to be a hoax; she wasn't more than eighty years old, he said. During the journalistic battles that followed, Barnum pitted reporter against reporter with alternate claims. The body at City Saloon wasn't Heth's at all. Her remains were now traveling Europe. Heth hadn't even died—she was living happily in Connecticut.

More than a decade later, now firmly established as a promoter and showman, Barnum learned of the remarkable voice of the Swedish songstress Jenny Lind. He seized the opportunity to manage her American tour of 150 concerts. The first was held on September 11, 1850, at Castle Garden in New York. From there, Barnum and Lind traveled south to Philadelphia and Washington City. A ship carried them to Charleston, nearly foundering mid-voyage. Lind played Havana and then set sail aboard the *Falcon* for multiple concerts at the St. Charles Theatre in New Orleans.

* * *

On December 10, 1849, Sims attended William Baldwin's speech before the Medical Association of Alabama. Baldwin spoke of the delusions flourishing amid the medical profession. He lashed out at steam cures and hydropathy, in particular. Sims seethed. Most of the men present knew he was in the process of purchasing a sulfur spring in Butler County, to be operated by his brother. It was yet another doomed attempt Sims was making to elevate himself to the ranks of Montgomery's well-to-do.

The speech got worse. Baldwin turned to quacks—men of dark and crooked counsel, calculating sycophants who sought distinction by advocating the vilest falsehoods—and surely every man in the room recollected the paper Baldwin had published condemning Sims's lockjaw cure. Baldwin dismissed what the better men of the profession accepted as their due—that the honor it afforded was like the honor bestowed upon conquering heroes. Baldwin preferred martyrs. The doctor's march was lonely, he said, and often he walked on stormy and starless nights. Yet a physician needn't worry if his own star seemed to set or even fall from the sky, for stars only seem to do so. In fact, as genius is immortal, a star that appears to have set has but risen to beautify the skies of other lands.

Four days later, the capitol building in Montgomery burned. Once again, Sims knew his ambition was too large for Alabama.

He had turned to water cures, for himself, shortly after the success with Anarcha. In the aftermath of his victory, he sank into his own violent case of the summer complaint, the illness that had killed his son and his first patients in South Carolina. Seeking a cure of his own, Sims took several of the still-fistulous slaves with him to the springs in Butler County that he would soon purchase. He was well enough to maintain a taxing schedule of surgeries, but the diarrhea would plague him for years. He existed on diets of oysters and pork fat, without salt, but was left dehydrated, drained of pounds and energy. In 1849, Sims borrowed $500 to travel to New York for the remainder of the summer. The city's famed Croton water seemed to act as a balm.

A hundred thousand southerners descended on the city every summer. Most ignored Governor William Seward's 1841 change to the slavery laws, prohibiting slaves entirely in the state of New York. The rule was only loosely enforced, and there were rumors of pending improvement. The Fugitive Slave Act was being debated in Washington City. If it passed, southerners traveling with their servants were at little risk of losing their property.

In 1850, Sims made additional visits to water cures in Alabama and New Orleans. In Louisiana, he happened to come across a fistulous slave, a difficult case that rivaled even Anarcha's injury. He offered the girl's master a cure, at no charge if the procedure failed. The man wouldn't budge, and Sims was forced to buy the young woman to bring her to Montgomery for additional experiments to perfect his procedure.

Sims and Theresa returned to New York that summer. He made quiet local inquiries. Fistula treatment in the city was so primitive as to amount to doctors suggesting that women stuff bottles of India rubber into their vaginas to staunch the flow of urine. With 750,000 people—ten times the size of any city Sims had lived in—New York surely had many fistula sufferers hiding in plain sight. More arrived regularly aboard the immigrant ships that deposited thousands daily onto the city's shores. If Sims were to move to New York, he reasoned, the exploding Irish population would supply material for experimental work almost as readily as the slave population in Alabama. This notion offered the chance for Sims and his family to skirt the threats of illness and slave insurrection, as well as the growing specter of secession.

He set out to rub shoulders with New York's great medical men Dr. John Francis and Dr. Fordyce Barker and Dr. Valentine Mott and Dr. Alexander Stevens, who was highly regarded even though he'd been outed as one of the early leaders of the Kappa Lambda cabal. In general, doctors in New York were in line with Sims's view of the profession. He heard it noted more than once that even the great Galileo had been a medical student before turning to astronomy. It was not uncommon to hear affirmations of the profession from classical times. Hippocrates said a philosophical doctor was like a god. Homer claimed a wise physician is worth more than armies to the public weal. And numerous others—Pliny, Cicero, and Rhazes the Persian—similarly exalted the divine origin of the profession. Sims attended a talk in which it was asserted that medicine in America would succeed precisely because of Americans' commercial and eclectic character. The American impulse for that which was new and exciting meant that we should not be so quick to brand novel methods as quackery, the speaker claimed. Might not a measure of wheat be gleaned from the harvest of the quackish chaff? The light of truth may be obscured by false doctrine, opined the speaker in conclusion, but brilliant discoveries achieved through the fearless collection of facts would beam from the darkness as clear and distinct as the morning star.

An institution devoted to fistula—a larger version of his backyard clinic in Montgomery—had already begun to take shape in Sims's mind when a pamphlet calling for a new hospital was distributed throughout New York. There was a want of provisions of relief for the sick poor, the pamphlet claimed. Bellevue had 550 beds, the New York Hospital 350, and there were only scattered others. By comparison, London had 3,200 beds in half a dozen hospitals. Paris had 3,580 beds, and 2,410 more in specialized hospitals, for a city of 1.3 million. Death rates in New York were skyrocketing, not even counting the recent cholera outbreak that killed six thousand. The pamphlet hoped to raise $10,000 and secure annual subscribers at $100 per year for a new institution. The scheme was similar to rumors that Sims heard of a hospital for women being proposed by Dr. Elizabeth Blackwell, who the year before had become the first woman in the United States to be awarded a medical degree. Blackwell too was hoping to raise $10,000. But no one was sure whether a hospital for females could be sustained by voluntary contributions, or that such an institution, if it *was* sustained, could also function as a school of medicine. Sims was relieved to hear that, for now, Blackwell had settled on the goal of a wing for women in a larger hospital.

For Theresa, who was always supportive of her husband but never particularly interested in his work, the time in New York fed the flames of her desire for experience of the cosmopolitan world. In late 1850, back in Alabama, word came of the imminent New Orleans concerts of Jenny Lind. The woman's voice was a global sensation, Theresa said. She insisted that her husband pay the outrageous fifteen-dollar ticket price. Sims agreed—there was opportunity in the journey. They could pay another visit to Cooper's Well, the Louisiana spring that had done wonders for him the previous year. Even better, he could book a room at an opulent hotel near the St. Charles Theatre, where Lind would perform, on the chance that Lind and her manager, the brilliant promoter P. T. Barnum, might also have taken rooms there. Sims's calculation proved accurate.

* * *

Even before the prospect of New Orleans, Sims had noticed a certain parallel in their manly spirits and innovative careers. Barnum first made his name with the display of a slave woman before the medical community. Now Sims hoped to do the same. His cure of Anarcha could be used to make his name, just as Barnum had managed to advantage the life and death of Joice Heth. Given the chance, perhaps Barnum would recognize that Anarcha too could be transformed into a sensation.

Barnum staged Lind's appearance in New Orleans beautifully. The newspapers gushed over the scene of Lind's arrival aboard the *Falcon*, a great seething concourse of humanity gathering on the wharf as she disembarked. A veritable carnival had sprung up in the lot next door to the theater. Lind's act was juxtaposed with stalls where, before and after the performances, concertgoers could pay to see mammoth hogs, five-footed horses, and a grizzly bear in chains. Barnum himself was a freakish figure, with a broad nose flaring out beneath his eyes, a great silken cravat hung noose-like around his neck, and two curly tufts of hair winging out from either side of his head like the outrageous wig of a clown.

Sims seized on his chance. On the morning of the concert, as Barnum strode through the hotel lobby, Sims called out a burst of praise for the genius of the Heth episode. The great showman paused. He agreed to sit for a moment with the forthright physician. Barnum admitted that the tale of Heth's birth in Madagascar in 1674 had been wholesale invention; she'd been born in Virginia. One must acknowledge the corn, he chuckled, when one has had a hand in picking it. Similarly, the stories of Barnum yanking out Heth's teeth to make her appear even older weren't true, but the rumors had been useful, so he'd done nothing to dispel them. Barnum was already at work on his autobiography. It was crucial to have your story told, he said, either by your own hand or by manipulating the pens of newspapermen to tell it for you. His whole being as a showman was dependent on newspapers and controversy, he said. The one needful thing to understand, so as to exploit both, was that reporters and newspapers were in competition with one another.

Sims blurted out a little of his own story. The slave Anarcha, and the many operations that had cost him so much in treasure and health, leaving him nearly crippled. Barnum waved a hand. Do not describe your sickness as weakness, he said. Rather, it is strength. It is the price of your genius and the evidence of your sainthood. And do not claim to have solved problems with reason and insight alone. Suggest, rather, the intervention of a divinity that, as with priests, proves your humility and exalts your sanctity.

The showman rose to his feet. He shook Sims's hand. Above all, he said, understand that the particular quality of the story you tell—its luster and pathos—dwarfs by orders of magnitude its veracity and its nature, whatever that may be.

When Sims and Theresa returned to New York in the summer of 1851, his brother-in-law had had enough. Sims was now only nominally from

Alabama; he wasn't doing his part to keep up the B. R. Jones dispensary. Sims's father intervened when the dispute was formalized in the courts and became the subject of local gossip.

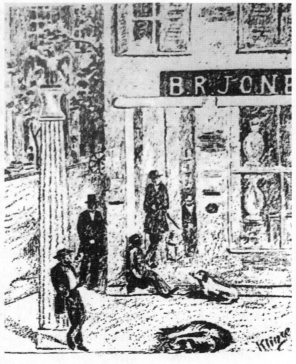

Sims again relapsed into his digestive complaint, and this year the waters of New York did little to sooth his recalcitrant bowel. He felt at home philosophically in New York, but interpersonally, the city doctors were as disagreeable to him as it was said they were to Elizabeth Blackwell. Socially, they erected a blank wall of professional antagonism. That said, word of Sims's fistula success had managed to escape Montgomery. He'd exchanged edifying letters with a number of physicians, including a young man in Boston, Horatio Storer, who had witnessed the famous Hayward's fistula cure. Sims met Storer after he and Theresa left New York in 1851 for Portland, Connecticut. They paid a visit to Sims's old typhoid patient Dr. Jarvis, who had been so fond of Anarcha and was thrilled to learn that the girl had been cured.

Jarvis facilitated several meetings. The first was with Storer, who had fascinating ideas about the roots of mental disturbance in women: they were of a reflex character, he said, arising from pelvic irritation. This suggested possible surgical remedies for conditions previously thought untreatable, by knife or otherwise. Next, Jarvis introduced Sims to a wealthy couple from Springfield, Massachusetts, James and Caroline Thompson, who were keen to hear of Sims's plan for a hospital for females. Sadly, their enthusiasm was born of Caroline's affliction with a uterine tumor that she'd been told was inoperable. Most likely, it was.

The meetings underscored the financial potential of the institution Sims envisioned. However, doctors in New York, Sims now understood, were impervious to anything that did not offer them something for the trouble of their attention. They were as unimpressed by his scattershot vision of a hospital as they were by his publications. His work had appeared in impressive journals, to be sure, but did he really think that what had distinguished him from country doctors in Alabama would set him apart in New York City? What could he give them, they wished to know, here and now? Barring an answer to that, their doors were closed to him.

After Connecticut, Sims and Theresa tried Brooklyn, but the water did not compare to New York's. They traveled to Philadelphia, and on a buggy ride through town they found an agreeable home on Vine Street where they could keep all the windows and doors open, quite as if it was Alabama. Sims still had friends in Philadelphia from his medical school days, but the remainder of the summer of 1851 was difficult in both spirit and health. They stayed on into the fall, which turned out to be a stroke of great luck, as Sims happened to learn of a new fistula cure being promoted by a doctor named Pancoast.

Sims rallied from his sickbed. He found the journal in which Pancoast had detailed his method, in 1847, when Sims was deep in the middle of his own experiments. Fortunately, the article was another small affair, and Pancoast's surgery was a needlessly complicated ordeal employing the four-bladed speculum of Charrière and an unwieldy tongue-and-groove suture. Still, the writing was on the wall: if Sims did not publish his method now, someone else would publish an elaborate cure and all his work would be lost.

He took a friend's advice to approach Dr. Isaac Hays, the Philadelphia editor of the *American Journal of the Medical Sciences*. Hays had published Sims a number of times now, but Sims had not visited him that summer. He was another of those whose vision had been corrupted by association with the Kappa Lambda men; Hays had gone so far as to help draft the AMA's code of ethics.

Sims played his emotions close to his vest. Hays agreed at once to a lengthy article. It was high time for such a thing, he agreed. Sims thought of Barnum as he sat down to dictate his article to Theresa, in a rush because

Hays hoped to run the piece in just a few months' time. How would it be best to tell the story of his cure? The problem was the clamp suture, the thing to which he hoped to attach his name. It cut out too often. In Alabama, his assistant Bozeman was already suggesting that the clamp suture was suited only to the most perfectly situated fistulae. It failed entirely in cases of multiple fistulae, or when the fistula was awkwardly positioned near the cervix or urethra. Worse, it worked only in conjunction with silver wire, and silver was not Sims's invention at all. It was LeVert's, and the man appeared to have no desire for the honor that anyone would judge was his to claim.

Barnum had said it must be a story. But for now, Sims resolved to establish the technique for the profession, and to do so in a fashion more expansive and with more woodcuts than he or anyone had used before. He would present only the perfection of his success. He would be vague about his failures and inspirations. If he hinted at predecessors while shrieking out claims of originality he would inoculate himself against inevitable criticisms. He would acknowledge the use of silver wire but downplay its importance to the efficacy of his method. The Sims position, the Sims speculum, and the S-shaped catheter—these were his cure and his glory, and they would plunge his name deep into the profession. The time for the luster and the pathos, for the story of Anarcha and the others—that would come later, in New York, and by then the goal would be so much more than a fistula hospital for women.

* * *

In May 1852, Sims attended the fifth meeting of the American Medical Association in Richmond, as one of three representatives from Alabama. He was encouraged to discover that doctors from all over the country had read "On the Treatment of Vesico-Vaginal Fistula," which Isaac Hays had published in January. There was a Dr. Holmes in Mississippi who was already attempting Sims's cure. There was Dr. Pope—Pope would soon be elected to the presidency of the AMA—who was seeking fistula patients in his home city of Saint Louis. And Charles Bell Gibson was already performing clamp suture surgeries at Richmond's impressive new Egyptian Building. Gibson was the son of Dr. William Gibson in Philadelphia, the very doctor who, decades before, had achieved renown with his double cesarean case and had feuded so fiercely with Sims's mentors.

In addition to these new confederates in his cause, Sims enjoyed encountering his old professors from South Carolina, Frost and Moultrie and Prioleau. Sims told his teachers the story of Mrs. Merrill, whose inverted uterus had called to mind Prioleau's lesson from so many years earlier. The group chuckled heartily at the tale of the struggling seamstress as Sims worked blindly to apply the position and procedure his professor had prescribed. There was a great lurch of laughter and joy at the moment when the trapped air burst out of Mrs. Merrill, like a horn shrieking an announcement of Sims's inspiration. The moment was so jolly, Sims resolved to work it into the tale of his success. The incident was an amusement, but also, as Barnum had suggested, it was tinged with evidence of the divine spirit that was subtly working to ensure that fate itself passed through the humble hands of Dr. J. Marion Sims.

The AMA conference stood in stark contrast to that year's gathering of the Alabama State Medical Association, which Sims did not attend, though he received the printed transactions early the next year. The doctors of Alabama were preoccupied with nonsurgical medicine. Now it was insane asylums. There were ongoing efforts to convince the state's picayune legislature to sign on to the vision that enthused philanthropist Dorothea Dix had propounded when she visited Montgomery in the winter of 1850. Worse was the year's valedictory address, "Report on the Diseases of Mobile During the Year 1852." The speaker's conclusion was even more foolish than his subject matter. A physician should not expect the popular promotion that is the award of successful labor in other professions, he said. Politicians and statesmen may receive their due meed of praise. They may be crowned with honors, their pathway strewn with flowers. The physician too will receive plaudits, but he must accept a silent crown that is more glorious than popular applause, and which rises heavenward like a fragrance from the domestic hearth.

Nonsense. Regardless, disease was the final straw in Sims and Theresa's decision to leave Alabama. The colics and dysenteries and light vernal fevers marching north from the bayous—to say nothing of the murderous yellow fever, and cholera, and the malaria that would surely kill Sims if a chill struck him for a third time—these had snatched from the celestial sphere not a few of their friends, and more of their friends' children. In April 1853, Sims's vision finalized with the healed bowel of the doomed, stabbed slave. A New York hospital would use fistula as its primary mission, but secretly it would aim its sights at far more glorious and profitable avenues: cancer surgery and penetrating investigations of the final frontier, the peritoneum. The hospital would be a laboratory. Who knew what other innovations he might discover? Sims and Theresa resolved to leave within the month, and he called on his friendship with Bozeman, who purchased his business and home. Rather than sell their servants, Theresa arranged to lease them to good families. The leases would form part of their income in New York, and if they struggled, she would return to extract their investment. They left the state midyear, not long after Nathan Harris traveled north with Anarcha.

Before they moved into the city, investing the bulk of their scant resources in an impressive but lonely home on the edge of town, Sims and Theresa and the children summered once again with Jarvis in Connecticut. They were barely fifty miles away when word came of the terrible train disaster at Norwalk. It was ghastly. Had Sims attended that year's AMA meeting in New York, he might have been on the train himself.

For the first time, but not the last, Sims tapped the tumor of Caroline Thompson that summer to buy her time. He wasn't yet confident enough with silver wire to use it to attack her growth, and Mrs. Thompson was far too valuable a member of society to risk such an experiment. In New York, the Irish would provide plenty of opportunity to perfect such investigations.

In the city, he arranged for many copies of "On the Treatment of Vesico-Vaginal Fistula" to be printed and distributed to doctors in both New York and Brooklyn. He found a silversmith on Duane Street, Mr. Berenbroick, who could make him wire of the desirable 29 gauge, and a toolmaker named Tieman agreed to fashion needles and a needle holder according to Sims's design. Tieman also made adjustments to Sims's speculum, deviating the curve of the blade from a right angle to enable greater leverage.

In Alabama, he had already begun to experiment with variations on the Sims position. White women refused to sustain the position for as long as the slaves he had experimented on. In New York, it became clear that white women preferred a left-lateral position to the knee-chest position. For most procedures, the left-lateral position proved equal to the task. Similarly, Sims invented a reclining chair for well-to-do women who were uneasy about being asked to immediately mount an examination table. Sims's chair was a modification of an invalid chair devised by a man in Charleston, but he made a note to take full credit for his ingenuity when the time came to do so.

Their savings didn't last long. They arrived in New York with $1,000; it quickly depleted to $116. Soon, Sims was accepting boarders in his home, patients from Alabama who had followed him north. Theresa was forced to cut up her dresses to make clothes for their children, and before long they were compelled to send their girls to public schools and were talking of selling their slaves.

Wherever he could, Sims begged for a fistula case to demonstrate his skills. But even when he got one, it was hardly the salvation they needed.

Dr. Valentine Mott, one of the founders of the Medical College of New York and a former president of the New York Academy of Medicine, brought him a curious case of a woman with a fistula of many years' standing. Mott had been trying and failing to cure her for years with the actual cautery. The case was curious in that the fistulous opening had come to act as a valve, releasing urine into the vagina only when the unfortunate woman reposed in certain positions. Sims cured her and published a brief piece about the case in the *New York Medical Times*. In the text of the article, he tried wooing his city brethren with a claim that the glory of the cure—the first in the history of New York—belonged to all of American medicine. He realized little reward. Other doctors asked him to assist in cases of lacerated perineum, or to borrow his tools for their own fistula work, and soon word was coming of successful cures from the city's various quarters. All the while, Sims's resources continued to dwindle.

At last, he resolved to reveal his plan for a new institution of medicine. He paid a visit to Mott's office. The man's impressive diploma hung on a wall, itself ornamented with a medal of the sort that was awarded to soldiers for valor. Mott, Sims knew, had spoken gratuitously of the opportunity afforded by disease. The illnesses arriving on ships from Europe, now quarantined at the Emigrant Refuge Hospital on Ward's Island, made the facility like a great medical laboratory. The profession might never again have so admirable a chance to attempt new cures and innovations, Mott had said. As Sims expected, Mott responded well when he described his vision of a hospital that would experiment with surgery rather than medicines. At once, Mott sent Sims to speak with the great Dr. Francis.

Francis had a storied career of successive specializations in materia medica, medical jurisprudence, and obstetrics. He too had served as one of the first presidents of the New York Academy of Medicine. When Sims arrived at Francis's home, he discovered that the man's wife was related to Francis Marion, the Swamp Fox, for whom Sims had been named. She had people in South Carolina still. It was likely they were distant cousins.

Like Mott, Francis glimpsed at once how the hospital Sims proposed might advance the causes of science and medical education. It could become a place where students would receive valuable clinical experience. In turn, Francis prepared for Sims a card of invitation to Dr. Alexander Stevens, the great physician whose greatness, as with Isaac Hays in Philadelphia, was marred by his Kappa Lambda association. Yet Stevens's influence could not be overestimated. It was said that the very idea for the New York Academy of Medicine had been his. Stevens's father had been among those who dressed as Indians to carry out the act of heroism that became known as the Boston Tea Party. Many years later, the great soldier's son had served as the second president of the American Medical Association.

Stevens greeted Sims warmly. They chatted at length about a case of inverted uterus that Stevens had had under his care for more than thirty years. He too was amused by the story of the seamstress Mrs. Merrill. At first, Stevens was as enthusiastic about Sims's plan as Mott and Francis were. He suggested organizing a meeting of the New York College of Physicians and Surgeons so that Sims could present his idea to the profession at large.

Trouble loomed, however, when Mott hedged on his support for Sims's plan. After several weeks of organization, Mott mysteriously announced that after long thought on the subject he had concluded that Sims's hospital would fail.

Dutifully, Sims had written out his plans in full. Stung by Mott's betrayal, he took the manuscript to Stevens, who revealed a greater horror. It wasn't only Mott. There was now widespread opposition to Sims's plan. Without knowing it, Sims had acquired unseen enemies, and with neither polity nor apology Stevens too retracted his offer to arrange an address under his auspices.

* * *

In the fall of 1853, when a comet again poked through the ceiling of the daytime sky, suggesting to some the star that had heralded the birth of the savior, Sims received a knock on the front door of his new home.

He was thrilled to encounter the Duncan girl from Alabama, whom he had known since she was perhaps six. She was in the company of a young physician. Sims was horrified to learn that Catherine Duncan and most of her family—and, remarkably, Anarcha—had plunged into the river in the dreadful Norwalk wreck. He could not fend off a fiendish thought. He had been set to tell the world of his cure of Anarcha, but he knew that by most definitions of the term she'd never truly been cured. What would have been better, Sims thought reflectively, was if Anarcha had died in the waters of the Norwalk. Her story would then have been marked by both victory and tragedy. Yet she had survived. Sims feigned relief at the news that Anarcha had returned to Alabama. He would have to hope that she would be heard from no more.

A few months later—with little progress on the hospital in the meantime—a distressing letter arrived. Catherine and the young doctor, Emmet, had become engaged to be married. Emmet had traveled to Alabama for their wedding, and he had encountered Anarcha and recognized her as Sims's "first cure." Emmet could tell that Anarcha's fistulae had recurred. Thankfully, he recognized the moment's delicacy, and Sims acted quickly in sending instructions that Anarcha be shipped to Richmond, where the younger Dr. Gibson could cure her quietly, with none of his New York brethren any the wiser. He followed his telegram to Emmet with a longer letter to Gibson, who replied at once that it would be an honor to operate on Sims's famous patient.

Sims suffered for a week in a dismal, crazy-making silence. Then—as if providence truly did smile on him—he received another knock on his door. An old patient who knew of his troubles wished to introduce him to a figure of particular qualities. This man, Henri Stuart, was a former newspaperman. Apart from that, it was difficult to say exactly what Stuart was—except that he was cut from the same clownish cloth as P. T. Barnum.

Sims's old patient claimed that Stuart had worked on the Atlantic cable and had suggested the site for what would become Central Park. He had launched plans for public schools in New York, and he had arranged for each to be supplied with a piano. He was a founder of the Normal College, and he was privy to the financial dealings of many great men, Horace Greeley and Cornelius Vanderbilt among them. Most recently, Stuart had aided in the founding of the Five Points Mission, which just the previous year had been established to provide aid to New York's most notorious neighborhood.

A meeting was arranged for that evening. The former patient and Henri Stuart arrived at Sims's home promptly at eight o'clock.

Stuart was tall and lanky. He had thin hair of a reddish-brown color and a nose that looked like a waxen spigot. Intelligence and energy emanated from him like the aura that spiritualists spoke of. He wasted no time in instructing Sims to relate his story. Sims did so—he told Stuart of Mrs. Merrill, Anarcha and the others, the years of toil, the victory and collapse from health, the plans for a hospital of wide-ranging purpose and innovation, the promise of a lecture in the city, and the betrayal by the very physicians who had benefited most from Sims's work, with no recompense to himself.

Stuart listened until there was nothing left to say. Then the lanky man burst forth with a plan. The idea of a lecture was a right one, Stuart said. It would carry the day. But Sims had been entirely lucky to avoid the medical clique of any particular hospital. Now was the time to think even bigger. Stuart knew just what to do. They would rent Stuyvesant Hall and advertise a lecture on the necessity of a hospital for the treatment of diseases of women, to be delivered by the much-celebrated surgeon Dr. J. Marion Sims, late of Montgomery, Alabama. All the leading doctors in the city would be invited, by special card. The sheer pomp of the event would compel them to endorse his plan. Stuart waved his hand when Sims mentioned the costs. Damn the expense, he said. Never mind the money. He would handle all that.

Stuart laughed aloud at the simplicity of his plan. If you don't make the damnedest failure that a man ever made in this world, he said, then in a month you will no longer be a beggar in New York but a dictator.

Fourteen

Emmet wedding—Leaving Alabama—A boy in France—Brown-Séquard—Experiments—A position in Richmond—Animal laboratory—Expelled from Virginia

İT WAS A SMALL WEDDING. THE YOUNG DOCTOR WHO CAME TO MARRY MS. Catherine Duncan wasn't a Catholic like the Harrises and the Duncans, so the wedding was not held at a church. After they said man and wife at Dr. Nathan Harris's house, the young doctor, whose name was Dr. Emmet, approached Anarcha, sought her out like he knew her and was looking for her, and when he got close his eyes squinted when he smelled her, but he did not flinch or exhale deeply or wave at the air in front of his face, so Anarcha knew he was a doctor who had seen many sick people. She was surprised to hear the name Dr. Marion Sims on his lips, though she knew that Dr. Sims had left Montgomery at about the same time she left Alabama for the first time. By the time she returned to Autauga County, word had spread by grapevine again that the Dr. Sims who cut off slaves' jaws and who had gathered together more women with holes—not just Anarcha and the others but more slave girls for even more experiments—was gone now. He had left Alabama, and there was no more need to worry about him roaming about the countryside like Raw Head and Bloody Bones.

Dr. Emmet asked Anarcha questions about Dr. Sims, about whether Dr. Sims's cure had been a success, and about how many babies she had. Anarcha said she had only one baby, Delia, but she wasn't a baby any-more, she was four and already carrying around other babies. Dr. Emmet said that he meant how many babies had grown inside of her and come out alive or dead, and the answer was five, some whose names she knew and some she didn't, and one who never even had a name. Dr. Emmet said there were people in faraway places, in New York, who knew about her, and it was strange that he knew that she'd been to New York, and that she was on the train that went flying into the Norwalk River.

It was a few days later that she was told she would be leaving Alabama for the second time. This time she suspected she was never coming back. She didn't ask whether she could bring Delia, she just announced it like it was her own decision. She knew that her missus wasn't coming, and she didn't know exactly who she belonged to anymore, but the slaves knew that when there were weddings or deaths there was often discussion among the white people about certain lands and negro slaves passing in ownership from one person to the next, and when they told her that she would be leaving with the young Dr. Emmet and the now Mrs. Catherine Emmet, she guessed that she was now owned by them, but no one said anything about a piece of paper in Montgomery, or any piece of paper anywhere, and she suspected there was no piece of paper, there was just white people who said what was true.

There wasn't time to bid farewell to any of the other slaves, though one or two learned of what was happening on the fast grapevine inside the plantation. Several managed to step outside their cabins as the wagon carrying Dr. and Mrs. Emmet and Anarcha and Delia bobbled off toward Montgomery, but by then the wagon was so far off that Anarcha couldn't see clearly which of the slaves—the men and women she'd tended with plasters and root herbs—had emerged to wave goodbye to them.

In Montgomery, they boarded a small steamboat that took them to Mobile and then along the coast to New Orleans, where Mrs. Emmet had many friends, including a man who had recently been named to the US Supreme Court, Mr. John Campbell. Justice Campbell had been a soldier before he was a judge, and he told raucous stories of having almost been expelled from West Point along with his friends Jefferson Davis and Robert E. Lee during the infamous "eggnog riot" of Christmas 1826. Then the Emmets and their servant and her child, which is how they had come to refer to Anarcha and Delia, took a much larger steamboat—almost as large as the *Pacific*, and very much like a floating city—up the Mississippi River. The ship was crowded with Louisiana planters heading north for the summer, or beginning even longer journeys to Europe. Everyone was dressed fine, but Dr. Emmet was quick to praise the captain and even the gamblers on board for the care they took with their toilet. Anarcha was leased as a chambermaid for the days they were on board. Delia stayed in a room beside the Emmets' cabin, and while Anarcha worked she saw fine ladies chatting with many men at once, speaking in different languages for each suitor. The slaves on board the steamboat acted like fine people too, more like house slaves than field hands, and there were firemen in the boiler room, and waiters, and cooks, and barbers, and deckhands. Rumors spread of runaways among them, either pretending to work on the ship or dressed up as freemen, walking about proud as though they weren't anyone's property. Anarcha was surprised when she was tidying someone's room and they arrived as she was finishing and the woman gave her a dime, and she was free to put it in her pocket, and she did.

The boat stopped at Natchez and Vicksburg, and sometimes Dr. and Mrs. Emmet got off to have honeymoon dinners and time alone without a servant and child in the next room. At night in the cities, and at stops in between, the steamboat paused, and plantation slaves from Mississippi toiled alongside the ship's roustabouts in the eerie light of burning pine knots to load sugar and cotton onto the lower decks, and as the boat got heavier it moved more and more slowly against the current heading north. It was a full two weeks before they reached Bolivar, and a leisurely week after that to Memphis, and that's where they got off and boarded a carriage to the train, first on the Memphis and Charleston line to Chattanooga, and then from Chattanooga on the Hiwassee Railroad to Knoxville, and from there the East Tennessee and Virginia Railroad took them to Lynchburg, and from Lynchburg the southern section of the Orange and Alexandria line shot up to Charlottesville, and from Charlottesville the Virginia Central Railroad scooted down to Richmond, and Anarcha didn't know that Richmond was their destination, at least for her and Delia, until they arrived and Anarcha was left in the care of Dr. Charles Bell Gibson, who was very pleased to meet her and didn't flinch, or even squint, when he smelled her. Rather, he smiled, and conveyed regards from Dr. Sims.

* * *

Early one morning, somewhere near Paris, France, a man woke to a ruckus coming from the bedroom of his fourteen-year-old son. The man found his boy up in his nightshirt, speaking incoherently and smashing all the room's furniture. The man threw his son on the bed; miraculously, the boy calmed. He reported that on rising to his feet, he'd felt something very odd. After that, he remembered nothing.

His father called for the family physician, who in turned called Dr. Charles-Édouard Brown-Séquard, a young phenomenon in the Parisian medical world. Brown-Séquard found the boy with a clean tongue, calm and cheerful. The famous doctor asked the boy to stand. His face changed the moment he rose, twisting into a spasmodic rictus. Brown-Séquard shoved him back onto the bed, and once again the frightened child calmed.

The case illustrated a principle that Brown-Séquard had been investigating since medical school. Disorders of the mind, he believed, could be linked to phenomena affecting the extremities. If proved, the theory could provide mechanical remedies for epilepsy, catalepsy, hysteria, even hydrophobia.

Brown-Séquard elicited from the boy the interesting tidbit that he had gone fishing the day before. He had removed his shoes to wade into the water. He suffered no injury, but Brown-Séquard asked him to remove his stockings anyway. The doctor discovered that pressure on the nail of the boy's right big toe caused him to break into the horrible grimace. Brown-Séquard used a pair of scissors to clip away a slight elevation in the nail, expecting to find a trapped thorn. There was nothing. Nevertheless, the boy was suddenly and entirely cured.

The truth was clear: a disorder of the mind could be caused by perturbation far from it. The condition could be relieved by eliminating the irritant.

* * *

Brown-Séquard was born in Port Louis, Mauritius, three hundred miles east of Madagascar, the product of a liaison between an Irish ship captain and a seamstress who was herself the product of a Frenchman and a native Mauritian woman. Brown-Séquard's father was lost at sea; his mother raised him. He had little formal schooling before they immigrated to France. She survived by embroidery work. He wished to become a poet. A man whose business was words—an author and librarian—convinced Brown-Séquard to study medicine instead.

FIFTY DOLLARS REWARD.—The above reward, and all reasonable expenses, will be paid for the apprehension and delivery to us in Richmond of a Negro Woman Slave, named MARIA, or, as she calls herself, MARIA PERRY, if taken 50 miles or more from Richmond, or thirty dollars if taken in or near Richmond.
Maria is of medium stature, with a round face, skin about ginger-bread color, a good set of teeth, full suit of hair, and a pleasant countenance. Her precise age not recollected, but she is believed to be about twenty-four or five years old.
PHIL. M. TABB & SON, Agents,
Office on Governor street,
mh 14—ts   Between Main and Franklin sts.

50 DOLLARS REWARD—For a Negro Woman, named MITTY HILL, who ran off from the subscriber on or about the 28th December last. I will give the above reward for her delivery at Cary street Jail, or lodged in any other jail so I get her. She is black, about 19 years of age, five feet one inch high, and has a small wen on one of her wrists. Her personal appearance is good.
ap 26 3t   THOS. BOUDAR.

FOR SALE—A negro GIRL, about 16 years old, to a city purchaser. She will be sold for less than her market value. Apply to
P. M. TABB & SON,
Office on Governor street,
my 6 3t   Between Main and Franklin streets.

He was drawn to experimental work. In medical school, he cut his finger while dissecting a corpse, caught sepsis, and was dangerously ill for months. His mother died shortly after he recovered.

He performed many experiments on himself. He swallowed a sponge tied onto a string, pulling it back up again over and over to study digestive juices. In 1851, a twenty-year-old man was guillotined in Paris. Brown-Séquard obtained the man's lower right arm and pumped half a pound of his own blood into it. Color returned, and the arm responded to agitation. The following month, Brown-Séquard repeated the experiment with the arm of another guillotined man. This time, a pound of dog's blood produced goose pimples and the impression of a pulse.

Mauritius had fallen under English rule by the time Brown-Séquard was born; he was not French. His black hair and brown-toned skin mattered little in seeking a medical education in France, and he was soon well known for a broad range of animal experiments. He once attached a dog's tail to the comb of a rooster and nursed the animal until the tail took root in the implanted tissue.

Not being French, however, meant that no matter how well regarded Brown-Séquard came to be, he would never receive a permanent appointment in France. A famous colleague, Dr. Paul Broca, suggested Brown-Séquard try America. Perhaps it was true, Broca said, that America had thrown aside the prejudices that had hobbled Europe.

Brown-Séquard sailed for New York City in 1852. He taught himself English on the voyage.

In New York, he offered obstetric examinations at five dollars per case at a time when the city's medical community was abuzz with claims that one of their own, an American, had bested the leading surgeons of Europe in the treatment of vesico-vaginal fistula. The pioneering surgeon was named Sims, a southerner. Brown-Séquard avoided southerners. When he couldn't, he fought with them about the abomination of slavery. He confronted them with the description of slavery cut from Jefferson's original draft of the Declaration of Independence: "A cruel war against human nature itself." The southerners scoffed and claimed that their slaves were much loved. Luckily, they mistook Brown-Séquard's hair and skin as evidence of Mediterranean blood.

His work on remote causes for diseases of the mind had homed in on epilepsy. He lectured on the subject in New York, Boston, and Philadelphia. He gave a talk to the Richmond Medical and Chirurgical Society in Virginia, close to the time of the 1852 meeting of the American Medical Association, held in the same city.

The evidence of slavery in Richmond saddened him, in particular the infamous and still-standing Lumpkin's Jail, which had been featured in a recent novel, *Twelve Years a Slave*. One had to work hard not to read between the lines of newspaper advertisements for the sale of damaged or sterile slave women. A sixteen-year-old girl would be sold for less than her market value. A fifty dollar reward was offered for the return of Maria, of gingerbread skin and a pleasant countenance. Another fifty dollars for the return of Mitty, who had a wen on one wrist. Brown-Séquard attended the meeting of the AMA and overhead Sims, the pioneering surgeon, describe his fistula procedure to a group of physicians. Sims had performed experiments on young slave women, just as Brown-Séquard performed experiments on animals. The two men did not speak.

Before he returned to Paris, Brown-Séquard became engaged to and married a niece of America's crusading antislavery senator Daniel Webster.

In May 1854, he received a surprise invitation to return to Richmond, to assume a professorship at a new medical school. He would offer lectures and be given use of a laboratory in the basement of the school's main hall, known as the Egyptian Building. Brown-Séquard was thirty-seven years old and had authored more than one hundred papers when he accepted the position and departed for America once more.

He sent instructions ahead for how his laboratory should be set up. The first sign that his appointment would be short-lived was the fact that when he arrived no accommodations had been made for his animals. There weren't even any animals! The basement of the Egyptian Building housed supplies for all sorts of investigations, but no cages had been constructed, no animals collected. The Egyptian Building's basement was home to its janitor and his wife, and there was a small space for a slave woman named Anarcha, and her daughter. Remarkably, Brown-Séquard discovered, Anarcha was one of the slaves of Dr. Sims's original fistula experiments. Horribly, she was now the subject of additional experiments in Richmond.

It was suggested that Anarcha help care for Brown-Séquard's animals.

He lectured upstairs in the Egyptian Building's main hall, and all told he would deliver sixty-five talks in four months' time, then tender his resignation. He sent his students into the streets of Richmond, to collect a vast caravan of dogs, cats, raccoons, terrapins, guinea pigs, rabbits, marmots, pigeons, mice, jays, ravens, and magpies. In courses, Brown-Séquard would wring off a chicken's head to show his students that even in death it would fly into fits. He would puncture the flank of a live dog to pump out its stomach acids and then dunk bits of bread into the liquid. Most of his private experiments built on his epilepsy work. He kept a cat alive for three months after destroying its spinal cord. He discovered that remote burns healed normally even in creatures whose cords had been severed. He learned what would happen if you tore asunder the facial nerves of rabbits. He began to wonder whether material drawn from the testicles of dogs could be used to enhance a man's virility.

He did not get on well with his colleagues. Once, he failed to attend a gathering thrown in his own honor. He heard rumors that American physicians were rushing to human trials with the results of his work, even as they criticized his animal experiments. It was said that he had been too directly influenced by *Frankenstein*, a novel that had poisoned the work of anatomists and galvanists. Brown-Séquard oscillated between rage and sadness at the hypocrisy of America. They lamented the fate of cats while the girl Anarcha lived in a basement, suffering procedures nearly as destructive. They gave her chloroform, but anyone could tell from her cough that its application had been too frequent, its delivery too inexpert.

Brown-Séquard challenged his colleagues with facts. It had now been two decades since England peeled off the scab of slavery. When would America acknowledge the scar that disfigured her face? Americans were obsessed with the political whirlpool into which they were being sucked, but they were blind to the scale of the conflict that loomed and appeared inevitable to an outsider. Brown-Séquard couldn't always check his tongue. The final straw—he left Richmond soon after, just as Dr. Sims was about launch his own hospital—came when he heard that his colleagues had openly begun to question whether all of his ancestors had in fact been of the white race.

Fifteen

The basement—Charles Bell Gibson—Chloroform—Lumpkin's
Jail—Setting the animals free—Washington City—UVA
speech—The naval observatory—The stars are always falling

THE SMELL OF THE ANIMALS MEANT THAT FOR SOME MONTHS, AT LEAST, Anarcha did not need to worry about her own odor.

She arrived in Richmond at the end of March 1854, and she and Delia were given a room in the basement of the strange-looking building that some believed had been brought from Egypt brick by brick. For a time, the building's caretaker and the caretaker's wife lived in the basement with Anarcha and Delia, but when slaves were hired from Lumpkin's Jail, three blocks away—which wasn't really a jail but a slave pen for slave traders—to build the cages for the animals, the janitor and the janitor's wife moved upstairs to get away from the endless ruckus that was like all the animals of the world gathered together in the boat in the Bible, but the story of the Bible boat didn't talk about the noise and the smell, and for some months it was as though Anarcha and Delia lived in dark woods so full of monsters all the forest animals screamed all night long.

When she arrived, Dr. Charles Bell Gibson experimented on her for a number of months, attempting to cure the holes that Dr. Sims had never cured, or had cured and they had broken open again. Dr. Gibson put her to sleep when he did his experiments, and she didn't know what position he put her into when he did his work because she was asleep, though on one occasion she knew that the experiment took place in the large chemical auditorium of the Egyptian Building. They pushed her into the chemical auditorium on a table with wheels, so that not ten or fifteen doctors could watch the operation, as in Alabama, but hundreds of men gathered all around, and the room was like a large funnel of the sort that slaves used to make lye. Some of the men were so high up they could barely see Anarcha, let alone see inside of her, which is what the Alabama doctors had done, taking turns to squat down behind her on Dr. Sims's stool while he pointed and explained his procedure. Dr. Gibson praised Dr. Sims to the class as a great champion of American medicine, solving a problem that doctors in Europe had failed to solve for hundreds of years, but he did not specify that Anarcha had been one of his patients. Dr. Gibson proudly held aloft the various tools that Dr. Sims had used on the cursed women in Alabama: the speculum that was what he used after he had used a bent ladle, the silver tube for the urine that he used after he had used the sponge that almost killed Lucy, and the silver wire that Anarcha saw only when it cured one of her holes and when Dr. Sims used it on the other cursed women before they were all either sold or sent to Autauga County.

Dr. Gibson told the gathered white men that he himself was trying to cure Anarcha now, even though her holes were thickened and indurated from all the previous experiments, and Anarcha didn't know what indurated meant, but it didn't sound like a good word, even though Dr. Gibson spoke of her as though she was an important person who lived in a basement with her daughter. Whatever Dr. Gibson did was lost to her because a different man who was maybe a doctor too poured some liquid onto a neckerchief and placed it gently over her face and told her to breathe, and it wasn't quite like falling asleep, but what else would you call it, and she woke in the black ward of the infirmary, and for six months the most she saw of Richmond was the free black people who paid four dollars to be treated for conditions that were not contagious, whereas white people paid five dollars and had private rooms. The wards in the Egyptian Building had nurses, and they knew a little but not much about how to care for women with closed holes, and Anarcha told them what she knew, and some listened and some didn't. Anarcha taught Delia, young as she was, how to do some delicate things with the tube that drained her urine, and while Anarcha was recovering from the experiments, Delia was sent down to the basement at night to care for the animals and to sleep, but every night after caring for the animals she sneaked back upstairs and slept with Anarcha, and sneaked back down in the morning before the nurses made their first rounds.

Dr. Gibson's experiments didn't work any better than Dr. Sims's experiments, but after Dr. Gibson's first surgery, Anarcha began her monthly bleeding again. Her bleeding had not come since she gave birth to a baby that didn't get a name before it died.

The chemical auditorium was over the basement, and when Dr. Gibson gave lectures the stories dripped down the funnel-shaped room and seeped onto Anarcha and Delia like lye. Dr. Gibson had to call out loudly to be heard. He had attended duels, he said, including one where a man was killed, and Dr. Gibson was splashed with the man's blood and he had to secure the pistols in the confusing aftermath because the killed man was hit in the head, even though true gentlemen never aimed above the knee. Dr. Gibson told his students that he had once treated a man who had been attacked by a circus lion, and on another occasion he described for his students the U-shaped cut he made around the scrotum of a man suffering from gonorrhea, for easy castration. There was a case of mysterious bone growth in the face of a negro boy, and there was a case of a growth in the gut of an old negro that required removal despite an incomplete history that made a full diagnosis impossible.

Dr. Gibson talked a lot about the deep parts of women, about the uterus, which was where babies grew. The neck of the uterus was a remarkable thing, he said, because it contained an infinite number of glands and follicles, and there were many things that could go wrong with that part, the cervix, if it was not left in peace: bad baby deliveries, abortion, and even hardened feces could rub against the cervix through the wall of the rectum and irritate it, and this could cause many of the ailments to which the fairer sex was susceptible, despite the claims of the recent lecturer in Richmond who had said that the union of mind and matter was best exemplified by the nervous system of the human female. It was very mysterious, Dr. Gibson said, because while a highly talented and famous doctor might report a bad cervix in three percent of the cases he saw, another famous and talented doctor might examine the same group of women and decide that eighty percent had bad cervices. The problem was that a great many women—he gave the example of one who was thrown from a carriage, and afterward grew sad and depressed and lost a great deal of weight—refused to be examined in ways that violated their modesty.

Last, Dr. Gibson explained to his students that the new chloroform was the best agent to put patients to sleep for operations, better than ether, also new, because he had looked at 1,400 cases, and no one had died from chloroform. It killed pain instead, and increased the chance that the surgery would succeed. Delia would have glanced wryly at Anarcha when he said this. Surely even Delia could tell that Anarcha was not being cured, and they had both noticed that Anarcha coughed frequently now even though she wasn't sick. Also, just inside her vagina, Anarcha could feel her bladder bulging, like a stone clenched between her legs.

* * *

When Dr. Charles-Édouard Brown-Séquard arrived in Richmond, Anarcha knew at an instant that he wasn't any whiter than she was black. She was convinced now—because after the Westcott plantation she'd seen a lot of slaves and a lot of free blacks—that her father hadn't been her father after all, and she may not have known for sure who her father was but he was white. Dr. Brown-Séquard recognized the same thing; they weren't blood but they were similar, and he talked to her, though it took her a while to understand the way he spoke, which was like snippets of what she'd heard from the ladies on the steamboat on the Mississippi River. Dr. Brown-Séquard told her that for most of his life he'd been known as Edward Brown, like his father, but when his mother died he added her name, and then he added Charles too because in France it sounded like he had a title. Anarcha never had a title—and one name instead of four suited her just fine. Like Dr. Emmet and like all curious doctors, Dr. Brown-Séquard asked her questions about the experiments in Alabama, and now the experiments in Virginia, and he shook his head and muttered words in French that obviously weren't good words, and he asked her to cough, which she did, and it caused a fit of coughing and a little blood, and Dr. Brown-Séquard shook his head some more.

Dr. Gibson had given up on her by then, so Anarcha and Delia were tasked, after the cages were built, with caring for the animals that began to arrive, screeching and terrified. It was Anarcha's job to feed and water them, despite her lame leg and her cough and the bladder like a stone that wanted to come out of her. After almost six months, the first she saw of Richmond was when she and Delia wandered out to gather food for themselves and the animals, so they could be kept alive until Dr. Brown-Séquard did his experiments on them.

There weren't any grapevines in Richmond. But there were newspapers to carry stories, and there were negroes who could read them, free slaves who weren't free, or free blacks who really were free, though they could be sent away from the state if the mayor or the state chose to send them away. These free negroes had a three-year contract to stay in the city, but there had been talk of reducing the contract to one year ever since Nat Turner saw a signal in the sky to kill fifty white Virginians forty miles south of Richmond, two years before the night the stars fell. Sometimes one of the free blacks that weren't free but could read, or the free blacks that were free and could read, would sit on a corner on Cary Street and read aloud from the newspaper, and others that couldn't read would linger nearby to hear the news even if they didn't know the one reading, and Anarcha and Delia paused as they walked past, or just slowed down and walked very slowly, taking care to give way to white people for fear of being shoved aside by a walking stick. They were going to the basin, or the inland sea, as it was called, that ran along Cary Street between Eighth and Eleventh Streets, near the flour mills and tobacco warehouses. They gathered water, Delia carrying some in both hands and Anarcha carrying some in one hand, her cane in the other, and this was how they heard news of the mayor of Richmond, who sat behind a desk and ordered stripes for slaves. Twenty stripes for a slave named Thomas who cut a white man with a saw. Thirty stripes for Edward, who stole a box of shoes. Fifteen stripes for Malinda, who obtained six pounds of fresh pork under false pretenses. Twenty-five stripes for John Hill, who was impudent and used insolent lan-

> IMPUDENCE PUNISHED.—John Hill, a negro slave in the employ of Mr. P. L. Woodson, was brought before the Mayor, yesterday, and ordered twenty-five stripes, for using insolent and impertinent language to Messrs. Wm. B. Hopkins and P. B. Law, on two occasions.

guage. And twenty-five more, and prison as well, for Amanda, who conspired with another slave to escape but failed.

There was news of slaves who succeeded in running away too. Henry and James escaped from their jobs at a bakery. Moses Harris, known as the black doctor, hired himself out as a free man, and his master was fined ten dollars. A slave kidnapper was arrested for bringing a boy to Richmond from Washington City to be sold. And a seven-year-old boy named George was found hiding in a gentleman's packages. No one knew who he belonged to, so he was sent to the poorhouse.

A famous white man in the North, Horace Greeley, proposed ending slavery days by replacing cotton with flax. White men were arrested for cases of wife whipping, and storms raged through Richmond, bringing peals of lightning that purified the air. Newspapers advertised medicines, including Carter's Spanish Mixture for Scrofula, Dr. Bardotte's Worm Sugar Drops, Dr. Brainerd's treatment for blindness, Stabler's Diarrhea Cordial, and Dr. M'Lane's Celebrated Vermifuge for Tape Worms.

Dr. Brown-Séquard gave Anarcha money for feed for the animals. Anarcha and Delia walked through the city past the Exchange, Columbian, and American hotels, where white people stayed when they came off the ships, and their arrival was always announced in the newspapers too. They walked past the Odd Fellows Hall where there were exhibitions of moving dioramas, and Metropolitan Hall where there were productions of *The Virginia Cupids* and *Cocoanut Dance* or performances by Kunkel's Nightingale Minstrels, and these were also announced in the newspapers and on the street corners. Anarcha and Delia made their way to Rocketts Naval Yard or the First Street Market, which was where free blacks could make a living and see no white people apart from policemen, and while it was said that there were forty thousand people in Richmond, eighteen thousand slaves among them, Anarcha had never been in a place where there were only black people, save the slave quarters of the Rose Hill plantation of Henry Lucas in Alabama, but even there you always knew the master was nearby in the main house, sitting up and eating his supper and maybe spying out his glass windows at you, and drivers and overseers were always coming around to check for noise and runaways.

Goods even cheaper than at the markets could be bought in secret stores in Richmond, though there was talk that free blacks would soon be sold into slavery for trading on black markets. The confectionary shop on Thirteenth Street between Main and Franklin was one such store, as close to the Egyptian Building as Lumpkin's Jail, and though the owner of the confectionary store had been arrested twice he hadn't ever been convicted. Anarcha and Delia walked past the Tredegar Iron Works. They walked past rows of chained slaves being escorted by dealers, who always dressed in black, from train cars and canal boats to Lumpkin's Jail. They walked past the First African Baptist Church, where a different kind of court was held to show that black people weren't guilty of the crimes that white people convicted them of. They walked past black funeral processions: a hearse drawn by two horses, followed by hackney coaches and men dressed in foppish extravagance on saddle horses, and the black gentry following behind in French clothes—embroidered waistcoats, patent leather shoes, silk hats, resplendent brooches, and kid gloves. Sometimes this was the cast-off clothing of white people, and sometimes it had been purchased from the Jews. They walked past the prostitutes on Cary Street, both white and black, and they once saw Ann Maria Dean, madam of a brothel and the most famous and important black woman in Richmond, and not only was she free, it was said that the mayor liked Ann Maria even more than he liked the white prostitutes who worked for her.

The slaves and free blacks of Richmond had been afraid of the Egyptian Building even when it was just a place of medicine. Then the animals arrived, and rumors began to circulate about devilry in the Egyptian Building basement, because the screams of the animals could be heard clearly from the street. Dr. Brown-Séquard told Anarcha that he could not use the painkilling chloroform on animals, as had been used on her, because the screams of the animals and the twitching of their ears was how he knew a signal was traveling from their extremities to their cortex, and when he said "cortex" he tapped the side of his head so that Anarcha knew he meant brains. Anarcha and Delia were seen coming and going from the basement, and soon people were afraid of them too, and they could not go to the cook shops where black people worked and ate.

For several months, Anarcha cared for a cat that Dr. Brown-Séquard maimed by cutting its spine and stitching it back up, and she and Delia kept it alive by holding it like a baby and letting it suck on cloths dunked in milk. The cat lived for several months, which the doctor considered a great success. She assisted in his procedures, holding the animals as they clawed and spit and bit, and Dr. Brown-Séquard patted the dogs on the head and whistled lullabies as he cut into them. One evening, Anarcha stepped out from her room and found Dr. Brown-Séquard collapsed in a corner of the basement laboratory, unconscious, covered from head to toe with dark, fly-paper varnish. It took her an hour with sandpaper and alcohol to remove it. Dr. Brown-Séquard said he had been trying to prove something about the action of human skin.

* * *

Dr. Brown-Séquard disappeared. He did not say goodbye, did not even wave. For a time, it seemed that everyone forgot Anarcha and Delia and the animals in the Egyptian Building basement. Dr. Charles Bell Gibson, the janitor and the janitor's wife, and the nurses in the wards had long since stopped visiting the basement due to the smell and the noise and the rumors. Anarcha and Delia might have slipped out into the city, might have run away, though of course Anarcha wouldn't have been running at all but limping with her cane. But she did not run away, because how far could a crippled woman get, with a girl to slow her down, and rewards printed in the paper, and dogs trained to track them? Anyway, she couldn't leave the animals trapped in their cages, to die. After a few days, when it was clear that Dr. Brown-Séquard was not going to return and there would be no more money for food for the animals or for Anarcha and Delia, she decided to release the animals—not the chickens, as they could eat the chickens, and not the rabbits or the raccoon for the same reason, and though she'd eaten many strange dead animals in the woods she wouldn't eat a cat or a dog, the kind of animal that would lick your hand.

She would release the animals slowly, otherwise it might be noticed. After a week, she carried the ravens' cage outside and opened its latch, and one raven hopped up on top of the wooden lattice and waited for the other to hop up as well, and then they took to the air and flew off together south, toward the James River, just as if they hadn't been locked in a cage in a basement for five months.

Next, she released the magpies, and the single jay that remained, and what was left of the pigeons, and she and Delia watched the birds ascend to freedom in bursts of feathers and sometimes a squawk or a coo. For the remainder of the animals, she waited until nighttime. She started with the cats—there were many cats—and she released them not outside but near the open door, and the cats were hesitant and weak and hissed when she picked up their cages, and when the latch was released and the door of the cage was open it took them a while to sniff the free air and tiptoe with careful, silent steps to the doorway, and then suddenly they slipped out into the night as though they had effected their own escape. She released one dog, which ran off abruptly toward the baying of other dogs far off in the city, and she planned to release the other dog the following night.

That day, however, a man in a crisp uniform entered the basement.

He was clean-shaven, like Dr. Sims, not shaggy on the neck like Dr. Gibson and Dr. Brown-Séquard. He had a limp and a cane, as Anarcha did. The brass buttons of his uniform shone in the dim basement light, and there were gold tassels on the shoulders of his coat that were of a sort she had never seen before, and at first she thought he was a policeman who would take her to the mayor for stripes, for releasing the animals. She began to calculate whether Delia would have enough food to survive by herself in the basement until Anarcha returned after her stripes. But the man did not apprehend her. He rooted around in the basement storage and asked Anarcha some questions about her leg and her limp. She explained a little, and like Dr. Emmet and Dr. Gibson and Dr. Brown-Séquard, it started to seem like the man knew who she was. He did not even ask her name. The newspapers or grapevines of white people had spread stories everywhere. Like Dr. Emmet, the man said aloud the name Dr. J. Marion Sims.

He left, and Anarcha stopped releasing the animals just in case, and she wrung the neck of a chicken and she and Delia survived on its limp meat for almost a week before the man returned, in a rush. He told her that she had been purchased. She and Delia were now owned by a man named Lieutenant Lewis Maury—not the man in the uniform—but he would take her to a place where she would meet her new master soon, and perhaps her new missus. There were some other things to be done first, the man said. Speed was of the essence. She should gather whatever things she had, as they would leave Richmond in the morning. He departed the basement.

Anarcha felt a weight lift from her, like the birds flying to freedom. Her leg wouldn't last, the stone between her thighs felt like it would fall out of her, her cough was persistent and the blood came and went, and even if she wrung the necks of all the animals in the basement, the meat wouldn't have lasted forever. How would she have gone on providing for Delia until Delia could provide for herself?

That night—because once they left, no one would again come to the basement of the Egyptian Building—Anarcha released all the animals that remained. The dog and the raccoon and the marmots first, and then the rabbits, the chickens, and even the mice. The animals rushed off into the dangerous night, to hunt or be hunted, to starve or be killed, but to be free for a day or an hour or a moment.

* * *

The man's name was also Maury, he was cousin to her new master. They were both sailors and lieutenants in the navy. This Lieutenant Maury was full of anxious energy, and he arrived at the Egyptian Building in the morning and hurried them to the train station, explaining on the way that they would take the train to Charlottesville, where he would give a talk to students and retrieve his young second cousin. The four of them would then travel to Washington City. They would stay the night in a building where there was a large glass for looking at stars, and in the morning the Maury cousin would take her by train back to Fredericksburg, and from there they would travel fifteen miles south by coach, to where she would live and wait for her new master.

He had a coach waiting for them outside the Egyptian Building. Delia looked back once at their strange home. Anarcha did not. On the train, Lieutenant Maury explained to the conductor that his nurse and his nurse's daughter had to travel with him because he was lame. Here was his cane as proof. The conductor frowned and glanced at Anarcha's similar cane, but out of respect for Lieutenant Maury's uniform he did not make Anarcha and Delia go to the part of the train where slaves and free blacks sat.

As the train began to move, Lieutenant Maury produced a sheaf of papers from his breast pocket and spent a long time looking through them, shuffling the pages and muttering aloud words and phrases written there, ignoring the white passengers who scowled at Anarcha and Delia but who, like the conductor, chose not to intervene on account of Lieutenant Maury's impressive blue uniform with buttons and tassels. One man recognized Lieutenant Maury, and excused himself to say that he had enjoyed the lieutenant's book very much. The men shook hands and chatted about three comets recorded in the year 1854, including one named for Euphrosyne, goddess of cheer, joy, and mirth. They went on excitedly about the sea, and the stars, and a display of aurora they both recalled from the year 1847, when a band of luminous matter scudded across the heavens very quickly, nearly blotting out Castor, the second-brightest star in the zodiac. Lieutenant Maury cheerfully noted an oddity. The star that was named for one of the twin sons of Zeus was itself a pair of twins, a binary star system. The stranger smiled, shook his head at the quirky majesty of the universe, and moved on.

Anarcha and Delia were sitting across from Lieutenant Maury, and they had little else to look at but the man in his uniform. He was revered by others, they knew now. Lieutenant Maury glanced between them for a moment, then returned to his papers. He had made only a moment's progress when a thought—a thought that would have been inevitable to a man who studied the stars—seemed to occur to him.

Had Anarcha been alive and in Alabama on the night of November 13, 1833, the night the stars fell? Like everyone who witnessed them, Anarcha would have remembered that night very well. If no one had previously asked her about the falling stars, this was the moment when all the stories she remembered could come falling out of her, in turn. Yes, she'd been alive but very young, she said. She remembered that children had laughed at the sight while their parents cried and prayed, and she remembered that she had known, though she was only Delia's age then, that the world wasn't ending. If you looked closely, she said, you could see that some of the stars weren't falling at all. They were fixed behind the moving ones. Maybe the night of the falling stars was not a warning of the end of all things, Anarcha said, but only the end of some particular thing. She didn't know what thing was ending. But weren't things always ending? Maybe it was slavery days that were ending, as the slaves and free blacks in the streets of Richmond had sometimes said.

She couldn't remember the last time she had spoken so long, particularly to a white man. She recalled Pheriba as she spoke. In the middle of her speech, she had stopped looking at Lieutenant Maury. When she finished, the train thrummed and churned. Lieutenant Maury gazed at her for a long moment, and then tapped his papers into a neat pile on his knee. He said there was something in Washington City he wished to show her.

In Charlottesville, Lieutenant Maury gave a speech to a literary society of students. Again, he used the ruse of his lame leg to bring Anarcha and Delia into the hall where he spoke. They were ushered to a balcony like the cramped upstairs row of seats where slaves sat in white churches in Alabama.

Lieutenant Maury preached to the gathered students about the glory of Virginia and America, goodly lands with wide fields, bright skies, and free people. American youths, he said, had an advantage over European youths in that they had no prejudice of class to overcome. A young man's superiors were those who had won their superiority with industry and virtue—hence the responsibilities of freemen. Young men should read newspapers, he advised, so as to acquaint themselves with the affairs of state and with the welfare of their society.

It was allowed that New York had beaten Virginia in the race for power and greatness, Lieutenant Maury said. But had it not been the South that sent the first steamship across the ocean? Did not the first locomotive blow its whistle into the warm air of a southern day? The wealth of the four largest of the nation's original states told the story. In 1850, the average value of property held by Virginians was $427, compared to $234 for New Yorkers. In Georgia, it was $652, compared to $232 in Pennsylvania. The difference could hardly be explained in terms of slavery alone. The question now was whether New York's reputation for civic improvement indicated a more enterprising native spirit among the Yankees. The battle was not finished, Lieutenant Maury said. The future would be won by those who mastered the material agencies of steam, the telegraph, and the printing press.

A great deal could be learned, he called out in conclusion, from careful study of the heavens. Viewed through a telescope, the passage of a simple star across the celestial meridian is exquisite, lovely, sublime. Such observations, however, reveal far more than the matter and the makeup of nature. The great law of the universe is progress, Lieutenant Maury said. Just as stars cannot keep their place and must always push forward, so should today's graduates recognize that their own progress is not complete. To stop learning is to forget all that you have already learned. To cease in the eternal quest of one's own forward motion is to be like a planet that is hurled backward toward its destruction.

* * *

Lieutenant Maury owned only a single slave in Washington City, an old woman who cooked for his family. Anarcha and Delia were shown to the old woman's room, where they would sleep the night on the floor. Delia was left with the cook while Lieutenant Maury hurried Anarcha off to show her what he wished to show her.

The home was connected to the observatory, which was a large building with a round dome on top, like a cake that had baked and risen. The lieutenant took them outside, where it was already night. He gestured up at the Seven Pointers. What do slaves call the Big Dipper? he asked. The Seven Pointers, Anarcha said. Then he pointed again and asked what slaves called the constellation Orion. Ellen Yards, she said. She explained that slaves used both of the constellations to count time at night, and to find passage through dark forests in winter. Ell and yards, Lieutenant Maury articulated slowly, and he produced a notebook to write down what she'd told him.

He took her inside and explained that the whole of the building was about understanding the stars—a house for the heavens. A glass was really a telescope, he said, which was really a transit instrument, and he admitted that late at night, when his assistants had grown weary of nocturnal vigil, he came here alone to view the vault above, sparkling with brilliants, like a sheet of black cloth inset with diamonds.

He showed her the observatory's peculiar clocks. The Kessel clock in his office. The Molyneaux clock. And the Frodsham clock that featured a compensated pendulum with a knife-edge index that swayed between globules of mercury, which were connected by wires to a galvanic battery that served as a registering apparatus. Deep in the night, Lieutenant Maury said, he enjoyed the eternal dead beat of the clocks, their pendula clicking the escapements ever forward like the footsteps of time. With the clocks, he could predict the appearance of a star, invisible without the glass, as it marched to the music of the spheres, sliding ahead along its invisible wire.

They moved into the telescope room. The telescope looked nothing like a glass, Anarcha thought. It looked like a cannon aimed at heaven. Lieutenant Maury spoke as he consulted books and clocks, making careful calculations and adjusting the aim of the telescope accordingly. Though vast, he said, stars were like babies. The firmament was their mother. Sometimes stars were born singularly, sometimes they came in twins and triplets. As God had told Abram, Lieutenant Maury said, the infinite stars numbered the descendants that had been promised to the chosen people.

The stars ignore our existence, he said. The great irony of astronomy, which is the scientific study of the heavens, is that the vast progress civilization has made in its understanding of space had done nothing to diminish its awe. Nor had the legends and myths associated with individual stars been snuffed out. Today, we see the stars just as Job and the patriarch and the apostles saw them. The wing of the bird and the flaming path of the comet are each adjusted with equal nicety, and this is how we know the world is not designed by chance. Just as the stars pass predictably overhead, so did God compel ravens to carry bread and flesh to the prophet Elijah on the brook Cherith, east of the river Jordan.

His tuning of the telescope was complete. He looked at the clock and consulted his scribbled calculations. He motioned for Anarcha to put her eye to a small lens. At first, she saw only darkness. But then a roundish light appeared, blue in color, like the moon but smaller and brighter, moving steadily through her field of vision. She watched until it passed from one side to the next, and looked up at Lieutenant Maury.

The stars are always falling, he said.

Sixteen

Samuel Gilbert—Articles—Planning the lecture—Newspapers—
Stuyvesant Hall

IN JUNE 1849, AT ROUGHLY THE SAME MOMENT SIMS AT LAST SUCCEEDED
in closing one of Anarcha's fistulae, former Mississippi governor Tilgh-
man Tucker, who had retired to his Louisiana plantation, Cottonwood,
noticed a small growth on his face. Wedged between his nose and cheek,
the tumor resisted the treatment of several eminent physicians and grew
steadily over the course of the summer. After six months, Governor
Tucker traveled to New Orleans to visit a medical man with a mysterious cure for cysts, lumps, and excrescences of all kinds. This practitioner,
Samuel Gilbert, was not a regular member of the profession. In fact, many
considered him a quack. Even then, licensed physicians were lobbying the
Louisiana legislature to pass laws that would put so-called doctors like
Gilbert out of business.

By the time Governor Tucker arrived at Gilbert's clinic, the entire area
from the corner of his eye to the end of his nose had become a single lump
of fetid flesh. A new growth had sprouted on the opposite side of his face
as well. Gilbert pronounced it a case of eating cancer. He set about treating it with a procedure known only to himself—one that did not in any
way require the use of a knife. Within four weeks, the Governor's face was
entirely healed.

Sims first heard of Gilbert's practice, and of the case of Governor
Tucker, when he visited New Orleans for his ailing bowel and bought the

fistulous slave to take back to Montgomery for experiments. Professionally speaking, the governor's celebrity made him a good catch for Gilbert: flouting the ethical impropriety of medical publicity, Gilbert arranged for the details of Tucker's case to be printed in the *Daily Delta*. Controversy erupted when the *Delta* also printed accusations that Gilbert's cure was false. Rumors spread that Governor Tucker had already departed the corporeal realm. This played right into Gilbert's hands: the *Delta* was forced to print a retraction. Governor Tucker was not only hale and hearty, the editors wrote, he had recently visited the newspaper's offices. Unbelievers were welcome to visit him whenever they wished. Governor Tucker died several years later, not yet sixty years of age, likely succumbing to the cancer that Gilbert had never truly cured. Yet for years he lived on as a prominent citizen who offered scrutiny-tested evidence of the effectiveness of Gilbert's knife-free cancer cure.

Public accounts of the method were never specific, but all serious physicians knew that Gilbert was using caustics—sticks of silver or potassium nitrate—to chemically cauterize and melt away diseased tissue. Caustics had long been a mitigating treatment for cancers of the uterus and other female afflictions. Gilbert believed wholeheartedly in the authenticity of his method, and that was his appeal. Few of his patients were cured, but all were given the impression of effective treatment. It was even probable, Sims thought, that some of them experienced a measure of relief.

More instructive than the medicine—as Sims planned his own hospital—was Gilbert's business acumen. He offered free services to thousands of poor patients. When a particularly horrific and malignant tumor presented itself, he advertised operations that would be conducted before audiences of the doubtful. Charity cases made for compelling stories. He cured tumors of the eyelids in a slave of a feeble widow who had no other servant. He cured an ulcer that had collapsed the right lung of a boy who begged his way from Tennessee to Louisiana for treatment. Celebrated members of society were even more valuable. Captain Miguel Lopez was cured, after his liberation in Cuba, of a growth that began as a pungent sensation in the lower left corner of his mouth. Wealthy landowners from Texas and Alabama signed their names to breathless tributes to the eminent skill of Samuel Gilbert.

The key, Sims noted, was that it was all in the service of charging exorbitant prices to those who could afford it, and who could not find relief from licensed practitioners of medicine.

* * *

In 1852, Gilbert established an office in Memphis. He now offered cures for scrofulas—tuberculosis of the lymphatic glands—and chronic female complaints, in addition to a new cancer method that enabled him to treat even deeply seated tumors, if taken in proper time. Gilbert moved again the following year, to New York, just as Sims also was arriving in the city. A newspaper article retold the whole of the Governor Tucker episode, inoculating Gilbert against criticism. Another article boasted of the cure of a patient whose affliction had foiled eighteen years of attention from Jefferson Medical College's latest professor of surgery, the famous Dr. Mutter. Gilbert derided the amputations that were performed by the regular medical profession. He boasted of complete cures in eight out of ten cases. His business thrived, but the profession refused to accept him. Licensed doctors who were found to be in league with "Gilbert & Co." were shunned, socially banished, and denied acclaim.

Before Henri Stuart appeared in New York, diarrhea and bitterness had left Sims physically depleted and emotionally fragile. He'd been every bit as abused as the cancer quack. But while the quack realized a fortune in a clinic on Broadway, Sims suffered. His fistula method had been lifted from him by unscrupulous physicians, to cure paying patients they had been seeing in private practice for years. He'd been left flailing toward poverty, with a paucity of patients, mostly women complaining of painful menses. He had been treating them with the guaiacum tincture of Dr. Dewees, who claimed that his mixture prevented the buildup of a particular uterine membrane, enabling the free flow of menstrual matter. The mixture's downside was that its odor was even more noxious than the smell of urine and waste leaking from the vaginas of Sims's fistula patients. He was never able to compel a woman to persevere with it.

Sims's health deteriorated until he formed foot drop, like Anarcha and the others. Twice, he collapsed in the streets of New York. On one occasion he was mistaken for a drunk. On another, only his stiff top hat saved him from a frightful injury.

He continued writing his own story, as Barnum proposed, though he had no access to newspapers—and such a publication might have gotten him censured. Instead, he published accounts of fistula surgeries in New York medical journals, detailing cases that had come to him in Alabama, after he cured Anarcha, or were offered to him in New York. In January 1854, the *New York Medical Gazette and Journal of Health* published two cases. The first was a tiny slave named Amy, aged sixteen. It was the only time Sims cured a woman with a single surgery, and she was thus enabled to return to her master's plantation and wifely duties. The second was a forty-year-old white woman who was unable to bear the knee-chest position but was cured regardless, only to die a short time later of undelivered placenta. The following month, the *American Medical Monthly* published a remarkable case in which Sims found that the cervix of a middle-aged white woman from Wetumpka was poking through her fistula, emptying its monthly matter directly into her bladder. Her parts resisted all efforts to return them to their natural orientation. As her cycles would end soon anyway, Sims opted to accept the artificial diversion, and closed her fistula around the neck of the misplaced cervix.

Last, just before Sims met Henri Stuart, he finished the writing of a piece for the *New York Medical Times* about the valvular fistula case he had cured for Valentine Mott. He added the detail that the fistula was the product of a twenty-four-hour labor that resulted in craniotomy on a baby that weighed twelve pounds even after its brain was removed.

* * *

Stuart claimed that a public lecture would transform Sims from a beggar to a dictator. That would be fine, Sims thought, as long as a charity hospital established his reputation for procedures he could charge handsomely for in private practice, like the cancer quacks.

Stuart was younger than Sims, but for all his worldliness and confidence in plotting to navigate the city's juggernaut of power, he made Sims feel like a child. In the moment following his claim that Sims would be a dictator, Stuart produced a small almanac filled with his indecipherable scrawl. Flipping through the weeks, Stuart recited a host of public meetings, anniversary celebrations, and official gatherings that they should take care to avoid in planning a lecture to announce Sims's hospital. He chose May 18, still a month away, to ensure as large a crowd as possible. It was well before the gentry of New York would begin scattering to summer resorts and Europe. In the morning, he said, he would travel to Broadway and Bond to rent the lecture hall of the Stuyvesant Institute, then famous for an ongoing exhibition of more than two thousand Egyptian antiquities.

Stuart asked for paper and ink to draw a sketch of an invitation card that he would have printed and delivered across the city. Once again, Sims broached the subject of the expense. This time, he noted that the hospital would in all probability result in lucrative business for himself. Could Sims offer Stuart interest in a partnership?

Stuart did not look up from his intense sketching. He repeated that the expense was not a concern. However, he said, there was something Sims could do for him. A favor. An appreciation. He asked that two beds in Sims's hospital be reserved for cases that were judged by himself to be— he searched for the proper word—deserving.

Sims did not reply. Only then did Stuart twist his head to look the doctor in the eye.

I shall never ask anything of you unless I need it, he said. But then—if you can—grant it.

The request remained a mystery for month, until the day prior to the lecture. Stuart arrived at Sims's home unannounced, early in the morning, and brusquely instructed Sims to gather his coat and hat. They would be visiting the places of business of a variety of newspapers, he said. It was the ease of access that Stuart had to the offices of the city's great media men, and their familiarity with him, that told Sims all he needed to know about why Stuart might wish to have access to beds in a hospital for women. Sims resolved never to speak of it again. But he did offer up a tepid objection to Stuart's plan to visit the newspapers. He explained that the medical community frowned on brazen self-promotion. Sims thought the stricture foolish, he said, but what if no one came to the lecture because it had been advertised?

Stuart scoffed, waving a hand to hurry Sims into a hackney. It was not advertising if they did not pay for it, he explained. And they would not pay a cent! If doctors objected, Stuart said, Sims should simply tell them that he had been played for a fool by a craven newspaperman, like a card in a game of whist. But that would not happen. Only the naïve were unaware that doctors all over the city jostled like chickens to find journalists to write about their procedures and surgeries. Stuart winked, as though he was somehow aware that the week before Sims had met with a writer from the *American Phrenological Journal*.

When Stuart revealed the day's first stop, Sims choked on a lump in his throat: they were to call on Horace Greeley, the influential editor of the *New-York Tribune*. Sims had glimpsed presidents from afar and he had rubbed shoulders with senators, but he had rarely encountered a great man so perfectly poised to advance his own career. Greeley had served a term in Congress, and it was said that he would one day seek the highest office in the land. In the hackney, Stuart instructed Sims to speak to the media men as plainly and clearly about his plan as he had a month ago at his home. But as they ascended the stairs to the *Tribune*'s offices, a thought gave Stuart pause. He took Sims by the elbow. It was best, he explained, if they steered clear of the subject of slavery. Greeley was an abolitionist, and Stuart had assisted him with his abolitionist efforts. The subject should be avoided entirely. Sims nodded. Also, Stuart added, don't mention Vanderbilt. The two men were great enemies. Sims nodded again. And don't mention Henry Raymond, either, Stuart said, or the *New York Times*, or any of the *Tribune*'s competitors, most of whom they would be seeing that day. Sims nodded once more, and Stuart nodded a confirmation in reply.

The *Tribune*'s offices smelled of ink and sweat and teemed with harried writers and young pages weaving haphazardly through a warren of desks. They were shown at once into Greeley's office, which was notably small. Greeley's bald pate and crown, with wispy strings of hair hanging from his temples and from the back of his head to his shoulders, recalled the shiny dome and storied locks of Benjamin Franklin. Greeley's desk faced the wall; he faced the desk. He did not divert his attention from a printed galley sheet. Stuart moved alongside him and announced that this man Sims here was to deliver a lecture, tomorrow evening, on the origin of an enterprise that was surely to be of great benefit to humanity. At this, Greeley gave the diminutive Sims a doubtful glance. Stuart prompted Sims to explain, but he made very little progress in his story—he arrived only at the first utterance of "suffering womanhood"—when Greeley interrupted to instruct Stuart to write out whatever notice he wished and send it in. Back out into the newsroom, Stuart scribbled four or five lines

DR. SIMS ON A SPECIAL HOSPITAL.—Dr. J. MARION SIMS, late of Montgomery, Alabama, proposes, at the solicitation of members of the medical profession and others, to lay before the charitable of this City the propriety and necessity of building a hospital to be specially devoted to the treatment of the diseases peculiar to females. He will deliver an address on this subject this Thursday evening, at 8 o'clock, at the Stuyvesant Institute, No. 659 Broadway. Physicians and others acquainted with the professional standing of Dr. SIMS, will not be likely to remain absent.

onto a stray scrap of paper and placed it on top of a stack of copy carried by a weary-looking page boy.

Their next stop was the office of Henry Raymond. Raymond had once written for Greeley, but then, with the help of a banker, he'd broken off to found the *New York Times*. The *Times* was smaller, but its high moral tone made it influential in some quarters, Stuart explained. This time, Stuart told Sims not to mention Greeley, and not to mention his own southern heritage, though there was little they could do about his manner. The meeting went off much like the terse exchange with Greeley—Raymond gave Sims a sidelong glance when he noticed the lilt of his accent—and the result was the same: a quickly scrawled notice that would appear on the front page of tomorrow's newspaper.

Next was Frank Leslie of *Frank Leslie's Illustrated Newspaper*. The man was as much a Barnum as Barnum, and Sims resolved to befriend him, if he had the chance. Then came Frederic Hudson of the *New York Herald*, and Benjamin Day of the *Sun* on Publishing House Square. They crisscrossed the city to a total of fifteen publications, in each case gaining the audience of powerful men who received Stuart casually, as though his presence was regular and expected. Sims told a truncated version of the story he intended to deliver the following evening. As Stuart suggested—and as he had begun to do in his own papers—he emphasized the heroism and valor of his experimental subjects in Alabama, to offset the concerns of editors who might be wary of the sensitivities of their northern, abolitionist readership. In repeated, condensed retellings, Sims found that his story required a single prominent figure. As both his first patient and his first cure, Anarcha became the story's heroine.

Sims knew only fragments of the experiments that Anarcha was now being subjected to in Richmond. He had been right to trust that Charles Bell Gibson was a man vigorous enough not to shrink at human trials, but Sims had received only a single report detailing Anarcha's condition. Gibson was having difficulty. He was using chloroform, and that was a problem because an unconscious woman could not assume the knee-chest position that inflated the vagina. Sims sent along instructions for the left-lateral position he'd begun using on white patients, like the woman from Wetumpka, but he doubted it would work for complicated fistulae. Also, Gibson was having problems with the sheer number of experiments Anarcha had already endured. With each procedure, additional freshenings of the edges of the wound caused the fistula between Anarcha's vagina and her bladder to grow. Anarcha's uterus was prolapsing, and her bladder was threatening to push through her fistula into her vagina.

Given that she was now critical to Sims's story, Anarcha would eventually have to be dealt with. But she wasn't Sims's only problem. Doctors performing his surgery were reporting publicly that his clamp suture had required alterations to answer the needs of individual cases. They spoke glowingly of Sims, but the implication was clear: his device—the thing that was to make his name—was inadequate. Charles Pope heaped praise on Sims, but only for simple fistulae. He published a detailed account of a botched Sims procedure on a fistula that Sims had told him was inoperable. Even Bozeman, Sims's assistant in Alabama, had betrayed him with a piece in the *New Orleans Medical and Surgical Journal* that two-facedly celebrated Sims's victory while asserting that his method had been beset by difficulties.

The stakes of the lecture couldn't be higher. It was a final chance to build a lucrative career on the success of the clamp suture, and it was an opportunity to at last succeed in the eyes of family, friends, and acquaintances from South Carolina and Alabama, a number of whom had visited him in New York.

His quirky old teacher J. F. G. Mittag had turned up in Alabama several years before, to execute a series of portraits. After watching Sims operate, Mittag moved on to Tennessee, where he was proud to serve on a railroad commission with the navy man and self-made scientist Lieutenant Matthew Fontaine Maury. Mittag visited Sims again in New York, and Sims introduced him to the reporter from the *American Phrenological Journal*, who was impressed by Mittag's ability to locate morbid conditions in the human organization. For feature stories on both men—the magazine printed speculative profiles, like the writings of those who read the future in the movement of stars—Sims and Mittag posed for ambrotypes by a highly regarded photographer, Mathew Brady. Sims, however, balked at Brady's first likeness of him. He arranged for the man to do it again.

Josiah Nott visited too, on the occasion of the publication of his magnum opus, *Types of Mankind*. As the country had edged closer and closer to conflict over slavery, Nott had become more and more popular. He was now a vigorous defender of the supremacy of the white race. God had made the slave, he said, and no Yankee could bleach him.

Nott was followed by Reverend Milburn, the frontier preacher and adventurer, whose family Sims had treated in Montgomery. Milburn's most recent book included "An Hour's Talk About Women," in which he lamented the habits of girls between sixteen and twenty, preoccupied with their toilet. Enough time was wasted before the looking glass, Milburn wrote, as might acquaint them with the masters of classical literature. Beautiful feet were purchased at the price of bodily torpor. Woman should neither repose nor strive to keep up with man's triumphal procession. Light, heat, electricity, and galvanism had been made man's captives, chained to his galloping chariot. Woman should aspire to fulfill the duties of a lowlier sphere, whereby she would be advanced to one higher.

Sims's old friend Thornwell visited as well. After the young minister had convinced Theresa's mother to allow her daughter to marry Sims, Thornwell had become a professor and was now president of their alma mater, Columbia College. He had become a fire-breathing advocate of secession. Thornwell claimed that the position of the South was now like that of Greece, with the five millions of Xerxes stacked on the borders of the Attic peninsula. If the North was permitted to ravage, as Louis XIV had done in the Rhine Valley at the end of the seventeenth century, the wives and daughters of the South would find themselves subjected to brutal lusts. The slave would disappear like the red man. The whole country would become a blackened and smoking desert. If the South failed on the battlefield, Thornwell preached, they should fall back to guerilla resistance—every pass a Thermopylae, every plain a Marathon.

Sims agreed, but his own contribution to the scuffle would be advanced through the wealth and influence that would be bestowed upon him by the opening of his hospital for women. Of his visitors, the most pertinent and inspiring toward that effort was Henry Hilliard, the Alabama congressman whom Sims befriended only after he'd cured Anarcha. Hilliard was as resolved as Thornwell, but he took a more measured tone on the floor of Congress. He famously warned, just before he retired in 1850, that the South had a deep and settled feeling on the subject of slavery. Legislators should not suffer men whose vocation it was to agitate fatal measures. Like Barnum, Hilliard knew the value of a story. He advised Sims to one day pen his autobiography. But of more immediate use to Sims was the draft of a speech that Hilliard shared when he visited New York in 1854. "Woman—Her True Sphere" would be delivered in a few weeks' time, in Georgia, to the graduates of the LaGrange Female College.

The Bible tells us of the glories of the sun, the moon, and the stars, Hilliard wrote. But even more than God's book, it was the new science of the heavens, and what ingenuity had discovered of the object-crowded universe—the sublime scenery in which great constellations run their course—that best revealed the harmony that nature prescribes for woman in relation to man. Man is the sun. Woman is the morning star, glittering in pure and tranquil beauty. Man is formed for exploits. Woman is formed to celebrate them, and to illustrate the delights of home by sweet example. Instances when a man prefers the lute to his duty, or when a woman attempts to press into the empire that belongs exclusively to man—these incursions spoil the harmony of heaven and never fail to disgust. It is not because woman is inferior that she must not take part in the great affairs of the world, it is because she is more beautiful in her own gentle dominion. Woman has her own orbit, and she obeys it. She does not compel. She attracts, like the great spheres that populate dark, distant skies.

* * *

The power of the press was never made clearer to Sims than on the morning of his lecture, when fifteen notices in fifteen newspapers put his name before the entire city. Valentine Mott, who had told him he would fail, appeared at Sims's door before noon. He apologized for having doubted Sims's plan. He saw now that a hospital for women would most surely succeed.

Clouds rolled in that afternoon. Throughout the day, Sims tinkered with the draft of his speech, starting with Hilliard's characterization of women as tiny, brilliant morning stars. Investing his voice with Barnum's luster and pathos, Sims would say that the delicate twinkle of a woman's beauty was snuffed out by the scourge of fistula. The affliction that had frustrated the Old World for centuries had now been mastered not by a northern doctor, nor by a southern one, but by an American who offered salvation to depressed and afflicted women who were all too anxious to return to the service of their homes and their marriages. Beyond fistula, Sims would ask his audience, what other horrific female conditions might the physicians of a new hospital conquer for the glory of American medicine? Were not our lunatic asylums stuffed with women who had been left barren and nervous due to diseases that left them unable to fulfill their most natural duty? What honors awaited the doctors of the next generation, Sims would say, if they were afforded the chance to train and study in an institution dedicated to restoring celestial gleam to tarnished members of the more fragile sex?

At six o'clock, a great rain hammered the city, muddying every thoroughfare and ensuring, Sims feared, that his talk would draw only a light audience of naysayers and doctors anxious to steal his method. Stuart arrived at Sims's home in the midst of the downpour. He was untroubled by it, even as he had to raise his voice to be heard over the sheets of rain smacking the flooded streets.

They left for the Stuyvesant Institute early, to see that the hall was properly lighted. Sims took a seat near the podium to wait, glancing back occasionally as the doctors began to arrive. First they came in twos and threes, and then there was a steady stream of physicians, some saying good evening as they stepped past Sims, unaware that he was to be the speaker. He saw Elizabeth Blackwell in the audience, sitting with a young companion. It was said that Blackwell's sister Emily was studying in Scotland with the famous inventor of chloroform, James Simpson. Simpson, Sims had read, was experimenting with a surgery on the cervical canal—Sims was keen to attempt it. Thomas and Catherine Emmet approached to greet Sims warmly before they took their seats. Emmet was a concern. He knew that Anarcha had not been fully cured, and in a moment, Sims would be speaking at length about Anarcha. Emmet knew nothing of her progress in Richmond, but there was little that could be done about it now. The audience, swelling to the hundreds, contained members of all of New York's feuding medical cliques: the University Medical College, the New York Medical College, the College of Physicians and Surgeons. As the hour of the talk approached, the crowd murmured surprise at the sight of men known to be hostile to one another agreeing to sit in the same room.

For all his confidence as a planner, Stuart now appeared nervous. The size of the crowd, proof of his skills as a promoter, disturbed him. Sims had assumed that Stuart would rise to introduce him. But at the appointed time, Stuart only nudged him and nodded him toward the podium. The odd man feared speaking in public! Sims was nervous too, but there was no choice other than to simply begin. It was the final, critical moment of a plan nine years in the making, since the delivery of Anarcha's baby. Nine years of suffering—more if the speech were to fail.

He rose and assumed the podium. The audience did not acknowledge him at first, and Sims tapped the pages of his speech and adjusted his candle. He looked out into the dim room and recalled for a moment the night of his medical school days when his candle blew out in the dissection room in South Carolina. He had stood alone in the dark, in a dead room filled with lifeless, headless slaves. He had showed mettle then, and he would do so now.

Seventeen

*Nathan Bozeman—Fordyce Barker—Hospital boards—
Elizabeth Blackwell—Sarah Platt Doremus—The Board of Lady
Managers—First patients—Bridget Headley—First anniversary*

BY 1878, DR. NATHAN BOZEMAN WAS GRATIFIED TO HAVE SEEN HIMSELF described in European newspapers as "the greatest gynecologist in the world." Bozeman first traveled to Europe to demonstrate surgeries in 1858. In Coburg, Germany, he was invited boar hunting with Ernest II, Duke of Saxe-Coburg and Gotha. Bozeman and the duke took up positions on a forest scaffold, opening fire as the boars appeared between the trees. Bozeman was about to fell his sixth animal when one of the duke's attendants stayed his rifle. Each man had shot five boars. The duke should be permitted to shoot the most.

Years later, a painting of the scene hung in Bozeman's dining room in New York City. By then, he was on the staff of Woman's Hospital, founded by his onetime business partner Dr. J. Marion Sims. Bozeman and Sims, however, had been sworn enemies since 1856. And in 1874, Sims had been ejected from the hospital he created.

Bozeman was the ninth child of a family of Dutch descent. Bozemans had moved through Maryland, North Carolina, and Georgia and pressed on to Alabama—first in Butler County, then Coosa County, north of Montgomery, and then Autauga County, where they were neighbors to E. Y. Fair, Dr. Nathan Harris, and John Duncan of the Violet Hill plantation.

Bozeman was a large man, and he had been a large boy with a ruddy face. One day on the playground of the one-room schoolhouse where he took lessons from Reverend McAlplin, the minister inexplicably asked the young Bozeman if he wished one day to become a doctor. He never considered any other career.

He studied medicine in Kentucky, working with the famous Dr. Gross. He wrote his thesis on the hard, often fatal tumors of the body known as scirrhus. During a yearlong period of study with Gross after graduation—he administered chloroform for the doctor's operations—Bozeman delivered the anesthesia for the first successful case of anesthetized ovariotomy in America.

In 1848, Bozeman's father died in Autauga County. The family's slaves were left to his wife and daughters. Twenty-nine-year-old Silbey went to sister Ann. Twenty-five-year-old Claresy went to sister Elizabeth. Twenty-one-year-old Ester went to sister Martha. Sister Harriet received sixteen-year-old Lucy. Dick, Nancy, Tam, and Harry remained with the widow. Bozeman was left cows, a set of bedroom furniture, and the horse and saddle he'd already been given on loan.

In 1849, he moved to Montgomery, intending to set up a general practice. The medical community was preoccupied with the name of Dr. Sims, who after years of toil had succeeded in curing a case of vesico-vaginal fistula. There were rumors: Sims was a poor steward of money; he was hostile to the emerging trend toward medical ethics. Bozeman didn't fault Sims for his ambition, as some did—Bozeman was ambitious too—but he was as troubled as any by rumors that Sims had gained his success with the clinical assistance of the slave women who were his patients.

Equally troubling—as word went out that Sims was now seeking an assistant physician—was the fact that his success could not be corroborated. Many Montgomery doctors had witnessed Sims's early efforts, and they recalled the slaves upon whom Sims had experimented. By the time of the triumph, however, the physicians of Montgomery had left him. Sims's obsession with glory and notoriety had caused him to sacrifice honor, it was thought. Only the slaves had witnessed the historic surgery, and no doctor had examined the cured fistula in the girl known as Anaka, or Anarca. In fact, all the women that were supposed to have been cured were gone. The evidence of Sims's victory had vanished.

Sims was duly impressed when Bozeman presented himself for the available position, offering a letter of introduction from Dr. Gross. Sims read the missive at once. It seemed there had not been a rush of applicants. He inquired skeptically about Bozeman's experience with chloroform, appearing to have had little experience with it himself. Bozeman was surprised by how small and frail Sims was. Something afflicted him. It was apparent that he required an assistant not only because his fistula experiments were ongoing—details needed to be worked out before publication, he explained—but because he maintained a practice that would have exhausted even a fit man. Additionally, he announced that he would be traveling extensively in the next few years. Bozeman recalled remarks from dismissive colleagues about the quack water cures that Sims was said to be seeking out.

Sims offered the position before Bozeman left the office.

On their first full day of work together, Sims told the full story of his fistula cure. He excitedly described the initial inspiration for what he called the Sims position, and the Sims speculum. He hinted at various trials with catheters, many adjustments to his clamp suture, and he dramatically related the epiphanies of the split shot and the final success with Henry LeVert's silver wire. When Sims demonstrated his stitching methodology on a bit of torn denim, Bozeman could see that the rumors were true. Sims's fingers had a prodigious, lithe intelligence—so much so that he regarded as simple a procedure that was likely to be difficult for even an experienced practitioner to perform.

The rumors of Sims's cure—let out by Sims himself, Bozeman learned— had resulted in an avalanche of fistula patients, both white and black. For the most part, Bozeman's role was aftercare, the duties that Sims's first patients had performed for themselves. Bozeman began to assist in the surgeries, and it quickly became apparent which aspects of the procedure still required experimentation. It wasn't clear to Bozeman that the Sims position was required at all, unless you refused to employ an anesthetic. Even if it was necessary, why had Sims compelled the slaves to hold the knee-chest position at length when he might have devised a chair or a rest to make the position easier to sustain? Also, the blade of Sims's speculum was bent at ninety degrees. A more acute angle of seventy-five degrees would provide greater leverage and offer comfort to the patient. Last, the clamp suture—to which Sims was unfalteringly loyal—failed in multiple ways. In one case, the procedure to install the clamps went smoothly, but after six days the metal bars became so completely absorbed into the substance of the bladder only the lead shot remained visible. The clamps had to be dug out, through the wall of the vagina. In another case—a slave named Delia, purchased by Sims in New Orleans—the clamps cut out repeatedly, and a fistula that began as an oval 1¼ inches across grew in size over ten operations. Eventually, Delia was left with two fistulae instead of one.

It wasn't long before Bozeman recognized the truth: Sims was about as interested in fistula as he was in Alabama. Fellow physicians recalled for Bozeman Sims's initial aversion to the diseases of women, and now they took note of the fact that he summered in New York every year, leaving Bozeman to care for his patients. When he did return to Alabama, he occupied himself with experiments with silver wire, sometimes hinting that wire sutures might make for a revolution in the history of surgery.

The fistula procedure itself suggested new surgeries to Sims. In 1850, the backyard clinic received a thirteen-year-old slave girl, Lavinia, afflicted with a bladder stone. Sims speculated that if he could cure a fistula that resulted from obstructed labor—with extensive loss of tissue—then he could most certainly cure a fistula that was opened intentionally from the vagina into the bladder to remove the stone. Bozeman assisted in the first procedure. Sims made the incision, the calculus was seized with forceps, and the sutures were expertly installed and secured with silver wire. But even under ideal circumstances, the clamp sutures cut out. Lavinia was left with a gaping fistula.

Sims was not dissuaded. A short time later, another young slave, Louisa, age nine, presented with painful micturition and blood in her urine—another bladder stone. This time, Sims proposed a surgical deflowering—rupturing Louisa's hymen and dilating her vagina—prior to the procedure to remove the offending object. All went as planned, and a stone the size of a partridge egg was removed. Unfortunately, the clamp sutures cut out again, and Louisa was left with a fistula that had all the ill consequences of one that had arisen from tedious labor. Bozeman witnessed several of Sims's attempts to cure the girls, but then they disappeared, just as Anarcha and the others had done. He presumed that Sims was secretly making further attempts to cure them, taking care to hide his failures.

Early in 1853, Sims and Bozeman formed a partnership so that Bozeman could more fully associate himself with Sims's practice before he left for New York. Despite the fact that it was not a coveted property, Bozeman agreed to pay handsomely for Sims's home and office. By then, he was fully aware that Sims had been falsifying the success of his procedure. His celebrated article claimed the clamp suture never cut out; it did, frequently. Sims had attested to perfect results, but even assuming Anarcha and the others had been cured, the truth was half that. Last, while Sims had made quick mention of LeVert's wire experiments, the failure of his paper to fully acknowledge the work of his fellow Alabaman amounted, in Bozeman's view, to an adroit purloining of another man's labor. Strictly speaking, Sims was a thief.

Sims performed a final fistula procedure on his slave Delia before he left Alabama. He installed two sets of clamps and left the aftercare to Bozeman. Both sets cut out, and Delia was left in a horrible condition.

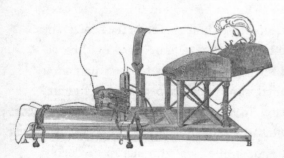

Within a month, Bozeman submitted a plan to a jeweler for a more acutely angled speculum. The following year, he invented a cushioned table to make the knee-chest position more bearable. He published his first fistula paper, about an operation performed on a slave named Emily, on the eve of a lecture that Sims was rumored to be delivering in New York to propose his own hospital.

The first of two revelations arrived early the following year, when a twenty-one-year-old slave named Matilda was brought to Bozeman all the way from Georgia. Not only was Matilda afflicted with *three* fistulae, her vagina was radically constricted by bands of tissue growing across the cavity. Matilda's case revealed to Bozeman that fistula surgery could succeed only if it was preceded by gradual preparation. He first incised her constricting bands of tissue, and then dilated the vagina for several weeks with a small oil-silk bag stuffed with bits of compressed sponge.

The exact position of Matilda's three fistulae demonstrated perfectly why Sims's clamp suture was inadequate. If they were all clamped at the same time, the bars would overlap, ensuring failure. If only one was clamped, the flow of urine through the unclamped fistulae would spoil the cure. Bozeman's first attempt to treat Matilda, limited to her lowest fistula, failed. So did another procedure. His second revelation came one day when he was buttoning his vest. The button itself suggested a solution. Rather than bars embedded in the vaginal tissue, why not a concave disk affixed over the sutured tissue, like a protective cap?

It made more sense to first attempt the button suture on a slave named Julia, who had a simple fistula that Sims had failed to cure two years earlier. The first button operation succeeded just days after word arrived that Sims's hospital in New York had opened its doors. Bozeman immediately set to attempting another button-suture procedure, this time on a notably tragic case.

The second pregnancy of an eighteen-year-old slave named Kitty had ended after three days of labor with the destruction of her unborn baby. Soon enough, she began to leak. Owing to her condition, she had been compelled to sit perpetually on a stool with a hole carved in the center; she dribbled into a vessel positioned beneath. Before long, she could barely stand. She became so emaciated her legs were barely thicker than chair posts, and the flow of urine resulted in profound sores on her nates and thighs. Inside, Kitty was little better. The walls of the vaginal cavity had begun to grow together; it was almost completely closed off. There was a fistula near the vaginal orifice, and another seated much more deeply, near her cervix.

The case would provide a perfect test for the button suture. If he closed Kitty's lower fistula first, urine streaming through the upper hole would test the protective quality of the button. The procedure was difficult; Kitty put up great resistance. Bozeman held out little hope, but at last he clipped the silver wires and removed the button. To his surprise, a perfect union had resulted. Over the next few weeks, Bozeman applied another button to her second fistula. Miraculously, the girl was completely cured.

The button suture succeeded again and again. A slave named Dinah, forty-seven years old, was cured of two fistulae of eighteen years' standing.

Another cure came in a case in which the entire septum had sloughed out. In autumn 1855, Sims's slave Delia returned to Montgomery for treatment. Bozeman cured her with two operations.

In early 1856—when he was already making plans to take his button suture to Europe—Bozeman published an extensive account of his experiments. He strained to acknowledge Sims's skill and perseverance. Sims was entitled to praise, Bozeman wrote. However, he then described the shortcomings of the clamp suture. He offered the button suture as an improvement.

Bozeman heard of Sims's reply before he saw it in print. Its viciousness was his mentor's final lesson in the profession of medicine. Sims told anyone who would listen that Bozeman was an ingrate and that his claims were false. Bozeman had appropriated for himself all the work that Sims had performed unaided. Bozeman was dishonorable in offering secret remedies that attempted to rob Sims of a discovery that would live as long as surgery was cultivated as a science. Worst, Sims accused Bozeman of stealing his implements, even as Sims appeared to have stolen Bozeman's improvement to the Sims speculum.

The button suture continued to succeed, regardless. In 1856, Bozeman cured several white women, one of whom Sims had failed to treat adequately. That same year, he cured slaves named Minerva, Amanda, and Ann. In 1858, just before he left for Europe, Bozeman cured the girls Lavinia and Louisa, whom Sims had left behind after creating their fistulae to remove bladder stones. Bozeman cured them all—all except Matilda, whose case had inspired the button suture. The procedure failed her, over and over. In 1858, Matilda returned to Georgia, and Bozeman never heard word of her again.

* * *

Sims had met Dr. Fordyce Barker even before he moved to New York City. Like so many of the doctors in Montgomery, Barker was younger than Sims, but he had more deftly carved his professional niche. Europe helped. A rugged Mainer, Barker had studied extensively across the continent before returning to America to assume the chair of midwifery at the New York Medical College. He'd been receptive to Sims's call for a new hospital from the start. He signed his name to the hospital circular that Sims had seen in 1850, and later he attested to particular concern for an estimated twenty thousand New Yorkers who lived in damp and filthy catacombs below street level. These grimy subterranean citizens generated a foul miasma that poisoned the air and sowed the seeds of disease among the inhabitants of the upper city.

In 1851, Barker told Sims that wherever a man goes he must forcefully *make* an opening for himself.

Three years later, Sims received sustained, enthusiastic applause at the end of his forceful speech at the Stuyvesant Institute. Then, like a fog, an awkward silence settled over the crowded theater. Henri Stuart had not planned how the lecture would begin, nor had he given thought to what would come after it. After a lengthy pause, one of the city's more eminent physicians rose to fill the void, suggesting that the gathering proceed henceforth like a meeting of a professional society. A secretary was appointed. A motion was made, and seconded, to establish a committee to explore the organization of a "Woman's Hospital," one that coincided to the utmost extent with the facility that had been so eloquently described by Dr. Sims.

Debate was vigorous. Naysayers claimed that anyone could apply silver nitrate through a cylindrical speculum. Astringent injections answered the needs of leukorrhea, and a metal globe was fully sufficient in cases of prolapse. There was no need for a hospital for women, and such an institution would upset the therapeutic monopolies that had been established among the city's existing hospitals.

Fortunately, these voices were in the minority. A motion to establish a committee of men to plan the Woman's Hospital—with Sims as lead surgeon—was passed.

Over the next several days, the men who would form the Woman's Hospital's first medical and governance boards were approached and agreed to serve. For the medical board, there was Dr. Edward Delafield and Dr. Horace Green, from prominent medical schools. There was John Francis, regarded as the father of obstetric medicine in New York. And last there was Valentine Mott and Alexander Stevens—Sims was forced to accept both men, even though they had betrayed him. For the governance board, there was the famed Peter Cooper, who had invented the nation's first steam locomotive. And there was E. C. Benedict, a well-connected banker who would give Woman's Hospital reach into the halls of city and state government.

In a month's time, Barker published a widely read piece praising Sims in the *American Medical Monthly*. Barker publicly chastised a doctor at St. Mary's Hospital in London who had been performing Sims's fistula operation without crediting either Sims or the Young America that had produced him. Sims's surgery, Barker wrote, was the only fistula surgery known with reason and science behind it. Most important, he praised the clamp suture as the singular feature of the cure. Without it, all the cure's other contrivances would be futile. Sims had produced a brilliant achievement of modern surgery, and words failed to capture the disgust that one felt for Old World doctors who lacked the manliness to acknowledge an American success.

* * *

Sims was well on his way to becoming a dictator. But as details of the hospital began to be worked out, Barker argued that for Woman's Hospital to come to pass, there would need to be a third overseeing board—one composed entirely of women. Henri Stuart agreed. The move would be more expedient than fundamentally necessary, Barker explained. There had already been talk in the city of a hospital for women, he reminded Sims, and of course it would be women who raised the funds and managed the day-to-day operations of Woman's Hospital.

On cue, four days after his lecture, Sims was visited by Elizabeth Blackwell, who had already heard rumors that Sims's first assistant was to be a woman. He placated her with talk of educating women in medicine and made a show of taking down the names of men she wished to propose for the board of governors. Otherwise, he politely insisted that the medical establishment in New York City was so firmly opposed to women studying medicine that the involvement of medical women would doom the project from the start. No—such an effort must emerge from the sphere of men.

He described his grand plan: he would raise $200,000 for a hospital that would occupy the recently built, castle-like Arsenal building, constructed to house munitions. On completion, however, the Arsenal had been seized by the city for the formation of what was to be called Central

Park. The Arsenal now stood empty. Blackwell recognized that Sims's plan was far more ambitious than anything she had envisioned. To appease her, Sims invited both Blackwell sisters to observe surgeries once Woman's Hospital opened its doors.

He summered in Portland, Connecticut, again with Jarvis, and recruited Caroline Thompson, whose condition had worsened—he tapped her tumor once more—as Woman's Hospital's first official donor. In the fall, he conspired with Barker and Stuart to form a plan of attack on the city's society ladies. Barker believed that a board of female or lady managers could be pulled together from his patients and the wives of prominent physicians. In this way, a measure of control could be exerted over them, remotely, as it were.

Stuart argued that care would nevertheless need to be taken in communicating to potential lady managers the precise purpose of Woman's Hospital. It wouldn't be as simple as it had been with the media men. Both he and Barker agreed that the dramatic tale of the slave girls banding together in Sims's backyard clinic would be effective in appealing to the women's charitable impulse. A story was the best weapon that Sims could wield in the campaign to win the ladies' compliance.

He spent the next several months traveling from house to house, describing a wholly different hospital from the one his lecture had laid out for the profession. Rather than a laboratory for new surgeries (though certain of the ladies intuited that benefits might accrue to themselves from experiments conducted on Irish girls), Sims characterized the Woman's Hospital as a larger version of his backyard clinic in Alabama, one wholly dedicated to offering a cure to poor women afflicted with the most unspeakable of maladies. Stuart and Barker proved correct. The story of the slaves in the North was not the scandal it had been in Montgomery. Rather, New York's society women were keen to hear of the slave women acquiring skills, becoming assistants and nurses. Sims cared little one way or the other. If Yankee ladies wished to believe the lesser races could be raised up from the low station that was prescribed to them, then so be it. The only thing that mattered was that his hospital be built.

The shift in fate was like another wink from providence—and just in time. Money had been dwindling. Theresa had returned to Alabama to dispose of their Butler Springs property and sell their slaves, a sacrifice that could not be avoided. He had trusted her to place them with relatives or in good homes in Montgomery, and he had written to her frequently of his progress with the ladies of New York. When the time came, he suspected, he would be able to charge as much as $1,250 for a fistula surgery on a woman of means.

His storytelling was effective, but the ladies' enthusiasm often dwindled when the talk turned to financial commitment. He met with the woman who ran the city's Home of the Friendless Campaign, and another woman who operated New York's lying-in hospital. They were reluctant to participate unless there were safeguards to ensure that the women who were admitted were of the proper moral character. Sims's list of names grew as ladies suggested other ladies to approach, and shrank again when more powerful ladies examined the list and scratched off women who lacked status or the necessary fortune. At the same time, Henri Stuart arranged introductions to aldermen and to New York City mayor Jacob Westervelt in an effort to secure a significant grant from the city's Common Council fund.

The break came when Sims secured a meeting with Mrs. Thomas C. Doremus, a small, frail woman with a reputation for indefatigable perseverance. In 1842, Doremus had laid the groundwork for the Isaac T. Hopper Home, to benefit women recently released from prison. In 1850, she established the New York House of School and Industry, to offer women an escape from crime and vice. In 1854, she assisted with the founding of the New York Nursery and Child's Hospital, which opened its doors just days before Sims's Stuyvesant Institute lecture.

He met with Doremus for what seemed like hours. By this point, having delivered his story dozens of times, he had begun seasoning the tale with exaggerations of just how immediately fatal fistula could prove to be. No matter—the ladies would never know the difference. In addition, he had discovered, and Barnum had suggested as much, that the women responded exceedingly well to the story of his own failing health following Anarcha's cure.

Doremus seized on the plan. At once, she further refined his list of names and insisted on several others to become the officers of what would be called the Board of Lady Managers. Within days, a meeting was convened at the house of Mrs. David Codwise to approve a constitution for Woman's Hospital. It became apparent that the Blackwell sisters, either before or after Sims's arrival in the city, had been in communication with some of these same powerful women. While granting Sims, as lead surgeon, his choice of first assistant—subject to the approval of the directress, Doremus herself—the ladies would not be dissuaded from an article of the constitution specifically stating that the surgeon's assistant be a woman. In return, Sims insisted that the language of the constitution hold that the hospital was not for fistula alone but for "diseases peculiar to women."

Stuart calmed Sims's fears. The language of the constitution was loose, he said. When the time came, they could interpret "first assistant" to mean the house matron; he suggested his own widowed sister for the role. Later, after Woman's Hospital had established its reputation, they would insist on changing the rule to hire a man. Similarly, the grand plan for a hospital at the Arsenal building was a vision for the future. After struggling with several landlords who balked at what their rooms would be used for, the Board of Lady Managers settled on a more modest location near Sims's own address. The four-story home at 83 Madison Avenue would be suitable for a hospital of forty beds. With remarkable speed, the lady managers hired nurses and chambermaids, and secured iron bedsteads, straw beds and mattresses, sheets, pillows, and towels. A parlor was neatly furnished with cane chairs, a settee, and a handsome table. The Ladies' Bible Society donated Bibles and testaments. The American Tract Society gave library books. The first patients, referred by doctors throughout the city, were ready a month before Woman's Hospital opened. Sims performed the first on-site operation in early May 1855.

* * *

The vast majority of patients were Irish. The first, Amanda Waldrop, twenty-two, had a fistula that was the result of sixty-eight hours of labor. She was discharged five days later, not benefited. Sims cured Mary Riley, Mary Cummings, Bridget McLaughlin, and Margaret Dillon—all in their twenties or thirties—some staying at the hospital for a month or two, others longer. He cured a twelve-year-old girl, Sarah Good. Mary Hallery, twenty-eight, had suffered a total loss of her vagina; she was sent away without treatment. Mary Smith, thirty-five, had worn a wooden float from a seine net in her vagina, as a pessary, for years. When Sims removed it, agonizingly for the patient, her bladder pushed at once into her vagina, just as he had heard Anarcha's bladder was threatening to do. Also like Anarcha, Mary Smith had had numerous pregnancies after acquiring her fistula. Sims would attempt to cure her only after the extensive excoriation of her nates and vulva had healed.

American women came as well, often not for fistula. Eveline Triesdale of New Jersey and Mary Stegher from Manhattan appealed for help with heavy bleeding during menses. Jane McRain, from Scotland, and another woman referred by one of the lady managers presented with the opposite problem, scanty menses. These latter cases hinted at a cause for a mysterious sterility that afflicted one in eight couples in New York, Sims estimated. Whatever prevented the egress of menstrual matter, he suspected, blocked the ingress of sperm, as well. Rich financial gain awaited whoever offered a cure for the infertility that threatened the city's powerful families and dynasties. In addition, Sims began employing a tube to augment the inflating action of the vagina in women who were either very young or very heavy. Happily, the tube also had the effect of rescuing respectable women from the embarrassment of air once again escaping loudly from their vaginas.

As he had suspected, Woman's Hospital brought the frontier of women's health to him. He began to glimpse remedies for a range of maladies, most of which had no treatment accepted by the profession at large. In the first month, the most promising case of all was an eighteen-year-old girl sent from the Home of the Friendless.

Bridget Headley was afflicted with a pedunculated tumor, a growth attached to the exterior of her womb by a tough stalk. It was the perfect chance to prove the theory about silver sutures that Sims had been dreaming of since Alabama. He could cut into her abdomen, remove the tumor, and tie off the stalk with silver wire. He invited the men of the Woman's Hospital medical board to examine the girl, but there was no agreement about what could be palpated beneath the skin. It might be a floating kidney, or a phantom inflammation. Sims convinced them

all, one by one, until only the troublemaker
Alexander Stevens remained. Stevens offered
a morose warning: if Sims succeeded, every
young doctor in the country would be inspired
to open the abdomens of every young woman
they could get their hands on. The meeting ended without permission to proceed.

Sims arranged to perform the operation anyway, at
night. Only the hospital's illiterate chambermaid—who
had designs to become a nurse—was in attendance.
Sims was correct: Bridget Headley had an ovarian
tumor. However, the girl died during the surgery, expiring even before he
had managed to fully separate the growth's adhesions.

* * *

The problem of how to record Headley's case in the Woman's Hospital
record book—until now, Sims had kept notes only for the purposes of
future publication—was solved when he struck on the thought of recruit-
ing Thomas Addis Emmet to be his first assistant. Two other young doctors had refused his advances. But when Sims thought of Emmet, the
benefit of keeping him close became apparent. What better way to keep
the truth of Anarcha's story quiet than to employ the one New Yorker who
knew she hadn't been cured?

Long before he managed to convince the Board of Lady Managers
to accept a man as his assistant—not difficult in the end, as by now he
knew how to charm society ladies—Sims made a show, late one snowy
night, of rapping on Emmet's door. He claimed that his car had derailed
just across Fourth Avenue; a long wait in the chill had compelled him to
seek the warmth of Emmet's fire. Emmet made a show of displaying for
Sims his careful documentation of his Ward's Island typhus patients. The
tallying work itself was not without interest. Sims wanted an assistant,
and if Emmet could take over the free fistula work—paying patients were
demanding more and more time—and also assume control of the record-
keeping duties of the hospital, all the better. Sims could then devote his
time to exploratory surgeries. On the spot, Sims insisted that he had just

the position for a man of Emmet's skills. If he would come to Woman's Hospital in the morning, he would witness a case of a sort he had never before seen. Sims would be operating on Mary Smith, the woman who had worn a fisherman's float as a pessary.

They made no mention of Sims's speech, and no mention of Anarcha, until Emmet showed Sims to the door. Here, Emmet paused. Was Sims aware, the young man asked, that the slave girl Anarcha, still very much in ill health, had now come into the possession of the well-known Maury family? The name rang a bell—hadn't Mittag served on the railroad commission with the famous Lieutenant Maury? Could that be why the Maurys had bought her? Emmet said he had heard the news while summering in New Rochelle with Roosevelts and Bullochs and Maurys, all navy folk. The Maurys of New York had been patients of Dr. John Francis for years. He noted this portentously, blocking Sims's path to the door. Anarcha was now tending to a young Maury wife, he said. She was acting as a midwife. And soon, Emmet said, she would be coming to New York City.

* * *

The opening of Woman's Hospital was not properly observed until February 1856. The first of many annual galas was organized by the Board of Lady Managers. A host of men rose to speak at Clinton Hall, on Astor Place, exalting Sims as rival to astronomers such as Newton and Rittenhouse. Or even better, perhaps, for what special benefit had come to man from the discovery of any new comet or planet? Every year, glasses of marvelous power mapped the heavenly spheres, but the glories of which those sciences partook remained starry and ephemeral.

No less brilliant, the speakers claimed, was that noble band of dutiful women who had succeeded in putting Woman's Hospital into operation. There are woman's rights and there are woman's duties, it was said, and when the latter are nobly performed there is little time to assert the former. Such were the industrious women of the Woman's Hospital Board of Lady Managers. Working as if penetrated by divine fervor, one speaker proclaimed, their names would never be forgotten: Mrs. David Codwise, Mrs. William B. Astor, Mrs. Ogden Hoffman, Mrs. Horace Webster, Mrs. Jacob Le Roy, Mrs. Thomas C. Doremus . . .

Eighteen

IN VIRGINIA, ANARCHA WAS NOT CALLED ANARCHA, BUT ANKEY OR ANKY, and patrollers were not called patrollers, they were paddarollers or paddy rollers, and the pass you gave them when you traveled, both slaves and poor whites, was not a pass, it was a remit. There were stories in Virginia of slaves preparing hot coals, packing mud into hollow logs before they were burned, to throw into the faces of paddy rollers who arrived late at night to break up meetings and frolics, and there was a story of a slave woman who was stripped naked and suspended from the rafters in a barn and then whipped while she dangled. There was a story of two young slaves who dragged a moccasin out of a tree. Its belly was swollen, so they beat it until a catfish came sliding out, and the catfish was swollen too, so they whacked it until a lady's snapper pocketbook came sliding out, and inside the pocketbook were two shiny copper pennies, one for each of the boys.

The day after Lieutenant Maury showed Anarcha the slow-falling stars through his glass in Washington City, he left her and Delia in the charge of his young cousin Richard. Richard Maury took them on the Orange and Alexandria railroad for twenty-eight miles to Brentsville, and then they switched to a coach for twenty-five miles to Fredericksburg. Richard was studying medicine in Charlottesville, and Anarcha had been correct to wonder whether people had heard stories about her, because Richard said that he had heard stories about her, and he was surprised to learn that she was still cursed with fistula, he said, and he asked a lot of questions about Dr. Sims. He revealed that Dr. Sims now had his own hospital in New York, and he was famous for curing women cursed with fistula holes and other miseries and ailments peculiar to females, he said. Alone with them on the train, Richard Maury talked a lot. But after they boarded the stage to Fredericksburg, with other travelers, he didn't talk so much, and in Fredericksburg Anarcha and Delia slept in the rooms of the slaves owned by the Fredericksburg Maurys, and in the morning a wagon arrived for Anarcha and Delia, steered by Jacob, who was a slave but also a driver, an overseer of slaves, and Jacob was going to take them to where they would stay until Anarcha met her new master and missus.

They were going to a place called Old Mansion, which was a very old home, almost two hundred years old, and Old Mansion had been built from bricks that had been brought all the way from England, Jacob said. It stood well back from the road that led into Bowling Green, which had two churches, two mills, a tavern that was called New Hope, and a Dr. McKenney who pulled slaves' teeth for a dollar per tooth. There were three stores, including Robert G. Allen and Co., which sold groceries, clothing, hardware, pottery, boots and shoes, hats and caps, and drugs and medicines of all kinds. There were three hundred people in Bowling Green—two hundred white people and one hundred black people—and some of the blacks were free blacks, and many slaves were hired out, or lent to newlyweds on the occasion of their marriage. Old Mansion was more famous even than Bowling Green, Jacob said, because George Washington had visited the home on his way back to Hooe's Ferry after traveling to Richmond to inspect the ports, and because shortly after Cornwallis surrendered, Washington held a banquet on the Old Mansion lawn for General Lafayette, who had sometimes camped with French soldiers nearby and who was the same General Lafayette, Anarcha realized, who had visited Alabama in 1825 for the grand fete that the slaves of Rose Hill and Bright Spot remembered for years. Later, Thomas Jefferson came to Old Mansion to purchase a horse sired by Diomed, a famous racehorse, also brought from England, in the year 1798. Diomed sired many horses for the racetrack between Old Mansion and the road, and for other racetracks besides. Jacob explained, as they came trundling up toward the house, that the champion horse had won the first Epsom derby, which was the most famous horse race in the world, and then Diomed won nine more consecutive races, and no one had ever heard of a horse winning ten races in a row. Then he came to Old Mansion, and to this day the Old Mansion slaves spoke and told stories of Diomed as though he wasn't a horse at all but an important person, like Washington or Lafayette or Thomas Jefferson, who rode his horse Wildair, son of Diomed, out into the countryside and greeted people and conversed with them without their ever knowing that he was president of the United States.

Old Mansion was owned by the father of Anarcha's new master, a man who was recently widowed. His wife had borne twelve Maury children, and almost all of them lived. He had bought the plantation because he wanted to try to be a farmer, but he wasn't a farmer, he worked for the railroad. Behind the racetrack and the house, there was a kitchen and a smokehouse and a lumber house, and there was a warehouse for tobacco that wasn't used anymore, and an icehouse that looked like a house that was all underground except for its roof. Cherry trees surrounded the racetrack, and there were two giant cedars in front of the house as well, and there were avenues of elms and aspens to the south and north. There was a great mulberry tree too, to the west, which was also famous, Jacob said. Everything at Old Mansion was famous except for its slaves.

To the rear, there were terraced gardens that were even grander than the gardens Anarcha had seen at Rose Hill, in Mount Meigs, and Violet Hill in Autauga County: plots trimmed with box hedges, with separate spaces for squash, potatoes, cabbage, asparagus, peas, beets, carrots, parsnips, mustard, kale, parsley, tomatoes, peppers, snap peas, butter beans, and cantaloupes. And beyond those there were flower gardens as well.

There were ghost stories at Old Mansion, Jacob said, but the ghosts were the ghosts of white people. After he died, the home's original owner, Colonel Hoomes, appeared to each of his descendants shortly before it was their turn to die. Also, there was a headless horseman who could be seen racing furiously around the racetrack in front of Old Mansion on the night before the death of an eldest son. The horseman had been seen recently, in 1855, when the oldest Maury boy, an important man and the mayor of Washington City, died, and then his mother died not long after him, probably of grief. And lastly there was a story of a white man who was married but had fallen in love with one of his slaves. When his wife fell ill, he made a hideous mask and put it in the window of her Old Mansion sickroom, and when she saw it she was scared to death. Ever after, Jacob said, the woman's ghost haunted the house, and you never knew when she was going to appear, but only white people saw her.

Many of the slaves at Old Mansion were house slaves, and Anarcha didn't see them often. There was a passel of Maury children and grandchildren, and when Old Mansion became stuffed with Maurys, some of them went to the Woolfolks, two miles away, who were relatives by marriage. At such times, Woolfolk house slaves came to Old Mansion to help. There were two dozen Maury slaves in all, and those that were not house slaves worked at growing food. The master at Old Mansion was conducting experiments with wheat and corn and oats. When the Maury slaves were not planting gooseberry bushes or making blackberry wine or mauling as many as one thousand fence rails in five days, they were instead furrowing corn, or laying fodder in the peach orchard, or spreading experimental mixtures of California guano and bone dust in the wheat, though often the experiments failed and there were very few bushels to haul to the train station at Milford. Anarcha rarely saw these slaves, because before she arrived a level for a small cabin had been sewed for her, far out away from the house, beyond the stables, and even beyond the collection of slave cabins that stood beside the south fields. Anarcha suspected that Lieutenant Maury had warned ahead of the smell of her curse. Anarcha and Delia lived in the woods, by themselves.

The Old Mansion slaves included John and Cady, and all of Cady's children, and there was Arena and Rhena, and Betsey and Betsy, and Louisa and Julia, and there were a number of babies: a Caty who was eighteen months, and another Caty who was eleven months, and Ednie who was seven months, and Milly who was five months, and Bellefield who was four months. The month after Anarcha arrived, she caught Betsey's second baby, and that would become her job at Old Mansion, attending to births and caring for babies in the daytime and watching after pregnant women until their troubles were over. Betsey's second baby was taken away and sold, because the elder Maury needed the money. He wasn't any true farmer, and he couldn't afford any more mouths to feed.

At hog-killing time, the Maurys took two-thirds of the pork, and the remainder was given to the slaves, and Anarcha's weekly portion was delivered by the mothers who brought their babies out to her house in the mornings. Along with the pork, Anarcha received meal, sweet potatoes, molasses, a pumpkin, and sometimes an opossum if *She plays out at Ankeys house* the men had hunted and there was more meat than the Maury slaves could eat. Rather than oyster shells or wooden spoons, Anarcha was given old courseware and stoneware that the Maurys no longer used, or that had been used by previous owners of Old Mansion, and when she arrived she found that they had left her bits of Chinese porcelain and pearl ware that had broken in spots—plates with cracks, cups with broken handles—and there was a mason's trowel that she was given and that she used as both knife and spatula. Sometimes, the young Maury mothers—the white children also came out to Anarcha's house to play games with the slave children— brought leftovers from the Old Mansion kitchen: baked custard, oyster soup, silver cake, jelly cake, and plum cake, and when disease moved in to Bowling Green, there was a dish called chicken cholera that had calomel and opium baked right into the meat.

Delia wandered in the woods. Sometimes she brought home old clay pipes that she found in the dirt, and once she found an old coin that had been cut in half, and then cut in half again, like a wedge of pie. One of the Maurys explained that it was a quarter dollar from the country of Spain.

It wasn't long before word spread that Anarcha knew about cures and female problems, and slaves began to visit her cabin from nearby plantations. Anarcha taught Delia how to search for the cures that grew in the Virginia woods, rat's vein herb and heartleaf and crowfoot leaf. Anarcha saw many slaves that could be cured, and she learned too of slaves that were not cured: Selah died of neuralgia. Bumerage and Garland and Fleming died of consumption. Chaplis died of brain fever. Courtney and Maria Bet both died of smothering before they were one year old. Overton died of dropsy. Lucinda and Elvira, mother and daughter, both died

of typhoid, and there were two men named Moses from the same plantation, and they both died of pneumonia. Pollux drowned. Matilda Ann and
Elizabeth were burnt. Patsy, Robinson, and Charity died just because they
were old. Brutus was old too, but he died because of a disease in his heart.

Slaves in Bowling Green trusted Anarcha with their ills, but otherwise
they did not trust her. It took time to learn why.

* * *

In Richmond, slaves and free black people spoke with reverence of Nat
Turner and the message he read in the sky two years before the night
the stars fell. In Bowling Green, slaves spoke with reverence of General
Gabriel, who decades earlier had raised an army on the edge of Caroline
County. His plan to take Richmond and free the slaves was foiled not by
falling stars but by a torrent that gushed from the same sky.

It was white people who made slaves of black people, and it was white
people who told black people they should risk everything they had, their
very lives, to revolt. Frenchmen in Caroline County urged slaves to rise up
against their masters. Early in the year 1800, a hulking ditcher named Jack
was among the first to organize, and it was Jack who recruited Gabriel, a
blacksmith widely known along the stage road between Richmond and
Bowling Green for having only months earlier bitten off a sizable portion
of the ear of an overseer.

Jack was a giant, six feet five, larger in some stories. The low hairline
on his brow hid a ghastly scar, and he kept his hair long and unruly, tying
it back in a queue like the tail of a horse, as English soldiers had done.
Gabriel was a blacksmith, almost as tall as Jack but years younger, and
silent stories were told by the scars on his face, by his two missing front
teeth, and by the brand of a "T," for "thief," near the base of his left thumb.

Gabriel could read and write. His shop stood near the road, and the
grapevine had carried the story of another slave on Gabriel's plantation,
Jupiter, who stole a hog and suffered punishment from a wantonly cruel
overseer until Gabriel fought back, gnawing off most of the man's ear. The
men were tried in court. Jupiter was found guilty and he was whipped
on a whipping post thirty-nine times in front of the judges. Gabriel was
found guilty too, but he was given benefit of clergy, which meant they

didn't kill him but instead burned the "T" onto his thumb even though it was Jupiter who stole the hog. The "T" ensured that if Gabriel was ever caught again for anything there wouldn't be any beneficial clergyman. He would be hanged.

General Gabriel was not frightened. He and his brother Solomon and Jupiter joined with Jack, who arrived with news of an uprising. Throughout the summer of 1800, the men made themselves captains and recruited an army at barbecues, at fish fries, at stolen religious meetings at hidden brush arbors in the woods, and at taverns and dram shops where men gathered to drink and play quoits. There were secret meetings in plantation quarters late at night, and at forges like Gabriel's, where scythes were broken in half and fashioned into two murderous swords that could lop off a man's limb at a single blow. Soldiers were gathered in Norfolk and Richmond and Charlottesville, and in the counties of Henrico and Chesterfield and Hanover and Caroline and Goochland. A list was kept, either of men's signatures or their marks. In this way, the troops came to include Gilbert, who stuttered, and Ben who came from Gabriel's plantation, and another Ben who went by the name of Ben Woolfolk, whom no one trusted but who traveled deep into Caroline for recruits and returned with instructions for how to make paper cartridges. Others came with the names Liberty and Moses, and George Smith and Sam Byrd, and Pharoah and Tom, and a number of slaves named Billy, including one known as Billy Chicken, and there was Scipio and Thornton and Sawney, and two Martins, and Isham, Isaac, Laddis, Watt, Abraham, and Jon Fells. One night, the core group of rebels gathered to choose their general, and Gabriel won a vote over Jack, because many knew him, and because he could read, and because he had bitten off a white man's ear and like a miracle he hadn't been lynched for it.

They pooled money both earned and stolen to purchase powder for guns, and liquor to persuade additional recruits. They made spears, fixing bayonets onto the ends of long sticks. They fashioned crossbows. Gabriel wore through two molds making bullets in his blacksmith shop. Jack acquired seven pounds of gunpowder, and more was purchased in Richmond. By August, they had twelve dozen swords, six guns and a pistol, and more firearms waiting at a tavern. Some of the army believed they were the chosen people. God would lead them to the Promised Land. Ben Woolfolk offered a warning: they didn't have anything like the angel that God gave to Moses when he led the Israelites out of Egypt.

The plan took shape as the end of the summer of 1800 neared. A contingent would slip into Richmond to set fires to wooden homes on the south end of town, drawing away firefighters and soldiers whose rifles and pistols were locked away because it was peacetime. While they were distracted, a larger group on the north side of the river would seize the magazine, and they would take control of the governor's mansion and Governor Monroe himself. They would kill the unwitting firemen as they wearily returned from having extinguished the blazes. Whites would be killed on the way to Richmond as well, men from the cradle up, women to be spared, and some argued for sparing Frenchmen, Quakers, and Methodists. Even plantation owners might be permitted to live, if they accepted the end of slavery days and were willing to part with a limb. Two weeks before the end of August, the officers gathered under the guise of a prayer meeting to debate the date of the insurrection. They needed to act while the weather held. If they attacked on a Sunday, more men from Caroline could make the trek south. If they attacked on a Saturday, they would have fewer soldiers, but it would be less conspicuous for slaves to be traveling along the stage road.

General Gabriel chose Saturday, August 30, 1800.

The rain began in Caroline early that morning. By evening, it was a deluge, a flood spilling from the heavens like a plague poured to Earth by a heart-hardened god. The swamp between Gabriel's plantation and Richmond became saturated, and the bridge that crossed it overflowed with waters that seemed like an omen, a conjure. Water was magic, the soldiers said. Spirits couldn't cross it, yet you could locate it with ellum sticks. Cats and ants knew when rain was coming, but had anyone seen, before the deluge began, a cat washing its face or a stalk covered with insects frantically searching for higher ground? No one had ever seen a storm so fierce and purposeful. General Gabriel canceled the attack. They would meet again tomorrow. His confidence that hard rain was just rain, not a command from the sky, failed to convince all those who had gathered on the wet, dark night of August 30.

Tom and Pharoah notified their master of the impending attack. A sweep found little—the rains had washed away the evidence of their rallying point. But two house slaves, both women, affirmed that the uprising had been delayed only by a day. It took little time before roundups of conspirators began, and even less time before slave agreed to testify against slave, with the promise of money, manumission, or both. There were quick trials. Men were lynched outside Prosser's tavern on the stage road, and at the crossroads near Four Mile Creek church, and at Gamble's Hill. The bodies swung until white people began to complain about public executions in full view of women. Twenty-six men, General Gabriel among them, dropped from carts with ropes around their necks.

The Old Mansion slaves, some old enough to remember it, recalled the trials that were held in Bowling Green after most of the executions had already taken place—some at the New Hope tavern, some in a courtroom made up in the basement of Old Mansion itself. The same Colonel Hoomes who became a ghost and appeared to his relatives had stood in judgment over the accused men. Ben Woolfolk was brought to Old Mansion twice on the command of Governor Monroe himself, to testify against his fellow conspirators. Years later, the Woolfolk slaves of Bowling Green denied he was their relative. Ben was spared the noose and later sold. Pharoah and Tom received sixty dollars per month, for the rest of their lives. Half the men tried at Bowling Green were convicted and condemned, but white people had seen enough blood by then—either that or executing a slave cost too much money. Regardless, the condemned men, Jack the ditcher among them, were sold to Richmond traders. They were taken farther south, to be resold at a profit, and no news arrived thereafter of what became of those men, not by grapevine or train or newspaper or any other means by which a story could travel.

* * *

Fifty years later, the slaves of Bowling Green told stories and sang songs about General Gabriel. They were slow to trust strangers, even slave strangers, and particularly a strange woman like Anarcha, as women had been among those who had betrayed Gabriel's army. Now, at Old Mansion, there were rumors of men and women who helped runaways, agents who conducted slaves north on what people called a railroad but was really just slaves running through the woods or hiding in the topsails of ships on the Virginia coast. No one knew of any such agent in Bowling Green. Anyway, there were slaves, particularly those at Old Mansion, who believed that even in the days of General Gabriel, when there were two hundred slaves at Old Mansion instead of twenty, and when the hot hours were spent picking grubs from tobacco plants in fields that ran right up to the New Hope tavern—even in those days, the slaves at Old Mansion had it better than slaves at other plantations, where there were beatings and brandings and where one master, it was said, had invented a machine to do his whipping for him, so that he didn't even get tired when he whipped his slaves. The new master at Old Mansion, the father of Anarcha's master and missus, was like old Colonel Hoomes, who was said to have detested slavery and wished it could be done away with, even as he owned slaves and sometimes coveted them. Wasn't it better, the Maury slaves said, to be owned by a man who used slaves but hated doing so than by a man who owned slaves and enjoyed it? They accepted that the life of a white man's racehorse, even a white man's mule, was more valuable than their own lives. Why risk what you had, they said, when you were given pieces of Chinese porcelain to eat from, and leftover jelly cake to eat?

Woolfolk slaves thought differently. After they recognized that paddy rollers and masters rarely ventured out to Anarcha's house, deep in the woods, they gathered there late at night to talk, sitting outside around a fire, and sometimes Anarcha and Delia were asleep while the Woolfolk slaves dreamed of escaping north on the railroad, and sometimes Anarcha stayed awake and sat with them. After she had been to New York and back—and was experimented on again by Dr. Sims in his new hospital— they peppered her with questions. Was it true there were schools in the North for black children? Was it true that black singers traveled about to give concerts, and that black speakers gave lectures, and that white people paid good money to listen to them? Was it true that thirteen slaves had been burned at the stake after a revolt in New York in the summer of 1741? Was it true that slaves were still being sent to Africa? Mostly, Anarcha didn't know the answers and, as in Richmond, she knew that a cursed woman with miseries in her feet, a cane to walk, and a bladder that felt like it might slip out of her couldn't run away even on a train with a conductor to help her. The Woolfolk slaves disagreed with the Old Mansion slaves. Worse than slavery, they said—worse than women forced to bear yellow children, worse than seeing your children taken away and sold, and worse than a machine that did a white man's whipping for him, like a thresher or a gin—was a master who convinced you with kindness and gifts that the value of your freedom could be measured in dishware and leftover meals. Those whose bodies had been sold, the Woolfolk slaves said, shouldn't be so quick to sell their souls along with them.

* * *

It was six months before Anarcha heard anything at all about her new master and missus. At last, word arrived that they had been married. They had traveled to England for their honeymoon, and now they were back in the United States, in New York City, where her master had work to do. Anarcha's missus was a very young woman, and she was pregnant. They had sent for her. Anarcha would go to New York to care for her missus during her troubles. Within weeks of her arrival, she was sent to Dr. Sims's new hospital.

She entered Woman's Hospital on a Monday, four days before Christmas 1856, and through the holiday her only company was a ferret. Several of the creatures had been released into the building to control rats.

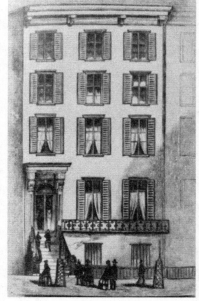

She was put into a room on the fourth floor, the top floor, and when she was shown to her cot, the Irishwomen in the other bunks gathered their sheets and pillows and dispersed to other rooms and floors. On the first night, she brought her plate back upstairs to eat alone. Almost tame, and distracted from its hunt by the smell of her dinner, one of the ferrets came sniffing into the room. Anarcha gave it a lump of baked potato and a stringy shred of beef. The little beast curled into a ball at the foot of her cot, but halfway through the night it was gone again. In the dark and quiet, Anarcha could hear the whispery screeches of its prey, scampering through the walls.

There was no sign outside to announce the existence of Woman's Hospital. It looked like every other house on the row. When Anarcha first arrived, she knocked on the wrong door, disturbing a woman who dragged her to the proper entry and complained to the house matron, who was annoyed both by the neighbor and by the slave girl, the first to be admitted to the hospital, who was now in her charge. A ward nurse gave Anarcha a tour. Through the parlor, on the first floor of the hospital, there were rooms for white women who were not Irish, and who paid money for treatment—three dollars, five dollars, eight dollars, or ten dollars per week, as some patients at the Egyptian Building in Richmond had paid. The nurse nodded to a pair of doors at the end of a hallway. The first floor was off limits to charity patients, she explained. The two rooms at the end of the passage were forbidden to everyone. The women who were treated in them were heard but never seen, and they never stayed more than a few days.

Dr. Sims's surgical theater was on the floor below, but he was rarely in the hospital, the nurse said. His assistant, Dr. Emmet, was now in Alabama. The women—there were forty beds—were alone for the holiday.

An open room on the second floor, full of beds and chairs, served as ward and meeting place for services that were held on Sundays, attendance required. It was also here that women gathered to do knitting that was assigned to them to help pay for their food and linens. Washing was done in the basement by chambermaids, some of them patients. At night, the women played lively songs on a piano, and sometimes they sang, but no one danced.

There was a white woman downstairs, Maria Sharp, who was very sick, sicker than Lucy or Betsey had ever been. It was said she was sick because she had refused to allow her clothes to be washed with the Irishwomen's clothes. The week before, she washed her own clothes outside and caught a chill. The others heard her vomiting at night in her room. She didn't complain, for fear that the operation to close her hole would be delayed.

Two days after Anarcha arrived, Maria Sharp died. Her body was carried out through the parlor, shrouded in linen.

Like Anarcha and the others in Alabama when the experiments began, the nurses at Woman's Hospital knew little of how to care for cursed women: how to throw water to clean the delicate parts, how to control the smell in the ward—the perfumes of the paying patients seeped up to the fourth floor—or how to care for women through the delirium of opium. As in Richmond, Anarcha shared what she knew. One of the patients was a large Irishwoman named Mary Smith, a favorite among the others because she was already working as a nurse, and because she could sneak liquor into the hospital. Mary Smith had been operated on a number of times, once just before Anarcha arrived. She was having difficulty with her catheter. Anarcha showed her how to turn the tube so that it caught more snugly behind the bone. It remained in place even when Mary Smith broke into laughter that was drunk twice, on opium and whiskey. Anarcha spent Christmas alone, but the Irishwomen soon accepted her, just as the Woolfolk slaves had eventually accepted her, and she spent New Year's Eve with a group gathered around Mary Smith's bed, sharing a bottle after the nurses had left for the night. They stifled laughter and sang songs softly so as not to disturb the women on the floor below.

It was lonely and cold in Anarcha's room, without Delia to sleep beside her.

She had brought Delia to New York. The young Richard Maury had once again escorted them on the train from Fredericksburg. A servant—an Irish girl—met them at the station and brought them by carriage to the home that the Maury family owned on Fourth Street, a mile from Woman's Hospital. At last, Anarcha met her master and missus. There was little resemblance between the Lieutenant Maury who was now her owner and the Lieutenant Maury who had shown her stars always falling through a glass telescope. Her master was thin, handsome, wore no uniform. His wife was barely more than a girl, barely older than Anarcha had been when she first became a cursed woman. It was still six months before her time would come, but her hands cradled her small belly like it was a baby already, and she fawned over Delia, practicing to be a mother.

For a room, Anarcha and Delia were given a corner of the attic, partitioned off with sheets. They were called downstairs every morning, but little was required of Anarcha apart from attending to her missus, feeding logs to the fire as she rested beside it, pouring her tea, emptying her pot if she became sick. The Maury home was filled with birds in large, domed wire cages. The birds were unlike anything she'd cared for in Dr. Brown-Séquard's laboratory—colorful and strange—and in the daytime they kept up an endless chatter of cheeping and screeching. Some of them were thick and frisky, with claws that gripped the wire bars of their cages like hands, but others were molting and sad, making sounds only when a like animal chirped from another room.

Members of the Maury family, young and old, came and went from Green's Farm and Tribridge Hall, Saratoga and Oyster Bay. They took walks in Tompkins Square park, attended matinees and plays, and worried that the temperature this year was too mild for cotton, or that ten dollars a barrel was too much to expect the poor to pay for flour. There were Maurys from the North, and Maurys from the South. Northern Maurys complained that the southerners were full of secessionist folly, and they worried over letters that arrived from loved ones that were not letters at all but sheets of politics of the sort you could find in any two-penny newspaper cried in the streets. Anarcha did not work in service, but the whole house could hear the Maurys passionately debating slavery over dinner. Southern Maurys claimed that slaves in the South were as happy and contented as any serf population in the world. Slave owners were as scandalized as anyone by a new, much-discussed book, *Autobiography of a Female Slave*. But to judge the whole of an institution, they said, by a single, likely dubious portrayal would be like judging New York City by the vilest creatures to crawl out of the muck of Five Points. Southern Maurys were amused by the reports of the many canes that had been mailed to proslavery congressman Preston Brooks after his cane beating of Senator Charles Sumner, in May, on the floor of the US Senate. The violent emotions dredged up by Sumner, and by Dred Scott, a slave who was then fighting for his freedom in the Supreme Court, proved that the only true way to protect constitutional rights was to extend slavery throughout the Union.

Northern Maurys responded with reports of antislavery conventions in cities across the state—Cortlandville, Binghamton, Owego, Ithaca, Elmira, Bath. Free states had twice the population of slave states, they argued, and three times as many schools, five times as many students, and ten times as many libraries. They argued that the relationship between the North and the South was like that of man and wife, and to proceed along some homogenous principle would be to suggest that man live with man, woman with woman! Madison, Jefferson, and Washington would have felt disgust at hearing a united nation divided by the vulgar names of Yankeedom and Slavedom. War was coming, the northern Maurys feared, just as quickly and surely as the comets that their famous navy cousin spied with his telescopes at the Naval Observatory in Washington City.

Other news came to Anarcha when she and Delia left the house at night for the final tasks of the day, emptying chamber pots into the sewers and fetching water for the morning. Servants lingered near reservoirs to share stories. Anarcha was warned of slave stealers, and of white people who would sell you fake freedom papers for twenty-five dollars. Did she know that the cowhide whips that were used on slaves in the South were fashioned in northern manufactories? Of late, there had been a case of a black man who was convicted of refusing to give up his seat on a train, and there was a story of a slave couple, separated during their escapes, reunited with the help of an underground railroad office in Syracuse. The price of slaves was going up in the South. Girls of fourteen and fifteen realized the best price.

As with the story of Gabriel's army, many recalled insurrections in New York City. In 1712, nine whites were killed in an uprising. Six rebels ended their own lives before they were captured, twenty were hanged, and three were burned at the stake. One was roasted for eight hours before he died, another was broken on the wheel, and the last, a pregnant woman, was held until she gave birth and then she too was hanged. Now, the papers told stories of black abolitionists calling for revolts across the South. In recent weeks, in Kentucky, a white family of eight had been poisoned by their cook. All of them died. In Louisville, a slave admitted to knowing full well of a plot to rise up at Christmas, but he refused to betray his fellows. He received more than five hundred lashes and died. For the same crime, another slave was whipped and then burned to death. In Virginia, in Prince William County, a whole family of slaves, grandmother, mother, and three boys, the youngest twelve, were hung for murdering their master on Christmas night.

There were further uprisings in Texas, Louisiana, and Mississippi. In South Carolina, thirty-five slaves were lynched after powder and muskets were found in their possession. Thirty-two slaves were arrested and lashed in Alexandria for gathering at a ball. In Tennessee, owners killed fifteen of their own slaves on rumors of an uprising in Perry, and in Dover eleven men were hanged on claims of a hellish and deep-laid plot. Among the condemned was a white man who had painted his face black to pass as a slave and instigate among them. He was spared the noose but taken to the woods for a sentence of nine hundred lashes. He died before his sentence was complete.

* * *

The Maurys arriving in the city for the holidays brought illness, and their illness brought a doctor, Dr. John Francis, to distribute medicine throughout the house. Dr. Francis too seemed to know who Anarcha was, this time even before he saw her or heard her story, and it was Dr. Francis who explained that Dr. Marion Sims would experiment on her once more. He would cure her, so that she would be clean to care for the missus and her baby. Delia remained with the Maurys. Anarcha was put in a hackney to Woman's Hospital.

In her first days, she was examined by other doctors, but these doctors did not seem to know her, and one remarked that it was very strange indeed for a slave to be treated at Woman's Hospital. She did not see Dr. Sims until after the new year. She was taken downstairs and told to undress, and when Dr. Sims came into the room with several other men it had been seven years since she last saw him.

He did not greet her or look her in the eye. He did not give any sign that he knew who she was. Dr. Sims spoke quickly. He asked her what her name was, and who her master was, and a nurse wrote down what she said. He asked her age, and she said she was a little girl when the stars fell on Alabama. Dr. Sims told the writing nurse she was thirty-two years old. He asked when her blood first came, which he had never asked her in Alabama. And he asked about her most recent baby, the large baby girl who died and came out with the use of tongs that were like the tongs Dr. Sims had used on her first baby.

He told her to climb onto the examination table. He explained to the other doctors that the position she assumed was the Sims position as he had used it in Alabama, before he began to operate on white women. The Sims position they used now, he said, was better suited to the forms of female diseases as they occurred in the higher grades of life. Anarcha expected a tug and the cold touch of silver, but instead she felt only a single finger move inside of her. She heard feet shuffling, men angling for a view. Dr. Sims explained that his finger had passed immediately into her bladder. The bladder was pushing through her fistula hole, he said, but luckily her womb had fallen out of position, as otherwise her bladder would already have come out of her body. Dr. Sims removed his finger and instructed a nurse to schedule a surgery for Monday morning. He was gone before Anarcha could either turn around or put on her clothes.

In three days' time, she was given a dose of opium before Dr. Sims arrived for the experiment. A nurse laid her down on her side. She heard Dr. Sims enter the room, but the drug had already begun to soften time, sever her from her cursed body. It had been years since she'd been awake for an experiment. The sharp pains that commenced brewed together in her mind with years of earlier experiments and pains, and with the brush of the cuff of Dr. Sims's sleeve along her leg, and with the subtle burn of the sunlight aimed onto her by a mirror, and with the gasps of breath that enabled her to stifle the impulse to cry out, and with the tears that squeezed out of her eyes and drew chilly lines down her cheek and neck. Imagine Anarcha, one part of her peeling up from the rest. Imagine her own imagination lifting from her mind like the lid of a box. Her thoughts flew, as perhaps the thoughts of all who take opium do. It felt, she thought, as it must feel after witches flayed their bodies and soared over the countryside, dripping down curses. Or, she ascended even higher, like an angel, and she felt weightless, as if among the celestial bodies, and it was she that sprinkled stars down to Earth, a trickling cascade of light. For a moment, she was not the one being experimented on. Rather, she stood alongside Betsey or Lucy, or any of the others, and she cradled their flesh as gently as if she was holding her white missus's baby, or she used the warmth of her breath to take the cold bite out of the blade of Dr. Sims's tool and kept it warm with her hands before it was slid into place. Then, oddly, she squatted down behind herself, performing the experiment she had seen performed so many times, and then it wasn't only her, it was all of the women from Alabama, and all of the knitting women at Woman's Hospital, all of them stitching closed holes, removing curses and conjures from many women, from white women and black women, all afflicted, all wet and noxious, but cured at last, and it was a vision that, like Anarcha, drunk on opium and outside of time, was not here and not now but was pleasant and quiet despite the pains and the callous voices behind and below her, and it was so distracting and transporting that she wasn't even aware when the experiment was finished, and she had no idea that this would be her final experiment, and that after Dr. J. Marion Sims left the room without saying either hello or goodbye she would never see him again.

Nineteen

New York stories—Blizzard of 1857—Thornton—
Return to Old Mansion—Cooking—Midwife—Lorenzo—
Sixth pregnancy

*W*OMEN'S HOOPSKIRTS WERE IN FASHION, UNION, LA SYLPHIDE, AND Skeleton skirts. Every week, a ton of cord, $6,000 in whalebone, and acres of muslin and crinoline were consumed in their creation, and the only difficulty they presented was how a gentleman should walk in the street alongside a woman whose dress measured fifteen paces around. New to America was the convenience of the mechanical arithmomètre, which after a few minutes of instruction made advanced calculations possible for even the most ignorant head. In Nicaragua, William Walker had seized control of the country, with the goal of transforming it into a slave society. And in the United States there was a new president, James Buchanan, who was the same James Buchanan that Senator William Rufus King had told Anarcha about in Alabama. In Washington City, free-state men from the territory of Kansas presented Senator Sumner with a cane of their own, its head depicting a hand strangling the serpent of the slave states.

In North Carolina, there was a fight over whether slaves, who could testify against other slaves in court, should be permitted to testify against white abolitionists. *Five Hundred Thousand Strokes for Freedom, Inside View of Slavery: Or, A Tour Among the Planters*, and *Slavery and Infidelity* had recently been published and were being widely discussed. A bookstore owner in Mobile, Alabama, was run out of town for selling *Uncle Tom's Cabin*, though the banished bookseller denied having done so. A

reverend sold a young female slave. Then he preached a
sermon on the grace of his actions. If he had sold her not
for chattel but for what young girls were more frequently
sold for, he could have gotten $300 more. Someone in
Richmond proposed selling south all of the state's fifty-
four thousand slaves, at $400 each, to raise $20 million
to improve the state.

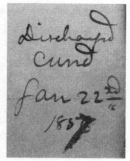

The nurses brought newspapers to Woman's Hospital.
The paper was used for kindling, and to stuff into the
cracks of windowsills, and for holes that the rats chewed in walls throughout the building. The Irishwomen who could read sometimes read aloud
scraps for those who were bedbound, and when the stories were about
slavery—and there were many stories about slavery—they brought them
to Anarcha's bedside. The stories blurred in her mind, blurry already from
opium. A doctor who was not Dr. Sims removed Anarcha's sutures on
January 13, and within a few days she was able to sit up in bed and climb
to her feet to urinate. One day, she rose when the Irishwomen rushed to
the windows to look out at the famous black minstrel singer E. P. Christy,
who had made a princely fortune from burnt cork and Ethiopian melo-
dies, the newspapers said. A great snowstorm had descended on the city.
Christy made a show and promotion of it, dashing through the white-
drifted streets in a magnificent sleigh pulled by a team of prancing snow-
white stud horses. The last bit of news to make it to the hospital was of the
roofs of four Brooklyn homes, blown off in the storm, one sailing several
hundred yards before crashing to the ground. The city crawled. Trains ran
on mail schedules a century old, and railroad crews fighting to keep the
lines open competed with crews from the stage lines working to bury the
tracks again. Villainous rowdies threw snowballs at the faces of ladies who
wandered into the street. By January 18, snowdrifts had climbed to eight
feet, too high for either ladies or rowdies. The temperature plummeted
overnight. Howling wind made melancholy music as it blew through
buildings and alleyways, like the insides of a musical instrument. Water
pipes burst, creating rivers that flowed into the streets and then froze.

Anarcha was improved—it felt as though the stone between her legs
would remain in place without her needing to clench it—but the cold made

her cough even worse. And she continued to leak urine. Nevertheless, after seven weeks at Woman's Hospital, she was discharged as cured on January 22, 1857.

* * *

A month earlier, on Christmas Eve, three slaves leased to a work gang on the York River Railroad had been detained in Bowling Green, Virginia. The men resisted application to search their persons. They were compelled to undergo examination regardless, and a letter was found in the pocket of a slave named Thornton, for many years a sailor on the Rappahannock River.

My Dear Friend,

You must certainly remember what I told you and you must come up to the contract—as we have carried things thus far. Meet at the place where we said and don't make any disturbance until we meet. Don't let any white man know any-thing about it unless he is trustworthy. The articles are all right, and the country is ours certain. Bring all your friends. Tell them, if they want freedom, to come. Don't let it leak out. If you should get in any difficulty, send me word immediately to afford protection. Meet at the crossing and prepare for Sunday night for the neighborhood.

Freedom—Freedom

Your old friend

W. B.

P.S. don't let anybody see this.

Sunday was only three days off. Word spread quickly, and a mob formed in Bowling Green, intent on murderous feelings despite the yuletide season. Thornton refused to detail the plot. Two hundred lashes did not compel him to betray his fellow rebels. He was not hanged. A magistrate sentenced him to many more lashes, to be delivered over a period of weeks, so that he would not expire before his punishment was applied in full. Thornton was still being whipped outside the Bowling Green courthouse when Anarcha returned to Old Mansion.

Anarcha and Delia and her master's two teenage daughters arrived in

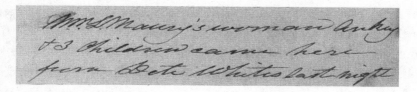

March 1857. Anarcha's missus followed two months later, shortly before her time came, and she traveled with one of the older Maury aunts from New York, and with Dr. John Francis. In May, all of them attended to the missus's birth. The pain lasted twenty-eight hours. To ease the misery, the Maurys and Dr. Francis discussed using chloroform. The Maury aunt, however, knew of a young mother who had breathed it in and then didn't know anything about her baby until it was five weeks old. She wasn't ever the same thereafter, the Maury aunt said. Two other women breathed the chloroform because they were afraid of miseries, and the drug killed the pain and their babies both. A woman named Mrs. Bainbridge didn't want to breathe the chloroform, but her husband was a surgeon, and he was very much in favor of it. She breathed it and her baby lived, but Mrs. Bainbridge died.

Anarcha's missus did not take the chloroform. At last, nature took its course and her baby lived and she was not cursed. In a few months, she was pregnant again. Soon thereafter, the Old Mansion slaves Louisa and Betsy gave birth as well, but there was no discussion of giving them anything to breathe for the pain. Anarcha caught their babies alone. Louisa's baby lived and it was a girl, but it was Louisa's third child, so it was taken away and sold. Betsy's baby boy lived too, and the boy was kept and he was named Charles.

Anarcha never learned to cook in Alabama—not when she was a girl, nor when she lived alone in the woods. In Virginia, she began to learn to cook the things that slaves cooked, for herself and for Delia, and for pregnant Old Mansion slaves and pregnant Woolfolk slaves too, and sometimes for the Woolfolk slaves who visited at night to discuss the whipping of Thornton, which continued for some weeks and then stopped, and then no one heard anything more about Thornton.

* * *

For ash cakes, mix two cups of meal with a teaspoon of salt and add water to make it sticky. Cover your hands with corn and bacon grease to shape the cakes, then wrap them in collard leaves or corn shucks and put them in the fire and cook them halfway. Sprinkle ash over them, finish the cooking, then take off the shucks and shake off the ash, and pluck out the splinters. Cook rabbit the same way, inside shucks and leaves. For persimmon beer, pick out the seeds, pack the fruit in a keg, and cover them with water. Add potato peelings and two cups of meal, and let it sour for three days. Mix with corn bread.

Corn bread is best when you can still see your fingerprints in it.

To keep your potatoes fresh, put them in a hole lined with straw. Cover them with earth and more straw. Irish potatoes make better pie than sweet potatoes. Cook your greens in the same pot you wash your clothes in. Anarcha sent Delia to the smokehouse to scrape up a mixture of salt and sand from the floor. She boiled the sand away and used the salty broth to season meat. In the Virginia summer, meat could be cooked on the flat face of a hot rock. To cook birds—any kind of bird—clean them, rub them down with lard, and let them sit. Broil them with pepper. As a chicken cooks, pound sixpenny nails into it to keep it tender. A possum is better when it's fattened for a time. Kill it, dress it, and hang it overnight to get out the animal scent. Then scald it for the hair, boil it to soften the meat, and lay strips of fatmeat over it as it bakes. When it's close to done, surround it with potatoes to soak up the gravy.

Remove the musk sacs when you dress a raccoon.

Make lye hominy and soap at the same time. First, make lye. Anarcha fashioned an ash hopper from a small barrel with corked holes in the top and bottom. She built a fire of oak logs, packed the hardwood ashes in the barrel, and poured in rainwater. After three days, she uncorked the bottom of the barrel and let the lye drip into a pot, careful because strong lye will take the skin off your hand. To make hominy, boil grain corn for a long time and pour the lye over it. Then soak the lye out with water and season it with salt and pepper. Cook it again in leftover grease from frying meat. That is lye hominy. To make soap, pour the lye in with fat and grease from a beef or a pig, and add turpentine if you'd made that too. Boil and stir until it's like jelly, then let it cool and cut it into squares. That is lye soap.

When the Maurys asked Anarcha if she knew how to cook, if she could come to Old Mansion and empty slops and do light cooking for Maurys who visited from Fredericksburg and Richmond, she said no, she never learned to cook and didn't know anything about it. Anyway, she couldn't cook when there were slave women with babies, and other slaves who needed tending until their troubles were over.

their light cooking & empty the slops

In fall 1857, there were horse races in front of Old Mansion. Masters brought horses and slaves, and when the races were run Anarcha and Delia could feel the pounding of hooves in the ground from half a mile away. The horse races offer the best explanation for how Anarcha met Lorenzo, an older slave from a plantation called Alto in King George to the north, owned by a man who also raced horses. One afternoon, Lorenzo visited Anarcha at her cabin. She did not know this man. But she knew what was in his eyes as she parched huckleberries in a skillet and pounded them up with a hammer to make coffee for them both. The next day, Lorenzo returned with a dead chicken and two live piglets she could raise on her own for meat. They baked the chicken and made dumplings by wrapping bits of meat in cornmeal and tossing them in with some boiling greens. For dessert, they had rock candy that Anarcha had made from molasses for the children, with Jerusalem weed in it for worms. It was sweet all the same.

By December, she was pregnant again.

Twenty

IN EARLY 1857, DUTCH PROGNOSTICATOR MATTHEW LÆNSBERG PREDICTED that a comet would destroy Earth that same year, on June 13. Decades earlier, in 1832, Lænsberg had suggested that another meteor would appear—also in June—to welcome an era of peace and calm. His error on the first occasion did nothing to prevent his direr prophecy, a quarter century later, from causing a global stir.

Adherents of the Anti-Development Theory claimed that the world was overdue for a catastrophe that would trigger the sort of radical climate transformation that geologists saw recorded in rock strata. Newspaper columnists quoted astronomers. John Herschel said a comet's entire tail might weigh but a few ounces. Jacques Babinet called comets visible myths. Pierre-Simon Laplace suggested that comets the size of small mountains had been enveloping the planet for as long as anyone could remember without their ever being perceived.

No major comets were seen in 1857. However, between 1854 and 1863, six were discovered by a young Florentine astronomer named Giovanni Battista Donati. The most significant of these was first glimpsed on September 6, 1858. A faint, curved extremity appeared. Over time, the comet's misty splendor grew and became visible to the naked eye as a fiery mass in a state of commotion, upheaved by violent internal forces. Donati's

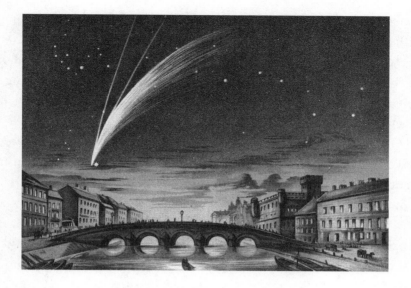

comet appeared to be in a race toward the horizon with the brightest star in the constellation Boötes, the herdsman.

In New York, Central Park was still under construction. The owner of a large telescope took up a conspicuous position on the park's unfinished east side to charge for close-up glimpses of the event. One day, Sims stood in a short line and paid six cents to mount a small ladder, place his right eye to the lens, and glimpse the nucleus of Donati's comet, surrounded by a pale light. It was not as if he was looking at something very large and very far away, but rather at something very small and pressed onto a slide, as some physicians had begun to do with what most, himself included, had considered to be a mere toy—the microscope.

In 1860, two meteors drew fiery lines above the United States, seeming to approximate the conflict that all quarters now regarded as inevitable.

The first appeared on July 20. Ship captains in the North were among the first to perceive an incoming projectile that grew to a disc twice as large as the moon before bursting into separate wedges that sketched colorful trails across the sky. From Brooklyn, the meteor presented as two burning balls, trailing sparks. From Long Island, it gave the appearance of a balloon afire, shedding flakes of flame. From Governor's Island, the meteor looked like a large gilt gas chandelier, all burners lit and shining with purple-tinted licks of light.

Two weeks later, a second meteor descended from the heavens above Kentucky, Virginia, and Tennessee. It burst in a great flash, appearing as two butter kegs tumbling across the sky. One glowed translucent red, the other green. Both gave off resplendent flashes.

On April 4, 1861, eight days before Confederate soldiers bombarded Fort Sumter in South Carolina, amateur astronomer A. E. Thatcher, using a borrowed 4.3-inch refractor telescope in New York City, discovered a comet situated inside the head of the constellation Draco, the dragon. A newspaper in Richmond called on Lieutenant Matthew Fontaine Maury to explain the phenomenon. Was it, in fact, the return of the comet that had roused dread in Charles V, the Holy Roman Emperor, in 1556? On April 18, Lieutenant Maury announced that he'd seen the comet from the Naval Observatory. It was one of his final acts as a member of the US Navy. Two days later, he resigned his commission to become a ranking officer of the nascent, and practically nonexistent, Confederate States Navy.

Visible to the naked eye by the end of April, Thatcher's comet sailed between the stars Athebyne and Zeta Draconis. By May, it had shuttled into the constellation Leo. A month later, it was streaking toward the horizon, leaving behind it an upright, fan-shaped tail that spanned a moiety of the azure field above.

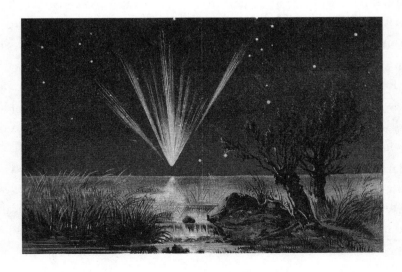

Would the United States end in just such an erratic blaze, observers wondered, once dazzling but now sinking into darkness? Or would it remain a fixed light, by which one might walk until dawn?

Southerners hoped Thatcher's comet would burst over Washington City and overwhelm the conspirators gathered there. A Charlottesville correspondent wondered if it would provide the same inspiration as the comet that had prefigured the assassination of Astorre III Manfredi in 1502. Wouldn't it be lovely if the celestial pillar signaled to some unknown hero to save the hour from Abraham Lincoln?

Sims took it as neither message nor harbinger. Nevertheless, he left the country. He booked passage aboard the *Persia* and sailed for Queenstown on July 17, 1861.

* * *

The previous few years had been a time of discovery and struggle.

The Board of Lady Managers, and even Sims's fellow physicians, had remained hesitant about his cancer cases. There were complaints about the devices he had invented to enable all sorts of procedures. His assistant Emmet voiced reservations about his curette: the ingenuity of man, he wrote, had never before devised an implement capable of so much harm. Valentine Mott objected to Sims's écraseur. The device had first been used in France, for the castration of horses. It worked by lassoing tissue with a loop of chain, which was then tightened and performed a crushing action. Sims's écraseur was designed to control bleeding as he cut stalks that connected tumors to healthy tissue. In 1860, a case offered him a chance to prove the value of the tool.

A woman from Connecticut was admitted to Woman's Hospital with a tumor the size of a Sicily orange. There was little hope for her. Nevertheless, Sims resolved to operate. It wasn't easy to convince the elderly Mott, five years from his own demise, to attend the procedure, but at last the old man agreed. Sims arranged to have the operation witnessed by a large concourse of medical gentlemen. He positioned Mott immediately to his right. The new Sims speculum was introduced. The tumor completely obscured the view of the woman's cervix. She was etherized—ether and chloroform were used regularly now, though Sims preferred the former—

and the loop of the écraseur was carried around the base of the tumor's unseen stalk.

Mott became agitated as Sims began the cranking motions to tighten the loop. He rose from his chair in objection. Sims had to fairly beg the man to wait but a few minutes more. Mott retook his seat. After a few more twists, the loosened tumor fell toward the mouth of the vagina. Most surprisingly, a sound of air began to emerge from inside the woman—not in an explosive burst, but in a gentle pattern. Sims and Mott exchanged a glance of horror as they recognized that the gentle pushes of breeze were timed perfectly with their patient's etherized breath.

Two or three more twists severed the tumor completely. It came free, and both men stared aghast at what was left inside: the entire rear of the woman's vagina was an immense, crescent-shaped cavity. Through it, they could see her detached cervix and uterus, and beyond they could see well into the peritoneum, where various organs gave the appearance of intertwined figures sketched over the points of a starscape. Her viscera gently heaved in and out, as though nudged by otherworldly winds.

Peritonitis was inevitable; the woman was doomed. The doctors quickly decided that reattaching her uterus was unlikely to extend her life; the organ was left to float in the peritoneal cavity. What remained of the cul-de-sac of the vagina was rapidly sealed. The woman lived for several months, until her cancer manifested once more.

* * *

After Emmet was installed as assistant surgeon, Sims requested additional doctors to free himself for further experimentation. He told the Board of Lady Managers that many incurable female diseases could be rendered curable—not only for the current inmates of the hospital, but others as well.

Beyond the fistula work, both at the hospital and in his booming private practice, Sims remained stuck for a time with many of the tools and tinctures and procedures that other doctors had invented: Dewees's tincture, when he could convince women to at least try it for cramps; uterine elevators—a lever on a stem—to return wayward uteri to their proper position; and awkward methods of repositioning prolapsed organs, followed by clunky fittings for pessaries. Sims was anxious to leave the bulk of the fistula work to Emmet, so he could explore uncharted territories.

They were exposed to baffling phenomena, the range of which underscored once more the richness of the vein Sims had tapped. Women arrived complaining of abdominal tumors and were delivered of healthy babies the next day, claiming never to have felt a single kick. One woman had nine children in fourteen years, having menstruated only three times. Others reported becoming pregnant from imperfect couplings, their husbands losing their semen early and depositing it only on their wives' labia. These immaculate conceptions suggested an ability of spermatozoa to travel far on their own locomotive power.

Sims saw five cases of complete absence of the vagina. In one, a woman had only a sort of blind pouch two inches deep. Neither she nor her husband was aware that anything was amiss. In another, the mysterious sloughing of a woman's cervix had resulted in a scar that clogged her entire vaginal cavity. Sims and Emmet encountered numerous cases of peculiar growths on the underbelly of the uterus. It was unknown to the literature, describable only as a cockscomb excrescence.

In 1856, they lucked onto the ability of sponge tents—compressed kelp that expanded when moistened, used to dilate the uterus—to annihilate growths. A young woman presented with persistent bleeding that left her waxy-hued and drained of life. A small sponge tent revealed a polyp, and Sims introduced a larger one in anticipation of receiving permission to remove the growth. The medical board failed to meet that week, and both Sims and Emmet assumed the other had extracted the larger tent. Days passed before the young woman complained of a rotten stench. Sims found the tent fully integrated with the growth and the tissue of the cervix. The only way to remove it was to pry around the uterine lining with his fingers, as he would with a tumor. The smell was so intense a nurse vomited. Nevertheless, the polyp was eradicated.

Most interesting was a pessary case in July 1855, just weeks after Woman's Hospital opened. The pessaries then available were Hodge's silver, U-shaped device, and Meigs's ring device, made of watch spring coated with gutta-percha. The woman's complaint was that the device she wore tended to become covered over with a rank, brownish crust. The case history included a conception after she had begun wearing the instrument. As the woman spoke, it became apparent that the device had not been removed during intercourse.

How was intercourse possible while the instrument was in place? Sims asked.

The woman was caught off guard by his frank use of language. It happened just so, she said.

Often? Sims said.

Now she blushed and put a hand to her throat. Oh, yes. Just as if there was no instrument there at all.

It was clear to Sims that the Hodge and Meigs pessaries could be improved upon by instruments fitted specifically to the particular dimensions of a woman's cavity. Before long, he was molding forms from block tin and sending the models to instrument makers for customized devices made from silver or vulcanite. This, in turn, led him to a new uterine elevator, one that moved on a rotating motion, rather than a motion on a single plane.

After fistula—profitable but limited—the most promising of women's ailments were painful menses and sterility, which his now extensive experience had confirmed to be a single ailment. A woman with a uterus that had flopped either forward or backward, or who was equipped with long or overlapping cervical lips, could be left with a canal that was blocked or crimped. Such anatomical irregularities hindered the escape of menstrual matter and inhibited a husband's seed from making the passage from vagina to womb.

For some time, Sims had been anxious to attempt the mechanical solution to the problem that had been proposed by Scotland's James Simpson: reorient the uterus, use blades to dilate the cervical canal, and install plugs as the wounds healed. Sims first attempted the procedure at his private office, but Simpson's practice of permitting women to immediately return home nearly proved fatal in several cases. The jostling rides across the city or to New Jersey resulted in sudden bleeding. In one instance, Sims arrived barely in time to save a woman he had incised hours earlier. He found her vagina filling with blood almost as fast as he could sweep it away.

In later cases, he kept women off their feet for at least a day, and devised a sponge probang to staunch the flow of blood. Soon, Sims and Emmet—not to mention the many young doctors who observed their procedures at Woman's Hospital—were shuttling all over the city to incise the cervices of women in their homes. The work was lucrative, if not quite so much as the cures of the cancer quacks.

The French had pioneered a different solution for too-lengthy cervical lips: amputation. The cervical opening could be made more accessible by the simple elimination of unnecessary tissue. Sims performed a number of such operations after Woman's Hospital opened, severing first one lip and then the other in separate procedures before discovering a patient who conceived between the two operations. Sometimes, the removal of a single lip sufficed. He had begun to envision an improved device—one outfitted with a blade, to be called a uterine guillotine, for the procedure's provenance—when another accident resulted in a fortunate advance. After a woman was etherized for amputation, Sims was informed that his guillotine was broken. He continued with scissors, and struck mid-operation on the thought of stretching a swatch of vaginal tissue over the ragged wound, just as flaps of skin were stitched over the stumps of amputated arms and legs. The woman became an unwitting pioneer.

Fear of surgery was an ongoing problem. Some women stormed off with mutterings of butchery when he explained the procedures for cervical incision and amputation. As often as he outfitted wives with pessaries their husbands never knew anything about, he performed operations on women who had no idea they were being subjected to surgical procedures. Thankfully, husbands knew their wives' best interest: they provided the consent that the dastardly new ethical constrictions placed on him. The trouble wasn't just timid women; Sims was sometimes forced to vigorously appeal to a husband's manly spirit—shaming them—to secure permission to operate. Doctors too remained fearful of attempting on live women what worked well on dogs and swine. The guillotine was a perfect example. He once removed a polyp with a stalk so tough it snapped a catgut guitar string. His guillotine would have made short work of it—if only doctors like Valentine Mott didn't shrink at progress.

In 1854, England's most famous surgeon of female maladies, Dr. Isaac

Baker Brown, published to acclaim a volume entitled *On Some Diseases of Women Admitting of Surgical Treatment*. Brown reported that he had been unsuccessful with Sims's fistula surgery. Nevertheless, he gave Sims's clamp suture all due credit. Sims thought of Brown as a potential ally. There were rumors that Brown was launching his own series of brave surgical experiments, for an operation based on long conversations with the Parisian physician Charles-Édouard Brown-Séquard.

Sims didn't know Brown-Séquard apart from what everyone knew: he'd been sent packing from Richmond after his corrupt heritage was exposed. Nevertheless, Brown-Séquard's work demonstrating that stimulation of the body's extremities could result in disturbing action of the brain was being incorporated into women's medicine by the likes of Isaac Brown and Sims's friend Horatio Storer. Brown and Brown-Séquard agreed: nervous conditions that saw women progressing from hysterias to epileptoid fits, and from there to seizures, idiocy, and death, were connected to the repetitive peripheral excitement of masturbation. The activity came about when women strayed from marital bliss; wayward women developed an unhealthy disposition for novel experiences and leaving home. Brown and Brown-Séquard differed only in their proposed treatments. Brown-Séquard advocated destroying the pudic nerve with the actual cautery. Isaac Baker Brown would take the bolder step of completely excising the seat of the mischief: the clitoris.

Following Sims's lead, Brown was on the brink of opening his own hospital devoted to women in London. This, coupled with Sims having been heralded in Brown's widely read book, surely figured in an invitation that Sims received, in 1856, to deliver the following year's annual address at the New York Academy of Medicine. It was a portentous victory. The event was only a few years old, but giving the address was already a great honor; the occasion would mark Sims's final conquest of the New York medical world. In four short years—just as Henri Stuart had predicted—he'd risen from nothing to near total dominance.

Twenty-One

The clamp suture—Mobile case—Foreshortening of the vagina—
Anarcha again—The Arsenal—The New York legislature—
"Silver Suture Lecture"—Artificial insemination—Vaginismus—
A Confederate spy

A PAIR OF THREATS AROSE, HOWEVER.

First, Sims's old assistant Bozeman published a paper attacking his methods. Bozeman complained that Sims had never detailed his experiments on Anarcha and the others. Furthermore, Bozeman claimed that Sims's clamp suture had been successful only half the time.

The problem was, it was true. The clamp suture was a failure. But it didn't matter, as the story of the device had served its purpose. Sims recalled how P. T. Barnum had handled the controversy over the fraudulent age of Joice Heth: he turned her autopsy into a new spectacle. Sims would do the same. First, though, he arranged, through Henri Stuart, to publish an anonymous response to Bozeman's article in the *New York Medical Gazette*. Not only was Bozeman wrong about Sims's procedure in Alabama, the notice claimed, Sims had made thirty perfect cures in New York, with no failures.

Next, inside of a week, he performed seven experiments using the so-called button suture that Bozeman had proposed as an alternative. The subjects included several women whom the clamp suture had failed. Predictably, Bozeman's button suture also failed. What Sims resolved to do, so as to poison the reputation of his former protégé, was deride the button suture in his upcoming address at the New York Academy of Medicine. But what exactly should the *focus* of the address be, if not his own clamp suture? One more clamp patient—a woman who had nearly died when a clamp severed an artery—offered a solution. Sims cured her with no device at all. That was the true revelation. All along, it was Henry LeVert's silver wire that had been the answer. The years of clamp suture experiments on Anarcha and the others had been wasted time. Silver sutures would solve the problem of his address. He would retain his narrative, but divert it so as to stitch a point of union between the story of Anarcha's cure and what he would now describe as the greatest advance in the history of medicine—silver wire as suture material.

The other threat was Anarcha herself. Unlike the clamp suture, Anarcha couldn't simply be snipped away from the tale of his success. He'd been concerned when Emmet first told him that Anarcha was coming to New York. The last thing he needed was for someone to learn that the central figure of his tale of heroism and perseverance had remained uncured. Fortunately, no one at the hospital knew her. And luckily, when she arrived to be treated, Emmet was in Alabama, attending to matters in the wake of the untimely death of Anarcha's former owner—Emmet's father-in-law, Nathan Harris.

And then, once again, providence seemed to intervene to turn the threat of Anarcha into opportunity.

* * *

In late 1856, Sims's old friend Josiah Nott sent him from Mobile a case of a dramatically anteverted uterus. The poor woman's organ was stretched out like a gourd. It lay radically out of position, almost flat along the top of her vagina. During an exploration of her cavity, Sims discovered that the organ could be entirely repositioned, with no pessary at all, if he simply seized her cervix with a tenaculum and tugged it forward. A surgical option was immediately apparent. The same tugging action could be achieved by the removal of excess vaginal tissue. An amputation of membrane would pull her parts into position, and a firm cicatrix would hold them in place. The operation proceeded quite similarly to his now clampless fistula surgery. The woman left New York with a perfectly positioned organ.

The procedure promised to become as useful and as remunerative as the incision of the cervix. As though on cue, Anarcha provided him with an opportunity for further experiment. All he knew of her condition, from Gibson in Richmond, was that her bladder was threatening to prolapse into her vagina. What if the foreshortening of the vagina to adjust misplaced uteri—as he had come to think of the new procedure—could work just as well to hold in check an errant bladder?

It was best if he saw her as little as possible. He left it to the house surgeons to perform her initial examination, just as he left it to them to perform the work of Stuart's two dedicated beds. These beds were now frequently taken up with abortion and syphilis cases, occurring in women whose characters Sims had intuited from the moment Stuart conditioned his assistance in establishing Woman's Hospital on control of two beds for women of his choice.

The house surgeons reported back that both of Anarcha's fistulae were gapingly open. There was little evidence that they had ever been treated. In addition, she was having difficulty breathing, likely the result of a too-frequent application of chloroform in Virginia. They advised turning her away as inoperable. Sims scheduled a surgery anyway, to foreshorten her vagina.

He was careful, when he entered the room, to give no indication to his assistants or nurses that he knew Anarcha in any way. He feigned surprise at the sight of a slave at the hospital. Out the corner of his eye, he could see the girl's puzzled expression as he ran through the series of queries that he posed to all new patients. For a moment, her voice in reply sounded identical to that of the young girl who had once dabbed his forehead during malarial throes. He was relieved when the opium took effect and left her dreamy and beguiled. He lifted the membrane of her vaginal wall, separating it from its attachment to the bladder to carve out a V-shaped portion. For his colleagues, Sims gave the impression only that he was performing another fistula surgery. Two weeks later, a house surgeon reported that the fistulae had failed to close, but there was improvement to her bladder. Sims arranged for Anarcha to be discharged after a blizzard hit the city. There was no need to see her again. In the months to come, the foreshortening of the vagina took its place as yet another weapon in his surgical arsenal.

* * *

He had wanted the Arsenal from the start.

As busy as the years were after the hospital opened, surgically speaking, the vast bulk of his time was spent lobbying for an even larger hospital, one of two hundred or even five hundred beds. The Arsenal was a perfect accommodation. Sims was drawn to the idea that the medieval architecture of the structure itself suggested the campaigns that had to be waged to conquer the dogged afflictions that assaulted the fairer sex.

With charity balls and benefit concerts at the homes of the wealthy and influential, Henri Stuart and Peter Cooper and E. C. Benedict and the Lady Managers had expanded the scope of Woman's Hospital's social and political influence. In 1857, a contingent made up of women reformers, physicians, and local politicians traveled north to Albany. They presented to the House of Assembly the case that the overwhelming success of Woman's Hospital at forty beds demonstrated ample need for a larger facility. The presentation's most poignant moment came when Sims read aloud the petition of Caroline Thompson, from Springfield, whose tumor had become more and more difficult to tap. Sims had not yet managed to convince the medical board to permit him to experiment with removal of the ovaries, the procedure Thompson desperately needed. Nevertheless— and to the brave woman's credit—she permitted herself to be recast as a fistula patient for the purpose of her speech, and to couch the stakes of a woman's health in terms laid out by Stuart and Sims. The case needed to be made in such a way that a man might fully appreciate the need.

How many of you, in your experience of life, Sims read aloud to the gathered legislators, have seen unhappy mothers and desolate homes? In many cases, the wife who had before been cheerful, useful, and happy, loses her health to some unknown cause. Her nerves are irritated, her mind clouded. When the husband comes home from his daily toil, the wife, suffering and nervous, fails to meet him with her usual happy welcome. She was once the light of his home, but now she seems to cast a dark shadow. Gentlemen, you all know that if home be not the brightest spot on earth to man, if he does not find peace, comfort, rest, and sympathy there, he will seek consolation and amusement elsewhere. Woe to the wife whose husband finds more attractive places than his own home can offer. Younger and fairer faces smile upon and welcome him, and in the excitements of society he seeks to forget his cares and drown his sorrows.

An act was soon passed—the funds necessary to transform Woman's Hospital into a state institution would be provided. The Arsenal, however, was denied them. Bureaucratic obstacles prevented any work from beginning until early 1858, when Woman's Hospital was granted full title to a plot of land at Fiftieth Street and Fourth Avenue. Construction would begin as soon as architectural plans were complete and the land was cleared. It had previously been a cemetery—decades earlier, upward of fifty thousand bodies had been hastily buried on the site during cholera epidemics. In some spots, victims of the disease were stacked eighteen deep.

* * *

By now, Sims hardly cared about the ethical strictures on doctors, particularly those that made it difficult for practitioners to seek business and acclaim. He had been more than happy to lend his name to advertisements for watchmakers and young ladies' boarding schools. It was remunerative, and an opportunity for his name to appear as equal with the likes of Peter Cooper, Horace Greeley, the gun inventor Norman Wiard, and the chess player Paul Morphy. Similarly, either Sims or Stuart drafted copy for the glowing portraits of Sims that appeared in the *American Phrenological Journal* and *Frank Leslie's Illustrated Newspaper*, whose editor he had succeeded in befriending.

He refused to be unduly disturbed by the outrage that followed his New York Academy of Medicine address. His critique of Bozeman, and the recasting of his fistula success as a victory for the silver suture, was met with attacks on his ignorance of the previous literature. Everything he had proposed, one writer claimed, had been known to others who cured fistula before him. Another reply in the *North American Chirurgical Review*—anonymous but probably penned by Bozeman, who had left for Europe—described Sims's discourse as an absurd plea for personal aggrandizement. The speech was full of forgettable frothiness and bombastic pretension. Bozeman chided Sims for suggesting that the occasion signaled his ascension to a presidential galaxy of previous speakers.

None of it mattered. A report on the AMA meeting of 1858 noted that not even just imputations of poor taste could prevent Sims from being heralded as a discoverer and inventor.

Perhaps it was the cavil on his presidential galaxy image—apt, if immodest—that compelled him, on a rare free day in the autumn of 1858, to stroll up the east side of Central Park. He walked past his much-coveted Arsenal building, now beyond reach, and continued to the telescope that had been described in some of the papers. Standing in line, he peered up at the curve of Donati's comet in the early evening sky. Sims did not anticipate that the telescope would invert the image—when his turn came, his vision was not of a falling star, streaking toward the end of the Earth, but of a climbing one. Given the nature of his work, was it surprising that the comet's well-defined head and nucleus, with a long, waggling tail that as far as anyone knew generated its forward motion, looked to him ever so much like a spermatozoon wriggling upward toward the womb, toward life?

The vision provided yet another God-granted insight—albeit one that came with a bite. What if the frequency of sterility among the married couples of New York was due not to wives' errant anatomy but to something amiss with their husbands? Many still believed, as his teachers had professed, that a woman's pains and sometimes her barrenness were penance for her original sin. But what if man too paid a toll for having nibbled the fruit he'd been offered? Only the toy microscope could reveal whether a man's seed was truly vital before it began its journey toward the egg. Or, because the vagina was a largely unhealthy environment for semen, as opposed to the womb that cradled it, perhaps a man's issue was extinguished before it could perform its life-giving act of penetration. The thrill of possible honor rose in Sims once more at the thought that he might again succeed where others had failed—in generating conception artificially. This time, however, the flush was tempered by a corresponding dread: if he was right, then he had already operated on a great many women with crooked wombs who had not required surgery at all.

* * *

The experiments were awkward, but how else could he husband the efforts of husband and wife?

It began with obtaining samples of men's fructifying fluid and subjecting it to minute observation. As he suspected, the source of sterility was sometimes a want of live organisms in the issue of vibrant men who could be accused of no lack of vigor in the delivery of their necessary ingredient. Men could be impotent but not sterile, or sterile but not impotent. Healthy sperm came in a range of mucous content, and he witnessed semen that had the proper odor but was afflicted with whitish mucosal flakes and lacked spermatozoa entirely. Normal semen dripped like water, but abnormal semen roped down off the end of a syringe. The observation of individual spermatozoa revealed uninjured swimmers darting sometimes to the left, sometimes to the right, occasionally projecting forward in a straight line across the field of his microscope's vision. Whenever they encountered an obstacle, they placed their heads against it as though trying to push it.

He could do little for men with dead sperm. But when he heard rumors from distant quarters of doctors etherizing women so as to enable insemination—another myth was the claim that fertilization was more likely if intercourse offered satisfaction to both parties simultaneously—it struck him that the best candidates for conception by artificial fructification were the women whose labyrinthine passages refused to submit to surgical remedies. The cases he'd already seen of virginal conception suggested a particular agency on the part of some women's bodies, so much so he theorized the existence of an unknown constrictor muscle in the upper part of the vagina. This muscle would cause the cervix to perform a vacuum action—like a suction bulb—to assist spermatozoa on their journey.

Confirmation of that particular discovery would have to be claimed by some other practitioner. Sims turned his attention to the opposite: women whose anatomies were hostile to procreation, either by architecture or by chemistry. In husbanding these afflicted couples toward the joys of family heirs, Sims prescribed sexual intercourse on the third, fifth, and seventh days after the monthly flow ceased, and on the fifth and third days prior to its expected return. He arranged to be present on these occasions. It was his charge—so as to determine the amount of semen to throw into the uterus—to swab a patient's cervical canal after coitus and examine it. Over two years, Sims provided monthly injections to half a dozen couples, at last achieving success in a barren woman afflicted with a dislocated organ and a contracted canal. Her conception was a remarkable success; none other had been recorded. Unfortunately, she miscarried at four months, after a fall and a fright.

* * *

For couples whose sterility was mechanical in nature, a surgical option was more appropriate—and more remunerative.

In May 1857, Sims encountered a baffling case in private practice: a forty-five-year-old woman of refinement and quality, married at twenty but a virgin owing to mysterious genital pain. He found her in nervous near-collapse. The slightest touch at the mouth of her vagina caused her to shriek and spasm. He managed to insert his finger to the second joint, but the resistance—wholly involuntary—was so great he lost feeling in his digit. The woman was highly sensitive to noise as well. Mostly confined to her sofa, she had for years given herself over to intellectual efforts.

He advised examination under ether. Apart from minor retroversion, the woman was anatomically normal and entirely healthy. He could explain neither the spasmodic reaction that made coitus unthinkable, nor why previous physicians' attempts to dilate her vagina with plugs had resulted only in agony. The solution was apparent enough: just as incisions of the cervical canal enabled a larger orifice in the interior of the body, so should it be possible to expand the exterior of the vaginal opening with blades. Incisions into the muscles and nerves flanking the vaginal orifice, followed by plugs, would create an opening that would enable intercourse. He could not explain the underlying mystery, but the likely culprit was motherhood denied. Pregnancy would result soon enough.

The couple begged for the procedure, but Sims balked. He explained that Woman's Hospital was intended as field of experimental observation. An untested procedure was unjustifiable on a woman of such high status.

It was fifteen months before he encountered a similar case. Another virgin exhibited the same dread of having her vagina examined, the same full-body seizure when she was touched. This time, surgery was justified: her husband had threatened divorce. Sims first attempted a cut only around the edges of the hymen. This offered no relief. In a second operation, he made incisions into the sphincter muscle, which manifested notable improvement. It was then, however, that the young woman's mother concluded that Sims was experimenting on her daughter. Of course he was! He attempted to explain what was at stake, given the husband's threat, but the befuddled mother yanked her daughter from Sims's care.

No matter; he'd learned a great deal.

A few weeks later—remarkably, as it was an unknown condition—another case fell into his hands, the wife of a clergyman. Then a fourth case appeared, and a fifth. He now conceived of a name for the condition: "vaginismus," reflexive spasms that prevented intercourse. And he devised a full cure: amputate the hymen completely, and then make several deep, two-inch incisions around the vaginal orifice, in the shape of a Y.

Practically speaking, the condition offered him a chance for publication. He'd produced only two articles since Woman's Hospital opened, and the vaginismus cure promised to be his most profitable innovation yet, as the condition seemed to predominately affect women of means. As the cases piled up—he sometimes had several vaginismus patients at Woman's Hospital at once—he set his sights on perfecting the cure before undertaking his own journey to Europe.

Two factors precipitated a trip that was long overdue.

First, Bozeman had sailed and returned, besmirching Sims's name across the continent. In England, Isaac Baker Brown had switched from the clamp suture to Bozeman's button. And in Scotland, James Simpson was criticizing Sims for having experimented on slaves without anesthesia. Sims needed to visit, if only to ensure that Bozeman did not secure the lion's share of credit for pioneering a field of medicine now widely known as "gynecology."

Second, the planning of the newer and larger Woman's Hospital hit a snag when Sims lost a vote on the nature of its design. Fortunately, the architect who was hired suddenly died. Sims seized on the chance to propose an Old World journey to study hospital design, to gather information for the replacement plan.

This last was merely cover for his true mission. The country was finally tipping into war; South Carolina seceded first, in December 1860. It was followed within a month by Alabama, Mississippi, and Florida. Louisiana and Texas came not long after. Sims had been correct to suspect that his success as a surgeon would provide him with opportunities to assist the emerging rebellion. The Confederate government took official form in February 1861, with Montgomery itself as its capital.

A message arrived through the Pratt family, known to Sims from his Alabama days. The father, W. H. Pratt, had been dispatched to Europe to seek loans of up to $50 million from European powers. His son Thomas, like Sims's own sons, Granville and Harry, had followed Sims into the health of women. In 1859, Sims had arranged for the young Dr. Thomas Pratt—who was now courting Sims's daughter Eliza—to take a position as house surgeon at Woman's Hospital.

The message instructed Sims and Thomas Pratt to travel to Europe together. Pratt was to coordinate efforts with his father. Sims was to establish himself as a surgeon of note in Ireland, Scotland, and England, and then travel to Paris, where he would receive further instruction. At last, Sims had the chance to fulfill his life's martial duty. Fate had determined that he would serve in a covert capacity, as his grandfather had once done.

Twenty-Two

Lincoln—Delia in service—War stories—Marriage—
Catching babies—Mary L. Booth—Anarcha's case record—
The Uprising of a Great People—*W. H. Pratt—*
"Hostile to the government"

ONE DAY, A PEDDLER VISITED THE PLANTATION OF DR. GRAVES IN DURHAM County, North Carolina. He was the ugliest man you ever saw, tall and bony with black whiskers and black, bushy hair, and a weird look like a dog that's been hit. The peddler sat on the porch and opened his pack full of items for sale: needles and thimbles, blankets and frying pans. The missus brought him a cup of milk. The peddler asked her, How many slaves does the master own? How many men do you have on the Confederate side of the war? What do you intend to do if your slaves are set free?

The peddler asked the missus what she thought about Abraham Lincoln. She told him she didn't want to hear about any Abraham Lincoln. He was nothing but a black devil messing in other people's business. The man chuckled, packed his bag. He thanked her for the shade of the porch and for the cool milk. He said maybe that old Mr. Lincoln wasn't so bad, and then he was gone around the bend.

Three weeks later, the missus received a letter from the White House. The peddler had been Abraham Lincoln himself! He'd been peddling all over the South as a spy, he said, to view the conditions of slave life on plantations. The missus got so mad she burned the letter and made her slaves throw the ashes in the river.

In Gallatin, Tennessee, Mr. Lincoln and his wife stopped at the Hotel Tavern, both dressed as tramps. After he was elected president, he wrote a letter to the hotel and told them to look between the leaves of the table where he and Mrs. Lincoln had sat. Sure enough, "A. Lincoln" was written there.

He traveled down the Mississippi on a flatboat. He rode through Alabama on a gray mule, not afraid of white people who said they would kill him if he ever set foot in their state.

In Falls County, Texas, Mr. Lincoln visited a plantation and slept in the missus's bed because it was the custom to give strangers a place to sleep. He saw slaves come up to the house to draw four pounds of meat, and he saw slaves whipped and sold. After he left, he wrote to the master and told him to look at the bedstead where he'd slept: "A. Lincoln."

Mr. Lincoln was a black man, some stories said, the son of a queen. Or, he was a medicine man who had said that every borned man should be free. He wanted to send all black people out west, to avoid allowing so many to sink into torment.

He came through North Carolina, and so did Sherman, dressed in rags. He was given food and tobacco to chew on. He attended meetings and dinners where white people talked about what they were going to do with the Yankees.

After he was elected, Mr. Lincoln traveled by ship to Beaufort, South Carolina, posing as a rail splitter. He ate dinner at a house called the Oaks. No one knew it was the president-elect of the United States. After he left, he wrote to those he had met and told them to give slaves three days per week to themselves, otherwise there would be bloodshed. He told them to look behind a certain door for a gold-headed cane he'd left behind. Please send that cane along, Mr. Lincoln wrote.

One day in Virginia, a slave girl named Lizzie saw a man walking up the road with her master. The man was dressed in overalls, with a red handkerchief around his neck. Lizzie knew it was Mr. Lincoln, but her master didn't recognize him. Mr. Lincoln picked Lizzie up and whispered in her ear that he hoped her people would be free pretty soon. He stayed in the home of Lizzie's master for three days.

Another slave in Virginia saw Mr. Lincoln wearing a big furred hat with an eagle on the front. He wore a long, lovely cape and he was riding a large black horse.

* * *

When Delia turned seven, she was put into service at Old Mansion to help care for Maurys. After Anarcha and Delia had returned from New York, Maurys began coming and going from Old Mansion with frantic regularity. Maurys did not watch their tongues around a girl as young as Delia, and Delia understood quite well. She brought her mother stories on a grapevine that stretched directly from Old Mansion, skipping past the huddle of slave cabins where the Maury slaves lived.

Lorenzo brought stories too. Lorenzo's master was Charles Mason, a lawyer and owner of a plantation called Alto, and on Wednesday nights, if Lorenzo could get a horse—and he often could because he was one of his master's favorites and Charles Mason was always telling him how fond he was of him—Lorenzo would ride the twenty miles from King George County, along the road that led to Hooe's Ferry. He would stay the night and ride back in the morning, and he would come again on Saturday night and stay until early Monday morning, leaving well before the sun came up because twenty miles took almost two hours at a trot.

Anarcha saw Maurys only rarely now. They came to her cabin to ask questions about cures and herbs, or they came when one of the slaves got pregnant, or when a Maury lady got pregnant. Anarcha's missus got pregnant again six weeks after Anarcha got pregnant by Lorenzo. That's how her missus learned that Anarcha was pregnant again, and she didn't ask any questions about how she got pregnant. She said Anarcha already had a daughter, a daughter who was liked and treated very well at Old Mansion, so when Anarcha's new baby came, it would be sold off as others had been sold off. The missus marched away, and Anarcha was not surprised, and neither was Lorenzo surprised. They did not speak of the baby because there was nothing to say that would be of use—and because they did not have to speak of a baby that refused to leave their thoughts.

It was only a short time later that Lorenzo, one night, asked Anarcha if she would confess that she wished to be married. She paused. There wasn't any reason that he said it—he just said it. Anarcha looked from his eyes to her lap. She replied yes, she would confess it, but only if he confessed it first.

Lorenzo said, I confess it, I wish to be married.

Then I confess it too, Anarcha said.

She didn't have any broom for them to step or jump over, but they counted it as a real wedding anyway, and as Anarcha grew with the baby that would not be their baby, Lorenzo was there to care for her. From that time forward, Anarcha always had a good husband to take care of her when she leaked or limped or coughed.

In the fall, as the end of Anarcha's troubles approached, a comet appeared in the sky, the same comet that J. Marion Sims glimpsed through a telescope on the east side of Central Park in New York City. From Virginia, from night to night near the end of September, dark outlines peeled off from the bright center of the comet. Four lines emerged from the main body, as if it was giving birth to a litter of puppies. The comet babies disappeared into its tail. Soon after, Anarcha's time came, and nature took its course, and she gave birth to another baby, and this baby girl was immediately taken away, just like her first baby, but this baby didn't die. Like the tail of the comet, the memory of the baby separated and glowed bright and lingered for a time, then began to fade.

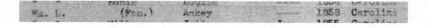

Six weeks later, Anarcha caught her missus's baby, and that baby was named Charles Walker Maury. In 1859, Arena gave birth to a baby girl, but that baby girl was sold even though Arena didn't have any other babies. For a time, Maurys were doing well because Anarcha's master was living at Old Mansion and he was doing carpentry work instead of sailing in the navy, and Maurys were planting cabbage seeds that had been sent to them by other Maurys in London, England, seeds ripened in the south of France, it was said. Anarcha's missus wanted portraits made of the two sons she now had. Then, in early 1860, she was pregnant again, and a few months after that a meteor came shooting out of a cloud over the South. It didn't have a train until it burst into two pieces, sparks shooting from the front ball to the hinder ball. The oblong bodies appeared connected by a scintillating cord of light.

In October, Anarcha's missus gave birth to a girl, Harriet Woolfolk

Maury, but she wasn't a healthy baby. Delia, now nine, returned at night from Old Mansion with news. As in Alabama, when the young Duncan girl died despite Anarcha's attempts to save her, the Maurys talked about how the baby girl Harriet had been caught. Delia said their master and missus wondered whether something had gone wrong with the catching, or with the cutting of the cord between baby and mother. Perhaps it explained why Harriet so often had boils all over her head and a fat, swollen neck.

By then, the war had started. It was the war that would free the slaves, Lorenzo said, and he worried from that time forward that he would have difficulty—remit or no remit—galloping horseback on the Hooe's Ferry road to see his wife. He said they should act natural and be even more polite with white folks. But in secret they should pray for freedom. Anarcha's missus knew Anarcha was married now but said little of it. The war didn't change much, for a time. First one Lieutenant Maury resigned from the navy, and then the other—Anarcha's master—did the same.

A new comet appeared, in the northern sky. For a time, it served as a point of reference, other than moss on trees, for slaves moving north through the woods at night. There were many runaways now, following that beacon of light. Sometimes Anarcha only heard them, as she had in Alabama when she was a cursed girl in the woods. Sometimes they stopped to rest a moment. She gave them food to eat and carry, but she was never a conductor on any kind of railroad.

In June 1861, Arena and Rhena gave birth. But nature refused to take its course, and both of those babies died as Anarcha caught them.

* * *

Before it began, Sims's career as a spy was almost foiled by a young, prodigious reporter for the *New York Times*.

Mary Booth descended from the Earl of Warrington and a man who once owned all of Shelter Island, at the end of Long Island. Booth was born in 1831. By then, the family money was mostly gone; her father was a schoolteacher in Brookhaven and worked part of the year in a wool manufactory.

As soon as she could talk, Mary Booth was able to recite poems and recount lengthy tales. She learned French and English simultaneously. Later, it was claimed she spoke and read Latin, Portuguese, French, Spanish, Italian, and German.

She read Plutarch and the Bible at five; Racine at seven; Hume, Locke, and Gibbon at ten. She accompanied her father to the wool manufactory and spent idle hours studying the intricate workings of old machines.

She was sent to school between ten and fourteen, first with Reverend Miles Tuthill at the Miller Place Academy, where astronomy, accounting, surveying, and navigation formed the practical education. At the Bellport Academy, she disliked mathematics but was determined to excel. She mastered Bourdon's algebra and Legendre's geometry.

In 1845, her family moved to Brooklyn, where an uncle worked as a night watchman. Her father established Public School No. 3; Booth tutored his students. Simultaneously, she attended Professor Abadie's Brooklyn Collegiate Institute for Young Ladies, where she was steered toward translation work.

It was said that Booth once fell in love with a young man. He signed on as a mate for a whaling expedition, set sail, and never returned.

At eighteen, she moved into New York. Her family kept two rooms available for her, a bedroom and a room in which to study and write. She found paying work in the city as a seamstress. She sewed vests in the daytime; her nights were reserved for study and writing. She began to perform unpaid translation work and produced unsigned articles and sketches, on subjects ranging from iceboats to the embalming of the human body.

In the 1850s, she became active in a number of salons and organizations, championing abolition, equal pay for women, and education for black Americans. The Alpha Club, a women's rights group, held meetings at the Booth family home in Williamsburg. Booth rubbed shoulders with Susan B. Anthony, Lydia Maria Child, Herman Melville, Elizabeth Cady Stanton, Harriet Beecher Stowe, Louisa May Alcott, and the poet sisters Alice and Phoebe Cary. She became a member of the Women's Rights Congress, the Society for Advancement of the Truth in Art, and the Anti-Slavery Society.

In 1856, she translated from French her first book-length work: *The*

Marble-Workers' Manual: Designed for the Use of Marble-Workers, Build-ers, and Owners of Houses. Her only payment was additional books to study.

Opportunity arose when Dr. Franklin Tuthill, brother of her former teacher, was hired as an associate editor at the *New York Times*. Booth became a reporter. She received modest pay for work that took her all across the city. Several years later, a friend suggested she produce a school-book for publisher W. R. C. Clark and Meeker, about the history of New York City. No such history had been written. In a year, she delivered an eight-hundred-page manuscript for *History of the City of New York: From Its Earliest Settlement to the Present Time*. Clark and Meeker redirected publication to a general audience. Published in 1859, the book elicited a letter of congratulations from Washington Irving.

Booth was twenty-eight years old.

It was the midpoint of a prolonged period of exhaustive production. *The Marble-Workers' Manual* had been followed in 1857 by *The Clock and Watch Makers' Manual*, which Booth did not translate but write, draw-ing on her fascination with mechanical devices. A translation of Joseph Méry's biography of poet André Chénier appeared in 1858, and the fol-lowing year Booth published translations of the *Thoughts* of Blaise Pascal and Victor Cousin's *Secret History of the French Court*. In 1860, she trans-lated Edmond About's novel *Germaine* and Jenny d'Héricourt's *Woman Enfranchised*.

Then, for reasons that remain unclear, Booth began working for Dr. J. Marion Sims. She took a room in his house as a boarder. She worked as amanuensis and accountant. She lived alongside Sims's family for the two years leading up to the Civil War. Why would a successful emerg-ing author, a humble reporter for the *Times* with clear sympathies for the North, agree to work for a southerner who had already been criticized for bombastic speeches and uncertain leanings?

Three years earlier, the *Times* had assigned Booth a story about the medical dispensary of Elizabeth and Emily Blackwell. The dispensary was about to expand into the Infirmary and Dispensary for Women and Chil-dren, an institution that became a necessity after Sims failed to accept either Blackwell sister as his assistant at Woman's Hospital. Modest in scale, the infirmary offered several beds and services for women, performed by female physicians. It was an institution dedicated to women, run by women.

Booth visited the Blackwells' home to interview them, but they were not present. Instead, Booth encountered Dr. Marie Zakrzewska, the Blackwells' confidante and colleague. Booth and Zakrzewska became life-

long friends. Booth's *History of the City of New York* noted the significance of the Blackwells' fledgling hospital but made no mention of Sims's Woman's Hospital, even though by then it was known across the United States and abroad.

It's unclear what work Booth did for Sims. She was alternately said to keep Sims's ledgers (she was not an accountant) and to have assisted him with a manuscript for a book project (Sims produced no books, and only a single paper, between 1859 and 1861). Most likely, she acted as a secretary and was employed in creating a legible set of case records from Woman's Hospital's earliest days, including a more neatly transcribed version of Anarcha's case. Anarcha's name was changed from "Anacha (slave)," in the old register, to "Anneca Maury—(a negro)," in the newer record.

Booth struggled to imagine ways to make a contribution as the war loomed. She settled on translations of texts from French intellectuals who wrote in support of the North. In thanks for the moral support provided to the public by translations of Augustin Cochin and Édouard René de Laboulaye, Booth received letters from Senator Charles Sumner, Secretary of State William Seward, and President Abraham Lincoln.

In early 1861, as war appeared more and more certain—and as Booth continued to live in Sims's home, less than a block from Woman's Hospital—she translated *The Uprising of a Great People: The United States in 1861*, by Count Agénor de Gasparin. Gasparin had fled France after refusing to support Louis Napoléon's constitution. Three years later, Napoléon III declared himself emperor of the Second French Empire.

Publisher Charles Scribner released Booth's translation of *The Uprising of a Great People* several months after the Civil War began.

The institution of slavery, Gasparin wrote, had always been dubious in a land where equality had been inscribed with éclat at the head of a celebrated constitution. America was an impressive nation. Its population had increased tenfold since the turn of the previous century, and it had produced personages of great accomplishment: Longfellow, Emerson, and Irving, to say nothing of scholars such as the navigator Lieutenant Matthew Fontaine Maury, or orators like Seward and Douglas and Lincoln.

Yet Americans had become habituated to the most odious of crimes. The passage of laws reducing to slavery every free black person who did not quit the soil of his home state had failed to raise even a murmur of disapprobation. The United States seemed on the brink of losing that faculty without which nothing can survive—indignation.

What would a victorious South look like? Fifteen states would soon be joined with Mexico, Cuba, and Central America, forming a colossal slave jail stocked by a renewed slave trade. The price of slaves would collapse, and the fortunes of southern planters would crumble. Immigration of whites to such a nation would be naught, and slaves would increase in all ways until the slave population far exceeded that of free men. Such a monstrosity had never before existed in the world, and such a nation would be at best a short-lived concern, representing slavery and nothing else, Gasparin wrote.

The ringleaders of Charleston and New Orleans were now claiming that sly men capable of presenting the cause of slavery in a seductive light were already being received sympathetically in England and France. England would be controlled through cotton, France through influence. But would the rest of Europe truly lend its hand to the most audacious attack ever directed against Christian civilization? Did it not recall the shudder that convulsed the world when the free nation of Texas was converted to a slave territory?

It was never in the compact of the United States that they would form a league only until it pleased some of them to leave it. In his farewell address to the nation, George Washington advised watching over the Union with a jealous eye. Silence and indignation should be imposed on any who dared renounce it, he said.

The election of Lincoln closed the past and opened the future, Gasparin wrote. A naval blockade would be installed to quash the rebellion, and the present crisis would regenerate the institutions of the United States. The principal consequence of the nineteenth century would be the elimination of slavery, in all its forms. Americans should take heart. The star-studded banner of the United States would be neither less respected nor less glorious should a few of its twinkling cluster of stars sour and fall away to Earth.

Installed in Sims's home, Mary Booth completed her translation of Gasparin one month before Sims departed for Europe as an envoy of the South. Whatever transpired between Sims and Booth at this time is lost. What came next was recorded in the records of the State Department.

W. H. Pratt of Mobile—father of J. Marion Sims's future son-in-law—was sent to Europe with instructions to procure $50 million in loans from European heads of state. To communicate with his superiors, Pratt requested return correspondence be addressed to a nom de guerre. One of his letters was intercepted at the United States' Dead Letter Office. His plans were revealed to Secretary of State William Seward, who promptly sent notice abroad: all American diplomats should do everything in their power to thwart the designs of W. H. Pratt.

Several weeks later, New York Commissioner of Police James Bowen received a bit of news about the private views of celebrated surgeon Dr. J. Marion Sims. It was a tip Mary Booth was uniquely positioned to supply. Sims was wholly secessionist in spirit, Bowen had learned. Only days before, he had sailed for Europe aboard the *Persia*, traveling in the company of Thomas Pratt, whose father was already there as an active agent of the South.

Bowen transmitted the news to Seward, who followed with another message to his staff: surgeon J. Marion Sims was on his way to Europe, and his purpose in traveling abroad was believed to be hostile to the government.

Mary Booth continued her translation work through to the end of the war. She wrote in support of the United States Sanitary Commission. Members of Woman's Hospital's Board of Lady Managers served on the commission's hospital ships, which sailed to battle sites to receive casualties.

After the war, Booth was offered the editorship of a new magazine, a publication aimed at an audience of women, to be called *Harper's Bazar*. She accepted. Within six weeks, the journal achieved a circulation of eighty thousand. *Harper's Bazar* included reports on fashion, domestic essays, short stories, brief accounts of significant events in New York, obituaries of persons of note, and so on. Booth remained as editor for more than twenty years.

The period of the joint lives and work of Mary Booth and J. Marion Sims was recorded in several sources. Yet Mary Booth never published a word about J. Marion Sims, and Sims's autobiography makes no mention of the much-celebrated Booth having once lived in his home. After his death in 1883, Sims was heralded in publications across the world.

Harper's Bazar took no notice of his passing.

Twenty-Three

Belgium—The Duchess of Hamilton—Edinburgh—
James Simpson—A death in London—Clitoridectomy hospital—
Velpeau—Paris—First case in France—"Malakoff"—
The little countess—The Kangaroo

IN BELGIUM, THEY ARRANGED THREE FISTULA OPERATIONS FOR HIM, BUT it was all a ruse to deflect suspicion. He performed all three surgeries in a single morning. A week later, one of the women died, his second death since arriving in Europe. This time, he blamed the nurse.

Alabama was well represented in Belgium. Years before, Sims's old friend Henry Hilliard had served as chargé d'affaires in Brussels, and more recently E. Y. Fair, from Autauga County, had filled the more senior position of resident minister. Fair resigned two weeks before Lincoln's inauguration, and he and his wife remained in Belgium to assume a similar post for the Confederate States of America once the continental powers recognized the new nation. By the time Sims arrived, Fair had returned to Alabama to tend to his property and slaves—including Anarcha's son Washington—but his wife remained abroad. In Brussels, Sims boarded at the Fairs' home. It was good to be among southerners again. He was provided with more than a room, as Mrs. Fair was an active secessionist, exceeded by no agent on the continent in activity to secure arms for the Confederacy and establish relationships with European heads of state.

Sims's contact in Paris, an Englishman in league with the cause, had arranged an introduction to King Leopold's personal doctor. Sims was invited to Belgium, where his surgeries, despite the death, were heralded by the medical community with a great banquet. He was nominated for the Legion of Honor. The real purpose of the trip, however, was to meet Princess Marie Amelie of Baden, the Duchess of Hamilton. She was cousin to Louis Napoléon.

The duchess arrived at the Fairs' home late one night, unannounced, taking excessive care because the new resident minister in Belgium, Henry Shelton Sanford, was employing private investigators to track the movements of dozens of Confederates and sympathizers across the continent. After a hasty introduction, the duchess explained that most of the French aristocracy, and both the emperor and Empress Eugénie, sided with the South. However, they had to take great care in how, and with whom, they shared their positions in regard to the American conflict. Even a breakfast invitation to an envoy could become international news. It was already the case that when the emperor wished to send private messages to the government of the United States, he arranged to have his teeth checked by an American dentist, Thomas Evans. Evans was a Union man and a longtime resident of Paris. He carried messages directly to the resident minister, leaving no paper trail. That was what was intended for Sims. What the emperor wished was that Sims take up permanent residence in France, so that he might be called upon to receive and transmit delicate messages to the fledgling Confederate government. Once he was installed in Paris, the duchess explained, she would take Sims into service as her private physician. If it became necessary, Sims would visit the emperor on the pretext of treating the empress, who was in any event keen on opening a hospital for women in Paris.

* * *

Six weeks earlier, the excellent news of the South's victory at Manassas had greeted Sims and the young Thomas Pratt when the *Persia* landed at Queenstown. Now the whole world understood that the war would not be a quick affair. Pratt immediately set off to Liverpool to find his father, and Sims traveled north to Ireland with a handful of letters of introduction from Valentine Mott and others. In Dublin, for a week and a half, he was feted to exhaustion by doctors and politicians alike, men anxious to observe the eating and drinking habits of an American only lately removed from the frontier. On one occasion, Sims fended off the advances of a wealthy Irish widow.

He traveled to Edinburgh, via Belfast and Aberdeen, and it was here that he was able to attend to the other reasons for his journey: the study of hospital design and the injury that had been inflicted upon his reputation by Bozeman's surgical grand tour, three years before. He witnessed ten days of surgeries in Edinburgh's Rotunda Hospital, and after years of performing James Simpson's incision of the cervix, he was at last able to question the man himself as to why American women seemed to bleed so much more heavily than European women. What Simpson revealed, by way of permitting Sims to observe a procedure, was that the operation in its originator's hands was an incision only by the most precise definition of the term. Sims later learned that deaths resulting from the procedure had been withheld from the medical journals. One woman died in Aberdeen, another on the Isle of Man.

Simpson had watched Bozeman cure a woman with his button suture; he was keen to see Sims perform a fistula surgery as well. But there were no cases available. The only operation Sims was asked to perform at the Rotunda was on a young virgin afflicted with a tumor the size of a pullet's egg. Sims had no trouble looping her growth, but its stalk kept breaking the wire that was meant to sever it. He was left craving his guillotine. What he most wished to share was the pioneering work he'd done on cervical amputation and vaginismus, but fistula was all the European doctors wished to hear about. Frustratingly, they lumped his own operation together with Bozeman's and called it the "American method." At least they gave silver wire to Sims alone—no mention of Henry LeVert. Within two weeks, he concluded that he would learn nothing new of surgery in Europe.

He did not operate on a fistula case until he arrived in London, where again he was warmly received. He met all the London greats—Wells, Savage, Routh, Wilde, and Isaac Baker Brown, who within the last two years had followed through on his plans to open a Woman's Hospital–inspired institution. Brown had left no mystery in naming his hospital. It was called the London Surgical Home for the Reception of Gentlewomen and Females of Respectability Suffering from Curable Surgical Diseases.

Sims performed his operation at the more modestly titled Samaritan Hospital. It was a difficult fistula, but not so difficult as to have signaled the tragic result—the woman died. The operation seemed to go well, and Sims impressed a crowded surgical theater. But the woman's aftercare was left to others, and Sims received no notice of anything amiss until the woman had perished. An autopsy left no doubt: despite having performed the procedure hundreds of times, Sims had inadvertently sutured closed her ureters. Her symptoms were identical to those of the all-too-familiar peritonitis; death resulted from kidney failure. To Sims's surprise, his colleagues appeared nonplussed at the loss, and they were no less impressed by his surgical technique. When he expressed concern that his European sojourn had begun on a sour note, he was blithely assured that no record would be kept of the case.

More notable—and ultimately more controversial—was a series of operations that Sims witnessed at Brown's London Surgical Home, a week before he departed for Paris. Brown revealed that there were already objections to his surgery to remove the clitoris, despite the clear indications of its efficacy, from Brown-Séquard and others. Mostly, the protests came from stodgy old physicians. Brown was already planning a book to document the procedure's many successes. Sims observed several surgeries—it sometimes resulted in frightful hemorrhage—and he heard various reports on Brown's cures. A seventeen-year-old girl had been taught to masturbate at boarding school, and excessive self-excitation had resulted in hysteria and catalepsy. A fifty-year-old woman from Newcastle upon Tyne had attacks that were so severe they could be triggered by the slightest brush against her dress. A thirty-nine-year-old woman was afflicted with a mania that gave great anxiety to her friends. She was always restless, constantly wakeful, and threatened suicide to every stranger she encountered. And a thirty-four-year-old woman was among the most eccentric of characters. She would go out to the country, alone, and walk for miles. She was irritable and passionate, and she had lost all of her gender's natural modesty in manner and speech. She was so forward at parties, gentlemen avoided her. She had never received an offer of marriage.

All were cured by excision of the true source of the trouble, Brown explained. Sims resolved to attempt the procedure when he returned to Woman's Hospital.

* * *

He traveled to Paris both to do his duty for the South and to find, despite speaking only rudimentary French, a wealthy clientele for his incision of the cervix, his amputation of malformed cervical formations, and his vaginismus operation. But it was fistula that would get him in the door—for both his role in the war and his private life. Theresa was already making plans to move the family to Paris for the duration of the conflict.

He had only a single letter for France, from Mott to Dr. Alfred Velpeau, whose incision of the cheek Sims had employed on the young slave George, fifteen years earlier. Velpeau had been among the first in Europe to assert that birth and midwifery should not be left to women, as had been the custom of humanity, but rather regarded as a true and distinct precinct of medicine. Sims took rooms on the Rue de l'Université, near Velpeau's Charity Hospital. He had little choice but to lurk outside the hospital walls, waiting for a way in.

One morning, he was beside the main gate when a young man approached, carrying himself a bit differently from the Frenchmen who wandered in and out of the hospital. The boy was likely a student, possibly foreign. Sims followed him into the grounds, where he overheard the student converse with a friend—his accent resembled Sims's own mangled attempts at French. Sims caught up to the young man just as he was fitting himself into a white apron for the day's surgical lessons. Sims tried a sentence. The student laughed. His name was Edmond. He was from New Orleans. Sims heaved a sigh of relief and explained that he was Dr. J. Marion Sims, curer of vesico-vaginal fistula, and he had a letter of introduction to Dr. Velpeau. Was Velpeau at the hospital?

Disappointingly, the boy didn't know who Sims was. Doctors in England, Scotland, and Ireland had all seemed well versed in his works. Edmond explained that what France knew of fistula came from the legendary Dr. Jobert de Lamballe, so renowned he was known simply as Jobert. As to Velpeau, he was away from the hospital but would return in two weeks' time.

There was nothing to do but wait. Sims invited Edmond to dinner, to gather information about Velpeau and whatever other Parisian physicians might be able to assist him in establishing his reputation. Edmond warned him against telling the story of his slave patients; it would most likely be met with ridicule. The boy observed that French doctors would probably regard Sims as a curiosity, a showman—something like P. T. Barnum.

Excellent, Sims thought. He said nothing of his portentous meeting with Barnum in New Orleans. Similarly, while he sensed that Edmond too had a rebel heart, he resisted the impulse to reveal the full purpose of his mission abroad. He'd been told to be careful. The boy seemed happy enough to sign on as his translator.

The days of waiting for Velpeau let him experience both the gaiety of Paris and its dirt. When the omnibuses weren't too crowded, Sims rode about the city, drinking coffee and listening to music at the Café des Ambassadeurs near the Place de la Concorde, or witnessing the five hundred jets of the fountains outside the Palais Royal on the first Sunday of the month. At three million inhabitants, London had been the largest city he had ever set foot in, but in England he'd scarcely had a moment outside a hospital or a medical society. In Paris, half the size, he saw it all. One morning, he witnessed a gang of servants cleaning a filthy street with water, like a surgeon flushing a wound. On another occasion, in the Latin Quarter, he strolled past a man offering tooth extractions on the street. Sims already felt an animosity to his counterpart, the dentist Thomas Evans—but it was no wonder that foreign dentists in Paris had been among the first to experiment with anesthesia. As the street dentist prized rotten molars from the recesses of patients' mouths, the Parisian crowds howled and applauded to mask their screams.

One night, Sims strolled across the Pont Neuf to the Île de la Cité to behold the Cathedral of Notre Dame, and to stand outside its adjacent neighbor Hôtel-Dieu, a hospital already a thousand years old.

After Edmond reported that Velpeau had returned to Paris, they visited Charity Hospital together at an appointed time. They caught the celebrated surgeon between a number of scheduled procedures; Velpeau took Mott's letter in a hand stained with his last patient's blood. He read it in English and then asked Edmond, in French, Well, what does he want?

Edmond had been right—there was coldness and derision in Velpeau's voice. Sims explained that he was the inventor of a new operation for the scourge of fistula, a procedure that had met with invariable success. If the professor would be good enough to procure a case, Sims would be delighted and honored to demonstrate a method that had improved upon centuries of failed efforts.

All right, Velpeau said coarsely. I'll get him one. He turned away with neither handshake nor nod.

It was some days before a case could be found. Every day, Sims dragged Edmond around Charity Hospital, imposing on doctors, appealing for patients. By the time a fistulous woman was found, word had spread to the Latin Quarter, and from there to the rest of Paris, that a young, bold American had arrived with a claim of success on a condition that had bested even the great Jobert. Anticipating a spectacle, the great surgeons of Paris, including Nélaton, Trousseau, Ricord, and Malgaigne, attended the operation—all except Jobert, who refused to appear.

Before the procedure, exactly as he had done with Anarcha and the others, Sims first demonstrated his surgery for an amphitheater of gathered physicians. He cut a hole in a piece of hard, thick cotton batting and expertly stitched it together again with the tools he would soon use on a young French woman, already positioned nearby on an examination table. Edmond translated Sims's speech nervously. He had never expected that as a first-year student he would find himself explaining procedures to the full congregation of French medical glory.

Sims hid his relief when at last he looked inside the woman and saw that the case was an easy one, a small fissure that did not touch the cervix or urethra. He was pleased to show the gathered doctors that the procedure could be performed without chloroform, and there was tentative applause as he announced the operation complete. Fearful of a repetition of the horror of what had happened only weeks before in England, Sims himself tended to the woman every morning. On the ninth day, the same physicians gathered for the removal of the sutures. Sims clipped away the wires. A French doctor stepped in to look inside, and then proclaimed with no little fanfare that the procedure of the American doctor had been a total success. Rather than Sims, the joyous crowd hoisted the young

Edmond onto their shoulders. No matter—Sims's introduction to France was complete.

The cases came quickly, then: a troubling fistula on a fat, obstinate woman at a private clinic on the Quai Voltaire; a case from Dr. Jarjavay at the Hospital St. Antoine, which Sims was encouraged to pursue even though he deemed the fistula inoperable; a case of a bladder poking through a fistula, and then from the vagina, brought to him by Dr. Vernier. Best of all, Sims was granted the honor of performing surgery in Jobert's surgical theater, at the Hôtel-Dieu. All the procedures were successful, and the cases created a furor in the Parisian medical community.

It was then that he was invited to Belgium. When he returned—the duchess now arranged the approval needed to operate on women of title and value in France—all the pieces were in place for the success of his missions. Not only would the duchess make him available to the emperor, an ongoing association with royalty would bolster his credentials. He began to suspect that in Europe he could charge thousands for a difficult fistula case. A practice that offered his full menu of surgeries, for a country and a continent that had never seen them, might earn him as much as fifty thousand per year.

Furthermore, he was now introduced to "Malakoff"—Dr. W. E. Johnston, an American physician who had long since traded the scalpel for the pen. Johnston produced pseudonymous dispatches from abroad—often with a medical tinge—for the *New York Times*. Years before, Sims had read Johnston's accounts of the siege of Sebastopol, and of the attempted assassination of Napoléon III by the scoundrel Orsini. Equally fascinating for New York doctors were Johnston's accounts of a physician who had infected himself with vaccine matter, resulting in the amputation of his tongue, and a man whose bony tumor of the eye socket grew until his eyeball was expelled and hung listlessly against his cheek. Like Edmond, Johnston too warned that Sims would be seen in Europe as a Barnum-like figure. With luck, Sims thought, he would repeat this for his New York audience in telling the story of Sims's reception in France.

Compared to Mary Booth, whom Sims had taken into his home in New York, "Malakoff" was a perfect compatriot. Booth had been a disappointment. She had never written a word about Sims—not even after

Mittag arranged for her to be profiled in the *American Phrenological Journal*. Worse, she had gone out of her way to assist the Blackwell sisters, who were now pulling patients away from Woman's Hospital.

* * *

Sims wrote to Theresa that his greatest success came on October 18, 1861, when Mungenier brought him a woman that Bozeman, during his brief time in France, had refused to operate on. It was a terrible case: the entire base of the woman's bladder was destroyed, and her detached ureters were exposed, squirting urine directly into her vagina in pulsing spurts. Sims promised a cure with a single procedure. Civiale, Baron Larrey, Campbell, Huguier, and others attended the operation at the Hotel Voltaire. The woman was cured with no fewer than twelve silver sutures.

Yet, Sims told his wife, the glory of this success was marred a month later, when at last he was asked to operate on a woman of class, a young, beautiful royal. The chloroform was administered, and all seemed to proceed well until the girl's skin began to turn blue. He froze. He had told them that he preferred ether, if anesthesia was to be used at all. He did not know what to do. The young countess's heart stopped. The gathered French doctors paused to let the American assert himself, but all Sims could do was watch the girl die. At last, Nélaton—who would soon become famous for an operation on Italy's General Garibaldi—leaped into the fray to tilt the surgical table upright, so that the young countess's head nearly touched the floor. The French surgeon explained that mice killed with chloroform could be revived with this quick action—holding them upside down. Sims stood to the side, as silent and dumb as a statue. After several tense minutes, life and breath returned to the countess's body. He continued his procedure, but the danger was not over. Twice more, the life of the young countess flagged, and Sims stood aside so that she could be revived by the quick-thinking French physicians.

After this, he was pleased to enter into the service of the Duchess of Hamilton. He played out his remaining time in France in repose. The royals behaved quite like normal people when they did not have to "put on their dignity" for visitors. He contemplated the career he would have in France after he returned home to fetch his family. Theresa—and his daughters—would be at home here. Perhaps, he thought, it was time to write a book of everything he had learned since Woman's Hospital opened.

There was some difficulty arranging his passport to return to New York. The North was requiring southerners to take an oath of allegiance. If he did so, he would sacrifice the property he still owned in Alabama. Furthermore, he learned that the Legion of Honor he had been awarded in Belgium had been held up—Henry Sanford, in Brussels, was refusing to accept it on his behalf. He would concern himself with that in America. For now, his missions were complete, and "Malakoff" would surely massage the story of the young countess for his New York audience. Sims expected to return home to a hero's welcome.

He sailed from Queenstown, aboard the *Kangaroo*, on Christmas Day 1861.

Twenty-Four

Raids on the James River—Maury sent to London—
Lewis a privateer—The Alabama—The career of the Georgia—
The Confederacy turns to Napoléon—A Paris ball

THE RAIDING PARTIES, EMBARKING ON DARK NIGHTS TO PLACE MINES alongside Union ships on the James River, used the light of Thatcher's comet to steer by. Its train lit the sky like a glorious flame and appeared to tug the stealthy craft through black and quiet waters.

Matthew Fontaine Maury was cleared by the "plucking board" in 1858. It was uncertain to what extent his cousin Lewis—Anarcha's owner at Old Mansion—had swayed the deliberations. Not only was Maury retained by the navy, he was promoted to commander. It hardly mattered. By then, *The Physical Geography of the Sea* had earned him worldwide renown. He would forever be known as the intrepid Lieutenant Maury.

He spent the years before the start of the war either ignoring its approach or doing what he could to avoid it. He traveled to England to promote his book. He attempted to initiate discussion between the North and the South. It was of little help. Thatcher's comet appeared, he sighted it at the Naval Observatory, and resigned. The comet grew over two months' time, until it was bright enough to light the way for the placement of his mines.

The mines were oak beer kegs stuffed with rifle powder, weighted to sink, and outfitted with triggers that lit a pressure-sensitive fuse. Designed in Richmond, the device worked swimmingly when it was demonstrated at size for the Confederacy's secretary of the navy, who in the early months of the war allocated $50,000 for a Torpedo Bureau tasked with crippling Union ships anchored outside Richmond. Lewis was given command of a battery at the mouth of the James, and the cousins worked in concert to perfect and manufacture mines. In addition, the Confederate navy took up Maury's plan for the rapid construction of a fleet of gunboats, which would begin to resist Lincoln's blockade.

The jury-rigged nature of the Confederate navy began to make itself apparent with the failure of the early, guerilla-style raids that Maury sometimes led on the James River, in the summer of 1861. The fuses of the mines failed to ignite, and pilots hired to steer the saboteurs through the comet-lit darkness showed up drunk. The raids mostly failed.

Matthew Maury kept up a hectic schedule of travel among Fredericksburg, Old Mansion, and Richmond, where Robert Maury helped to form the Virginia Volunteer Naval Company. Maury needed tact in negotiating his position in the new navy hierarchy; those who were now his superiors had been among the loudest of voices calling for his "plucking board" ouster. Lewis may have become collateral damage in those squabbles. He was ordered to oversee the construction of the gunboats, an effort that was similarly ad hoc. He was assigned thirty slaves to help perform the work, but they were all field hands. None of them knew how to hew a board.

In addition, Lewis was denied command of one of the vessels that the Confederate navy seized, reconstituted, and put into action in a ferocious naval battle off the coast of Virginia in early 1862. The CSS *Virginia*, an ironclad rebuilt from the hulk of a broken frigate, the USS *Merrimack*, rammed and sank the USS *Congress* and the USS *Cumberland*, and fought to a draw another ironclad, the USS *Monitor*, before being forced to scuttle herself to avoid capture. The battle was counted as a victory even though the *Virginia* was lost. Subsequently, Matthew Fontaine Maury was ordered to relinquish control of the torpedo effort and head for the Caribbean. Lewis was sent to Wilmington.

Maury rejected a covert appeal from Russia. He was offered an admiralty in the tsar's navy, with a salary of thirty thousand per year. The Russians promised him an estate for his family and the superintendency of the St. Petersburg observatory. He turned it down to fight in the war. Now, the order to sail south felt like a demotion. He didn't understand it until he arrived at the Charleston home of a man who owned a number of blockade runners, small vessels that specialized in threading the needle between Lincoln's warships. By then, a new vessel, the CSS *Alabama*, had launched from a port in London. Despite England's announced neutrality in the war, the *Alabama* had been stealthily designed and constructed with a single purpose: to disrupt northern merchant shipping. She escaped England before her true mission was detected, and by October 1862 the conquests of the *Alabama* were becoming the stuff of legend; she had captured and burned more than a dozen northern merchant vessels, mostly whalers.

Those were Maury's orders. He would sail to Bermuda, and from there travel to London to exploit his popularity as an author and scientist. He would assist with messaging of the progress of the war in the European press and work to procure additional ships to be converted to commerce raiders. He knew long before Lewis did that his cousin, who for the time being was still Anarcha's owner, was to become the commander of one of the new vessels.

* * *

Maury's first attempt to run the blockade failed. His ship was fired upon, but not hit. Three days later, poor weather permitted him to sail for Bermuda, but the slow boat's captain got lost. Maury reclined on the foredeck and used a sextant to navigate by the stars.

Bermuda was like a hideout from the pirate days of the West Indies. The crews of eight or ten other blockade runners all stayed in the same whitewashed hotel. They were men accustomed to salaries of fifty dollars per month, but now they were pulling thousands in gold for a single voyage. They debauched on champagne and tossed shillings from their balconies to the islanders below. Maury was feted first by the governor of Bermuda and then by the captain of the HMS *Immortality*, docked at Port Hamilton. After two weeks, he booked passage on the Royal Mail steamer for Halifax, where again he was hosted by the local governor, and by Admiral Milne of the seventy-two-gun HMS *Nile*. Milne gave Maury a meal and offered him a tour of the ship's gun decks. From Halifax, Maury arranged transatlantic passage on the steamer *Arabia*, plying between Boston and Liverpool. The voyage was smooth until the roaring forties, where the weather tested the ship's smokestacks. He arrived safely in England in early December and set to work to procure a ship for his cousin.

In Wilmington, Lewis Maury was laid low for a time by rheumatism. When he recovered, he was sent to Richmond. The wounded from Manassas streamed into the city; no one knew how many had been killed. At a hospital, Lewis happened upon the Maury family friend Dr. Charles Bell Gibson, who had fruitlessly attempted to cure Anarcha. It was Gibson who had made the arrangements when Lewis purchased her through his cousin. Now, Gibson was surgeon general of Virginia. He appeared exhausted—Lewis watched him operate on a doomed captain hit with a minié ball that had ricocheted around the inside of his rib cage. Lincoln must now thirst for blood, Lewis wrote to his wife. If the restoration of the Union was still the watchword, then there was no chance of peace, for among the southerners he had encountered there was a determination to be free or to be exterminated as a people.

One night, he was put into a room with two wounded men. One of them was dead by morning.

In August, he was sent to Charlotte, and from Charlotte to Jackson, Mississippi, to attend to a court-martial proceeding, and then back to Charlotte, and then to Mobile and Selma, Alabama. By November, he was back in Richmond, boxing up what items he had acquired to send to his wife in Milton, North Carolina. He did not have time to visit his family before he received orders from the secretary of the navy. He was to make haste to London, to report to Commander Matthew Fontaine Maury, and deliver a sheaf of cotton bonds. He would take command of a ship like the *Alabama*, a vessel of the sort that Lincoln had already denigrated as a privateer, a pirate ship—with a penalty of hanging if he was captured. He was ordered to enforce strict navy discipline. He would respect the rights of neutral countries and expect belligerent rights from any nation that hoped to have good relations with the Confederate States of America. He should seek to do the enemy's commerce the greatest injury in the shortest amount of time.

On December 16, 1862, Lewis signed documents selling all of his and his wife's property and slaves—including Anarcha and Delia—to his brother-in-law James T. White, who remained at Old Mansion.

* * *

Lewis spent Christmas at Charleston. On the rough seas to the Bahamas, one of the blockade-runner pilots was thrown overboard by a sudden swell. A rescue boat failed to find him.

A rumor among the islands claimed that a hunt was on for the *Alabama*, its havoc-filled career now tallying upward of thirty charred prizes. After the new year, Lewis set sail for Cuba on a ship he never would have imagined possible. It had a black captain and an entirely black crew. He did not know how they did it, but the captain and crew navigated by compass and stars alone. Never for a moment did they seem doubtful of their course.

From Havana, the steamer *Tasmanian* made three hundred miles per day. Lewis arrived in London on January 31, 1863, where he boarded with his cousin. He was promoted to commander the following month. His ship, a rebuilt merchant vessel to be called the CSS *Georgia*, struggled to escape dock in England just as the *Alabama* had. Off the coast of Ushant, in the lower channel, the *Georgia* rendezvoused with another vessel that supplied a crew of Englishmen. Most were no more than boys. They loaded guns that Lewis had ordered months before: two twenty-four-pound cannons, two ten-pound Whitworth rifles, and a thirty-two-pound Blakeley rifle that they had to move closer to the port of Brest to transfer from ship to ship, due to high seas. Once the guns were mounted, Lewis raised the Confederate colors and gathered the crew to explain the distribution of bounty. Each prize they took would be divided into shares, officers due two shares, crewmen one. He arranged passage home for those sailors who chose not to sign on to a Confederate man-of-war.

The *Georgia* took its first prize on April 25, 1862. Lewis had his choice of a number of sails on the horizon, and the *Dictator* was betrayed as a Yankee merchant ship by its skysail poles. He fired across its bow and put its crew in the hold. It was a struggle to set the *Dictator* afire, but they succeeded at last by first lighting her captain's quarters. Four days later, off Porto Grande due west of Africa, heavy with prisoners, the *Georgia* was sighted by the ten-gun USS *Mohican*. Luckily, she had let her steam down; they managed a tense escape. Next, in the equatorial doldrums, where squalls could come from every direction, they watched as a whirlwind formed on the surface of the sea, matched by the eddying of an ominous cloud overhead. A waterspout appeared, stretched between sea and sky, a column of wind and ocean twisting and writhing like a great serpent. As it moved toward the *Georgia*, the spout created a roar and an awe-inspiring whirlpool. Lewis was forced to spend powder and balls firing into the monster before it swamped the ship. The column collapsed and sank back into the sea, like a vanquished god.

They sailed west, flying mostly the stars and stripes, saving their colors and their coal for when they were in pursuit of a prize. By May 13, they neared All Saints' Bay off the coast of Bahia, Brazil, waters Lewis knew well from earlier voyages. The sighting of a man-of-war sent them to battle stations. It was the *Alabama*! The two vessels pulled into port together, and the crews joyously shared news. The *Alabama* had taken another twenty-five prizes off Brazil and had recently sunk the USS *Hatteras*, which fought until its guns were nearly on the level of the sea. In port, Lewis and the *Alabama*'s captain, Raphael Semmes, learned that the USS *Niagara* and the *Mohican* were hunting them. After a short respite, the *Alabama* and the *Georgia* broke the rules of port to escape once again. A mile out, the *Georgia* was fired upon from shore. For a nervous moment, through his glass, Lewis watched the cannonball skipping across the surface of the water toward his ship. It dipped into the ocean just short of its mark.

The *Georgia* transferred five hundred pounds of powder to the *Alabama*, and the two ships parted ways. They sailed south. In early June, Lewis sighted Sugarloaf Mountain off the coast of Rio de Janeiro. They seized the *George Griswold*, but freed it as it carried only wheat and flour, and they burned the *Good Hope of Boston*, which was stuffed with a cargo of Yankee notions: pianos, sewing machines, carriages, and furniture. On June 18, they spotted Trinidad and soon chased and captured the *Constitution*, ferrying coal and missionaries to Shanghai. Nine days later they seized the *City of Bath*, bonding it for $40,000, only to learn later that the wife of its captain had sewed $16,000 in gold into her dress. The crew of

the *Kent* submitted without a fight—they asked if Lewis commanded the
Alabama.

By the middle of August, the *Georgia* dropped anchor at Table Bay,
Cape Town. They were forced to leave at once because the day before,
the *Alabama* had taken a prize too close to shore. A swap of crewmen
with men ashore meant that for the first time the *Georgia* was manned
by a majority of American sailors. Heading north again, they bonded the
John Watt for $30,000 and then, almost at once, they crossed paths with
the USS *Vanderbilt*. Lewis spied through his glass the warship's rows of
eleven-inch Dahlgren cannons. Anticipating a battle, he advised his crew
to board the ship and die like men, rather than allow themselves to be
hanged from the yardarms. Miraculously, the *Vanderbilt* passed them
by—she was hunting the *Alabama*. They continued north. For several
days, the *Georgia* seemed borne aloft by a gigantic school of albacore and
bonito, crowding the surface of the water as far as the eye could see. At
night, the phosphorescent glow of the fishes' flanks lit the ocean as though
with flame, from horizon to horizon. In daytime, smaller fish frenzying
near the surface gave the water the appearance of a vast silver platter. The
albacore leaped sometimes twenty feet into the air to snatch at frantic
flying fish that left the water like ducks rising from a pond.

A long train of accumulated seagrass tailing behind the ship slowed
their speed from nine knots to five. Nevertheless, the *Georgia* took a
final prize on October 9, the *Bold Hunter*, itself slowed by a belly full of
coal. The ship was set afire, and as its masts and sails burned, it somehow tacked back toward the *Georgia*, as though steered by a demon.
The burning ship butted up against them several times. Lewis managed
to steer his vessel clear, but not before the coal in the hold of the *Bold
Hunter* burned holes in its hull and flashed them a glimpse of Hell, just
before the ship sank.

Dragging its thick, grassy crop, now in desperate need of repair and
provision, the *Georgia* sailed again into the English Channel in late October 1863, making for the port of Cherbourg, on the northern coast of
France. Lewis was uncertain of how they would be received. He dropped
anchor beside one of the great French ironclads, the 84-gun *Tilsitt*. Beside
the hulking warship, the *Georgia* looked like little more than a cockleshell.

The first word he received from land was that Commander Matthew Fontaine Maury was in France.

* * *

Six months earlier, in London, precisely at the moment the *Georgia* began its cruise, Matthew Fontaine Maury learned that his middle son, John, aide to yet another Maury military man, had gone missing near Vicksburg, Mississippi. He remained unaccounted for as Maury produced short pieces of propaganda for the local press, worked to secure loans, and helped to form the Society for Promoting the Cessation of Hostilities in America, a front for the effort to lure Britain to the side of the South. Through an intermediary, Maury purchased the HMS *Victor*, which would be converted into yet another Confederate cruiser.

Early in the war, Richmond believed—the Confederate capital had been transferred to the South's third-largest city—that England's declaration of neutrality was the weakest in Europe. If England sided with the Confederate States, then France, and perhaps Spain, would follow. By late 1863, foreign assistance had become an even higher priority, as news of the war was not good. There were always rumors that Charleston had been taken—it was unlikely, but the city remained imperiled—and there was word that Port Hudson had been starved out, the garrison keeping at their posts until the last mule was eaten. In Mississippi, both Jackson and Yazoo City had been sacked and burned. A great battle had been fought and lost at Gettysburg, it was said, though details of the scope of the defeat were scarce and untrustworthy.

Over time it became clear, despite royal sympathies, that English judgment had decided it would be inauspicious to interfere in the conflict. The navy shifted its attention to Louis Napoléon, who with queries about the effectiveness of southern ships had signaled interest in the South. France was now the better hope. Napoléon's voice spoke for an entire nation, and his ongoing war in Mexico—the French were preparing to install Archduke Maximilian of Austria as emperor—gave him a more than theoretical interest in the southern border of the Confederate States.

Maury was sent to France. He was to supervise the construction of four ironclad clipper corvettes of 1,500 tons, 400 horsepower. A shipbuilding firm in Bordeaux had offered to build the vessels, with only cotton bonds as payment. Such an arrangement could not possibly have been proposed without approval from the highest reaches of the French government.

Paris was overrun with sailors, agents, and associates of both the North and the South. Every southerner in Paris, civilian or no, was a spy of some kind. Confederate officials congregated at the Grand, a monument to opulence built to satisfy the emperor's desire for a hotel that would be the envy of the world. Maury dutifully visited the Louvre, the tomb of Napoléon I at the Hôtel des Invalides, and the museum of antiquities at the Hôtel de Cluny, and he attended one of the thrice-weekly balls in a garden along the Champs-Élysées, which at night was lit by a chain of gaslights half a mile long. Within a week, Maury had arranged to purchase and ship home five hundred phosphide fuses for his mines in Virginia.

* * *

Among the expats in Paris that Maury heard rumors of, *a violent secessionist* the strangest was surely Dr. J. Marion Sims. Maury had learned that Sims was in Paris the moment he arrived in France. The doctor, it seemed, had created a stir with the operation he had perfected on the slave girl—Lewis now called her Ankey—that Maury had brought to the Naval Observatory. Sims had quickly become a favorite of society, it seemed. It was said he was an intimate of Maximilian and his wife, Carlotta. It was even claimed that Sims had the emperor's ear at a time when the emperor was publicly ostracizing southern diplomats, to sustain the appearance of ongoing neutrality. Not that Sims kept a low profile—rather, he had a reputation as a violent secessionist, and his home was known as a meeting place for southerners of all kinds, navy men in particular.

Maury did not meet Sims until Lewis's ship, the *Georgia*, finished its cruise at Cherbourg. At last, the emperor had granted Confederate ships the right to

> A Paris letter in the New York Herald says that the house of Dr. J. Marion Sims, of New York, (a native of South Carolina,) is a great place of rendezvous of prominent Secessionists in Paris. Dr. Sims gave a ball at which Mr. Slidell and family and all the hightoned Secessionists of Paris were present. A number of paroled Rebel officers were in the party, and attracted great attention and sympathy.

dock at French ports for repairs. It was a subtle action, but it provoked strong remonstrances from the Lincoln administration.

Weary from his voyage, Lewis traveled to Paris from Cherbourg. The cousins reunited. Lewis was too ill to continue as commander of the *Georgia*, but he was well enough to attend a ball at the home of Dr. J. Marion Sims. Well into the evening, the two cousins had the chance to shake Sims's hand and inform him of their peculiar connection. Even more than the lives of men who traipsed freely about the world on warships and steamers, Maury proposed, it was this young woman—a slave, no less!—who demonstrated the smaller and more intimate place the world had become. Her quiet, invisible influence had vaulted itself through the universe. Was it not remarkable? Like a rogue star or a planet without a system, she had by turns fallen into the orbits of men who now offered champagne toasts thousands of miles from where any of them lived.

Maury was struck by Sims's response. At the name of the girl, he flushed as though he'd seen a ghost. He immediately asked if Anarcha was alive. Lewis said yes, alive and well enough, albeit sickly. Sims muttered something about the impossibility of her condition. Medicine was not magic, he said. He was even more surprised to learn that Anarcha was married, or thought herself so. For a moment, his eyes darted, as though news of the girl's ongoing life required something more of him than a simple nod to the vicissitudes of fate. He excused himself, claiming that someone needed to refill the glass of the beautiful French wife of the South's lead diplomat in France, John Slidell.

Lewis sailed for home. After the war, he was exonerated by an act of Congress. He moved to New York to work in the customs house and to make a home with his wife in Brentwood, on Long Island. Maury continued his efforts in Paris. He attempted to appeal to Maximilian to launch a naval campaign in California. A few ironclads that set sail around Cape Horn could induce California and her sister states in the west to act on what was already an impulse—to leave the Union and seek more profitable associations. Next, the South made an offer of a cession of Texas and a portion of Louisiana, if France intervened in the war. It was of little use—Napoléon betrayed them. In 1864, the *Alabama* docked for repairs in Cherbourg, as the *Georgia* had done, but within weeks the famed ship was sunk in a battle that many Parisians traveled to the coast to witness, from the roofs of houses overlooking the sea. The war was over in a few months' time.

The body of Maury's son was never found. It was determined that he had been captured after he borrowed a pair of field glasses and took a horse along a river for reconnaissance; he was executed behind enemy lines. Maury did not immediately return to the United States. First, he attempted to sell his mines in Europe, detonating a sample for Napoléon in the Seine to induce a purchase. He traveled to Mexico to establish a colony for displaced southerners. He left before the effort was dissolved, and before Maximilian—also betrayed by Napoléon—was executed by Benito Juárez. In the end, Maury returned to Virginia and accepted a professorship at the Virginia Military Institute.

No Maury ever saw Anarcha again.

Twenty-Five

Early months—Manassas—Fredericksburg—Lewis departs—
Woolfolk slave escape—Anarcha leased—
Charles Mason of King George

*A*FTER THE WAR STARTED PROPERLY, YANKEE GENERAL ULYSSES S. GRANT
rode up in a balloon to count the horses and mules in Confederate camps.
The North had many balloons. The South had just one, stitched together
entirely out of silk dresses donated by southern women. There was no gas
except in Richmond. The balloon was inflated, tied onto an engine, and
taken along the York River Railroad, to view up and down the line. One
day, the balloon was tied to a boat on the James River. The tide went out,
the boat was left high and dry, and the balloon made of silk dresses was
lost.

In Richmond, the price of coffee soared to $4 per pound. Tea was $20.
Butter was $2 per pound, and lard was $.50. Corn sold for $15 a barrel,
calico was $1.75 per yard, and a yard of muslin goods cost $8.

Women at Old Mansion made plaited hats out of rye straw, with wide
brims just like the hats they had ordered from Paris before the Yankees
cut off supplies.

Plantations stopped planting money crops, tobacco and cotton, and
planted food for soldiers instead. Food for slaves was rationed, and the
best food went to the hardest-working slaves. To steal milk, men sucked
directly from the udders of cows, so they wouldn't be caught carrying it.
Anarcha chipped up sweet potatoes, dried them and parched them, and
ground them up for tolerable coffee. They lived on hominy.

Anarcha's master left Old Mansion to manage a lumberyard where they were cutting boards to make ships. They worked so hard and so fast they had to put shoes on the oxen. For a time, Maury children and Maury slave children played at Confederates and Yankees. White children always played the Confederates.

For some time, stories continued to arrive. Fired anew with the spirit to flee, Woolfolk slaves gathered at Anarcha's house at night to trade news of the war's early battles. If you were far away, you first heard the faint sound of bugles and then the crackle of musket fire, and maybe you saw bombshells in the distance, candles flaring in the woods. If you were close, the first thing to come was the zip of musket balls passing you by, or hitting the ground around you like hail, and sometime after came the sound of the guns, and still later a riderless horse would gallop past you with its entrails hanging out, running until it got tired and fell down. If you were closer, you saw white bodies go up in the air and come down black—that's what powder did to white folks. Or you saw cannonballs sailing through the battle, and if a chain was stretched between them, they cut down the trees of the forest like a sword. You would see horses with all four legs chopped off by similar means, still alive and struggling to stand on their stumps.

In Arkansas, a slave family was about to sit down to a dinner of peas, ham hock, and corn bread when they heard the bugle calls and hid in the cellar. A white woman fell down the cellar steps and stayed hid down there with them, and they heard a wounded soldier crawl into the cabin overhead. He moaned and moaned from his wounds, until at last he stopped moaning.

A slave in Mississippi watched soldiers dump nineteen bodies into a well and fill up the rest with dirt.

Maurys came and went frantically now, north to Fredericksburg, east to Richmond, slaves sometimes traveling with them, carrying stories. Anarcha's master had been promoted. He was now Lieutenant Colonel Maury, and the other Lieutenant Maury was now Commander Maury. In Richmond, Commander Maury was conducting additional experiments on underwater mines, which made the slaves who helped him nervous. They carried small mines up and down the stairs and cleaned up the water after the explosions in the iron tub. Lieutenant Colonel Maury was ordered to the command of a battery at Sewell's Point near Norfolk. His letters home revealed that his force of machinists, carpenters, locksmiths, and shoemakers was too small and too sick to effectively man the fourteen guns that were mounted barbette to fire over the parapets. The enemy observed their camp from another balloon, and one night, three slaves took advantage of a soldier who fell asleep to steal a boat and make their escape.

A Maury office in New York was ransacked and relieved of $80,000 in stocks and bonds. Two Maurys were arrested while traveling between the North and the South, on charges of carrying correspondence across enemy lines. Letters arrived only by private post, erratically. Maurys requested in their letters that they not discuss how letters were sent, or how they arrived, as some were intercepted and read. By early July, the flow of stories began to trickle off. Maurys at Old Mansion and Fredericksburg craved news, but there was none—not even lies.

From forty miles away, they heard guns, like a low steady roar, from a battle fought in Manassas. Tin pans rattled gently in the cupboards, and it was several days before they could find the chickens and the geese. A Maury traveled to the battlefield and saw all the Union dead stripped of their shoes—the South had no leather. A northerner was spotted fleeing the battle in a buggy, with a congressman. The congressman beat off a young slave who ran alongside the buggy and tried to climb inside with them. Would any slave master do such a thing? Lincoln defied his promise to fight a humane war, declaring all surgical and medical supplies contraband.

After the battle, there was a curse of caterpillars so thick you couldn't take a step without crushing them. Then there was a wave of squirrels running south, thick like a carpet on the ground, and flocks of pigeons flying north, blotting out the sun like a cloud. Confederate men were seen fleeing the battle, and they were reduced to eating raw meat on the way. Eating raw meat makes men mean.

Lorenzo stopped arriving on Wednesdays and Saturdays. There was no word from him. The stage road that passed Old Mansion was soon crammed with wagons, some of them baggage wagons like long, ponderous machines, pulled by no fewer than six mules. The good wagons of the Maurys were stolen and replaced with broken wagons, and there was no telling if the thieves were from the North or the South. There were skirmishes between cavalry and Confederates, and Union soldiers stole wagons loaded with hams and rebel hardtack biscuits. The Union army passed right through Bowling Green, and Union officers were forced to order their men not to insult slaves. A lone slave man, passing a group of blue-coated soldiers, was met with taunting noises, cawings like the call of a crow.

Yankees moved into Fredericksburg. Yankee ice carts sold Yankee ice. Yankee boys cried Yankee newspapers. Yankees moved into homes with their families, Yankee businessmen took over Main Street, and Yankee soldiers worked to repair the bridge across the Rappahannock that Confederate soldiers had destroyed when they pulled back toward Richmond. Good southern women, looking as gay as you please in kiss-me-quick bonnets, avoided walking under the American flag hung in front of City Hall. When they caught Yankee soldiers admiring them, they turned up their noses and drew down their lips, like a tobacco chewer about to squirt his amber. They looked ready to swallow up the entire Union army.

There were debates about which currency was best, Union greenbacks or Confederate dollars, and trade settled on an exchange rate of seven of the latter to five of the former. Slaves in Fredericksburg demanded to be hired for their labor. A man named Dr. Hall wanted to hire his slaves, but he was prevented from doing so by his fellow whites. His slaves ran away. A black woman arrived at the home of the Fredericksburg Maurys to offer her service for a price, and it took only a moment for all of them to recognize that she was a slave who had run away from the Maurys in New York City, twenty-five years before. Stories limped to Old Mansion of runaway slave women arriving in Fredericksburg through the woods, carrying children, and of old men and cripples somehow making their way north to freedom. The runaways had heard rumors that their masters were planning to move south, and to take their slaves with them. They fled instead.

Maurys refused to go to church in Bowling Green if there might be Yankee fighting men present. The church was offering services for North and South every other Sunday. Union soldiers did not come south as far as Old Mansion, it was said. But one night, as the Woolfolk slaves sat around Anarcha's fire, discussing when and if to flee north—who would go, who would remain, and how they would again find one another after freedom came—a Yankee soldier stepped out of the forest with a rifle in his hands. He made a gesture to others behind him, secret soldiers who remained hidden in the black woods. The largest man among the Woolfolk slaves, Moses, as strong as any man in the county, climbed to his feet and went to speak with the soldier. Every eye watched the two men, but the popping fire drowned out their voices. After a time, Moses nodded, and then the soldier nodded and turned back to the forest.

There was a Confederate army camped nearby, Moses explained. The soldier told him where. All they needed to do, Moses said, was run to the north and sneak past the camped army. There would be food for whoever arrived across the line, jobs for the able-bodied, and guns for men who wished to fight for the freedom of those they loved. That night, the Woolfolk slaves resolved to flee when the time was right. Those who voted to run included Moses and Mack and John Finny, Mike, Anthony, Henry Ray and George Robert, Annie and Charlotte and Aggy and Marthy Ellen, and Minor and John Calhoun.

At the end of the summer, Old Mansion became a house of sickness for Maurys and Maury slaves alike. Anarcha's missus and her two sons shared measles. Two slaves came down with diphtheria—Anarcha treated them with wild burdock root and potash. Lavinia got sick and lost a baby that wasn't born yet. In November, the missus's baby Harriet succumbed to her boils. Delia told Anarcha that as the Maurys brushed the hair of the dead baby's head they remarked on how much she looked like the bust of her dead grandfather. Charley Maury asked if Harriet desired her playthings in Heaven. His brother said he wanted to run into the rain so he could catch croup and go see his sister.

It was still months before they would leave Old Mansion, but Anarcha later recognized that this period of pain—when the missus was torn between hating the place that killed her girl and not wanting to leave the earth in which she was buried—was the moment when all their fates were sealed.

In the winter, sabotage along the stage road made travel impossible for wagons. Riders inched their way between cities, circulating a rumor that New Orleans had fallen. There had been a rash of rebel prisoners taking an oath of allegiance to the North, it was said. After the new year, seventy-five bullet holes were discovered in a monument erected to George Washington's mother. Six thousand Yankees were captured in retreat from Richmond. Stragglers and deserters roamed the countryside, and Yankee families and soldiers once again departed Fredericksburg. An army of 35,000 Union soldiers camped nearby for the cold months, and only ten miles away an army of 30,000 Confederates camped between Bowling Green and Fredericksburg. One night, the rebel magazine exploded, throwing the leg of its guard thirty feet into the air. The railroad that ran a few miles to the west of Old Mansion carried supplies and more men north from Richmond. Into spring, there were skirmishes at Falmouth, to the west of Fredericksburg, and at night, soldiers from either side were snatched from their posts. The city loomed as a battleground.

After Lieutenant Colonel Maury once again departed to fight the war, Delia was caught listening in on the missus. The Maurys were planning to leave Old Mansion with their slaves. They would go south, to Milton, North Carolina. A number of good families were gathering there to skirt the brunt of the battlefield. The missus seized Delia by the arm when she caught her eavesdropping. She threatened to clip her ear if she revealed anything of the plan. They'd all seen slaves with clipped ears. Regardless, Delia ran home and told Anarcha everything she'd heard.

The Woolfolks made similar plans. On the morning of August 2, 1862, the Woolfolks instructed their slaves to have their breakfast and then gather their clothes for a journey. Instead, twenty-five of the Woolfolk slaves met at Anarcha's cabin. There was Moses and Henry Ray and John Calhoun, and Aggy, Charlotte, and Marthy Ellen. They planned to walk until noon, stop, and hide until nightfall. Then they would complete a journey around the Confederate army to a narrow point of the Rappahannock, west of Fredericksburg. With luck, the river would be low.

That night, the Maurys told their slaves that two of the runaways had changed their minds and returned home. As to the others, they chastised the women who had preferred freedom to their duty. There were now nine children left behind, motherless.

Anarcha expected they would all go to Milton soon. She was almost right. Fearful of another escape, the missus saved the news until the Maury horses and buggies were packed with what the road could bear. What good was a nurse, the missus asked Anarcha, if she couldn't catch live slave babies, or cure the white ones that fell ill? She explained that Anarcha had a new master, Charles Mason, of King George County. Delia was going south, to Milton. Anarcha was going north, toward the war.

The missus climbed into her buggy seat. You're lucky, she said. You are losing a daughter but gaining a husband.

Twenty-Six

Clitoridectomy—Henry Raymond—
The woman from Faubourg Saint-Germain—
Napoléon

SHE WAS TWENTY-FOUR, FROM MASSACHUSETTS, AND SHE HAD FIRST BEEN admitted to Woman's Hospital for painful and scanty menses, and leukorrhea of many years' standing. Her skin had a greenish-yellow tint, she had been bedridden for six years, and she was subject to constant hysterical convulsions. Emmet incised her cervix in July 1861, just after Sims departed for Paris, and after the summer, she improved such that she could walk, unaided, for up to sixty feet. The nervous convulsions continued.

She was readmitted to Woman's Hospital on January 3, 1862, a week before the *Kangaroo* docked in New York. Sims returned to work. The woman's case appeared to be a perfect opportunity to test the theory of Isaac Baker Brown. On February 21, Sims divided her clitoral sheath with scissors. Her clitoris appeared in no way remarkable. Per Brown's method, he seized the clitoris with forceps and applied the red-hot iron of an actual cautery, severing the organ with a cutting and sawing action. He closed the flaps of the wound with two sutures. The operation had little effect. She remained weak, and the convulsions continued—particularly when she was subjected to examinations. They continued to apply unguents until Sims returned to Paris. He never learned whether the woman's condition had been in any way improved.

The time in New York was fraught. As he had hoped, the *New*

York Times heralded his return with an unsigned story—surely, it was "Malakoff"—detailing the widespread celebration of his skills, a record of which all Americans could be rightly proud. But New York was no place for a southerner during the war. When the fighting started, Thomas Addis Emmet traveled to Montgomery to offer his services to Jefferson Davis directly. He was admitted to the president's office, but Davis politely told him the South had enough surgeons. Go home, and care to the needs of women, he said. Now, both Emmet and Theresa told Sims that their mail was being monitored, their servants were likely reporting on them, and southerners were loath to set foot in a northern home.

Woman's Hospital was struggling. Emmet complained that the Board of Lady Managers had become assertive in Sims's absence. They were threatening to close the hospital completely, and they'd had the audacity, Emmet said, to insist that he consult more regularly with the Consulting Board of Physicians and Surgeons, as though the ladies knew best which treatments should be performed! For his part, Sims focused on his plans for the new hospital on Fourth Avenue, likely to be constructed only after the war was finished. He began work on his book, corresponding with the French artists who would produce its illustrations. The volume would simultaneously appear in England, France, and America. As to operations, Sims performed Brown's clitoridectomy just once during his months in New York, choosing instead to focus on cervical amputations, refining the procedure for France. Even surgery was a disappointment. In one instance, his failure to properly grasp the remarkably thick stalk of a uterine growth terminated fatally. The woman caught a chill and died before he could devise an instrument suitable to her case.

More important, he formed a plan to clear up the tangle that had delayed his Belgian Legion of Honor award. Secretary of State William Seward was known to be a close associate of Henry Raymond of the *New York Times*. The closest Sims had ever got to Raymond was the day Henri Stuart shepherded him about the city, preaching the news of his lecture to whoever would listen. But hadn't Raymond served the hospital well on its administrative boards, and wasn't his wife an active Lady Manager? Hadn't the *Times* sung his praises only weeks before? Sims asked a friend to throw a dinner party and invite the Raymonds. He would broach the subject of his award at an opportune moment.

When the evening came, he waited until after dinner had been served. The guests spread through the house to smoke, drink, and converse. Already, Sims had sensed a stiffness in Raymond, not so different from the chilly reception he'd first received from Dr. Velpeau in Paris. At last, he made his approach. Initially, he noted his connection to the *Times'* "Malakoff" in France, describing a particular operation Dr. Johnston had attended. He omitted his more significant connection to the onetime *Times* reporter Mary Booth, whose loyalty was doubtful. Sims acknowledged the unavoidable fact that he was a southerner, but he insisted that he was as loyal to the Union as any man in New York. Then he shifted to his request. He regaled Raymond with the injustice of an honorable award denied and suggested the ease with which the error could be undone by a gentle suggestion that would bring renown to all Americans. Would Raymond do him the favor of reaching out to Secretary Seward?

Raymond paused, then squared his body to Sims. I don't think any man, he said, who holds the sentiments that you do has any right to expect favors of any sort from our government.

He walked away.

On July 18, 1862, Sims and his family sailed from New York aboard the *Great Eastern*. This time, he did not know when he would return.

* * *

Thornwell died in South Carolina, in August. In Lancaster, Mittag's son was tried for and acquitted of murder, and Mittag would lose everything during the war. Sims's father enlisted to fight, in Texas. In New York, Henri Stuart took up the cause of gunmaker Norman Wiard, threatening Lincoln's secretary of ordnance with a sale to the South if the North didn't purchase Wiard's artillery rifles. In Massachusetts, Caroline Thompson finally succumbed to her tumor.

Sims and his family settled on the Rue Balzac. Theresa and their daughters immersed themselves in Parisian social life; Carrie, the eldest, became a lady-in-waiting for Empress Eugénie herself. Granville, the first of Sims's two sons to study medicine, along with Harry, began studies at

Charity Hospital. Daughter Fannie entered a school near Fontainebleau, and now Eliza was all but engaged to Thomas Pratt, whom Sims took on as a partner in the practice he established in Paris.

The duchess introduced him to the most influential people in France. For a time, he thrived. In September, a woman of high position who had begged off cervical incision for sterility because Dr. Nélaton had told her it could be dangerous relented and quickly conceived. Word of the success spread, and soon Sims was traveling outside the city to perform the operation at dozens of country châteaux. A few months later, he was brought a case of fallen uterus, and he returned to his foreshortening of the vagina, now finding that excising a trowel-shaped portion of mucous membrane worked better than the V-shaped excision he had used on Anarcha. A number of similar cases soon followed.

In early 1863, he was baffled by a young couple who failed to conceive despite all his efforts. They assured him it was not a case of premature ejaculation. First, Sims examined the wife's cervix for signs of sperm the morning after copulation. Then, eight minutes after. Finally, he performed an investigation just a minute after completion of the nuptial joy. He failed to find even a single spermatozoon properly installed. This could indicate nothing else: elongated vaginas, with the cervix entering the canal closer to its midpoint than its cul-de-sac, had a kind of evacuating power, a springing forward as the husband removed himself. The vagina ejected the husband's seminal fluid, without regard to the vigor with which it had been deposited.

His European career proceeded smoothly enough, until he was approached by a young, beautiful woman with ancestors in two of the most important families of Faubourg Saint-Germain. It was a case of severe vaginismus. Abroad, his cure for vaginismus had been the most coolly received of his procedures; English doctors, in particular, had been hostile when he read his paper on the subject before their medical society. There were open challenges to his claims that the condition was unknown, that it did not appear in the literature. That wasn't a problem—he would eliminate the claims when the lecture was prepared for his book. But the incident did trigger greater scrutiny of his work. Spencer Wells questioned whether his silver sutures were necessary, and Brown faulted his denuding method.

Simpson published a book reminding the medical community that Gosset had done Sims's fistula surgery long before him, and he pointed out that after Sims abandoned his clamp suture, all that remained was Mettauer's procedure. Equally dismissive was Goldsmith, who questioned Sims's process for cervical amputation. Surely, he wrote, the operation would be reprobated by English doctors, and rejected by English ladies.

Hints of these duplicitous attacks escaped England. When Sims returned to Paris, he learned that certain French physicians had objected to his being granted approval to perform operations in France. Nevertheless, permission had been granted. The vaginismus procedure, however, nearly derailed his European career.

Prior to the woman from Faubourg Saint-Germain, he performed the operation only once in France. It produced no effect. He was undaunted, and when the well-bred beauty from Faubourg Saint-Germain presented with the classic symptoms, he did not hesitate. This time, the procedure went as planned. Within three months, she had conceived. Her pregnancy, however, was attended by severe emetic action, far more than the usual vomiting associated with the early stages of pregnancy. Further examination revealed that her uterus was poorly positioned. Sims adjusted it and fitted her with a pessary.

By then, he was following the duchess on her frequent visits to Baden-Baden. When he next departed for Germany, the young woman from Faubourg Saint-Germain and her husband traveled with him. Six weeks of baths did nothing to prevent the vomiting, or arrest a precipitous decline in her health. Sims advised therapeutic abortion. The young lady refused. He traveled with her back to Paris, and left her in the care of a renowned accoucheur, a man who was confident that he could safely bring the baby to term.

Two weeks later, word traveled back to Baden-Baden: the woman was dead. Worse, Parisian newspapers were filled with lies about her demise, attributing the tragedy to the young American surgeon who had arrived in the city of late and who was performing ghoulish, ghastly operations. Worse, the vile press attributed the death not to his vaginismus procedure but to his incision of the cervix, which was far more central to the profitability of his practice. It was yet another reason to keep trusted reporters close.

Perhaps, he concluded, it would be better to sequester himself for a time among the duchess and the royals, where he could work unimpeded on his book.

His call to duty came just a short time later. On the morning of May 5, 1863, the duchess wrote to inform him that the emperor expected him at the palace at the Tuileries at two o'clock. Sims had some idea what it was about: the war had begun to turn. After Manassas and another debacle at Antietam, Lincoln had replaced his top general for being unwilling to engage the enemy. Initially, Sims had been delighted to learn that this general was the son of George McClellan, his old professor at Jefferson Medical College. It was the selfsame boy to whom Sims had gifted coins for taffy in Philadelphia. The young McClellan had grown up to be a southerner in almost every respect. Was it any surprise he was hesitant to fight southern generals who had been among his former school chums? Regardless, after McClellan was replaced, the tide of the war had seemed to turn, and now, to avoid antagonizing representatives of the United States, the emperor was keeping at arm's length John Slidell, the Confederacy's man in France.

Sims had made Slidell's acquaintance in his own home. In Paris, he and Theresa had made a point of putting on gatherings and banquets for displaced southern diplomats and officials. Somehow, Slidell knew of Sims's arrangement with the duchess. They never spoke of it directly. But one evening in early 1863, when they had a quiet corner to themselves, Slidell offhandedly instructed Sims—if and when the time came—to give the emperor the impression that, as error travels with lightning wings, reports of Union victories were exaggerated. The North was prevailing only in conflicts where its navy conferred upon it a decided advantage.

Sims arrived at the palace. The emperor was waiting for him. He was not a tall man, but he was taller than Sims. More remarkable than his height was the size of his head; its great weight alone seemed to account for a crooked tilt to his countenance. Louis Napoléon had heavy-lidded eyes that brightened only when he seemed amused, and his face appeared lengthened by the imperial goatee, with its neatly waxed mustache. He spoke near-perfect English, with a slight German accent.

Indulging in the artifice of their meeting, the emperor first spoke about his mother's death, the suffering of her final days, and the exact manner of her passing. Unlike other royals who donned and stripped away their dignity like a cloak, Louis Napoléon appeared permanently perched between pomp and informality. Even his gentleness had a ceremonial scriptedness. At last he segued into political affairs. France was then a year into its speculative Mexican venture, he said. He revealed that Lincoln had offered recognition of a French-ruled Mexico, on the condition that France not deal with the Confederate States of America. Also, the emperor had been warned that giving safe harbor to southern ships in French ports could be regarded as an act of war. With a casual, offhand manner, he mused about the position of the Confederacy on the subject of belligerent rights. Was it true, he asked Sims, that the sentiments of citizens of the United States had been depressed by the exploits of the *Alabama*, the *Florida*, and the *Georgia*?

Sims revealed what he had been instructed to reveal. The South had won glorious victories at Manassas, Antietam, and, since then, Fredericksburg. Lincoln's proclamation of emancipation had been delivered prematurely; it would be rescinded. As to the war's progress, it was clear to any objective observer that the only battles in which the United States achieved even muted success were those in which it enjoyed a maritime advantage. With a potent navy, a southern victory was inevitable. In the future, the Confederate States of America, with inexhaustible supplies of coal and iron, would recall with gratitude any nation that provided assistance that saved lives and money and foreshortened the war.

The emperor grinned. Was it true, he asked, that southern ships were manned almost exclusively by English crews? That they had never docked at an American port?

Sims said he was not privy to the details of naval tactics.

Napoléon paused. Then he allowed—as though speaking only to himself—that what France most wished to know was whether the administration of Jefferson Davis would be amenable to southern states acting as bases for France's ongoing struggle in Mexico.

Now it was Sims's turn to smile. Of course, he himself would be amenable to such an arrangement, he said. He promised to see to it that the proposal would be considered at the highest level. Inwardly, Sims marveled at the emperor's savvy. He was arranging his contacts with the North and the South such that he would be rewarded regardless of the outcome of the war. As a southern surgeon who had founded a hospital in New York City, Sims understood only too well the need to navigate to one's own benefit the bereft territories suspended between antagonistic forces.

The emperor concluded their meeting with an invitation to Sims to spend a fortnight at the Château de Saint-Cloud, with the empress and her entourage. Of course. If they were to sustain the impression that Sims was treating the empress for some condition, he needed to be in attendance upon her, particularly when the emperor was conducting business at Vichy. In a way, it was payment for the favor of Sims's role as secret courier. It meant that for the rest of his life, he could advertise the fact that his patients had once included the last queen of France.

Twenty-Seven

Saint-Cloud—The ghost of Anarcha—Granville—
McClellan's son—Dr. Gream—
Clinical Notes on Uterine Surgery—*Eugene Tilt*—
A modest satire—The trial of Isaac Baker Brown

HE VISITED SAINT-CLOUD AS A GUEST OF THE DUKE DE BASSANO. THE empress and the duchess were present, as were Maximilian and Carlotta. They spent time driving about the expansive grounds of the château, chatting under its trees, and visiting the grand cascade of Antoine Le Pautre, two hundred years old and the center point for festivals that could be viewed from Paris, just across the Seine. In the evenings, they explored the empress's private library or viewed the château's many paintings, which included Winterhalter's famous portraits of the emperor and the empress, though Sims preferred Vinchon's *La Mort de Madame, Duchesse d'Orléans.*

He delivered the emperor's message to Slidell and was not called on in an official capacity again. He believed he had succeeded in befriending both Napoléon and Eugénie. He returned to his practice in Paris and moved his family to the Rue de Surène. By the fall of 1863, southern ships had been granted port access for repairs and coal at Brest and Cherbourg. By then, the news from Gettysburg and Vicksburg had made it clear that the war had turned. The emperor's decision to at last permit southern privateers to dock at French ports was an act of strategic duplicity. It could not be said that Napoléon had denied assistance to the South, yet there was little risk of the North acting on threats of reprisal in a conflict that it now appeared likely to win.

Sims settled into a comfortable career. He performed an ovariotomy for Nélaton, and though the woman died, the postmortem demonstrated—as it had with the slave who had been stabbed in Alabama—that his silver sutures performed admirably in the peritoneum. At Mittag's request, he sent money to South Carolina. He received a letter from Charles Bell Gibson in Richmond, requesting funds for the production of prosthetics for the South's war wounded. Sims had not heard from Gibson since Anarcha arrived in New York. Before he could arrange for funds to be sent, he learned that Gibson had died—he had succumbed, it was said, to the exhaustion of the war's medical work.

Curiously, not long after, the ghost of Anarcha reared up before Sims once more. Thus far, he'd been fortunate that the English doctors now scrutinizing his procedures—since then, French doctors had labeled him too bloody, too American—had not questioned the fable he had erected atop the fiction of Anarcha's cure. With Anarcha gone, his story was safe. But was she truly banished? In late 1863, Sims put on another gathering for southerners, decorating the rooms of his home in Confederate colors to welcome naval officers fresh from their cruises. The ball would repeat in the spring, when Eliza at last married Thomas Pratt.

The evening proceeded joyously enough. There was little sign of what all of them knew—the turn in the war was decisive, regardless of whether there was a Confederate navy. Of course, Sims recognized the great scientist of the seas Commodore Matthew Fontaine Maury when he arrived with a fellow commander. He was caught off guard when the two men approached him and shook his hand with surprising ease, as though they somehow knew one another.

In a sense, Maury explained, they did. He established that his colleague was actually his cousin, another Maury. This cousin was the latest owner of the girl, Ankey—or Anarcha. It was Maury himself who had purchased her through Dr. Gibson in Richmond. Was not Anarcha the celebrated patient upon whom Sims had performed his famous experiments?

Sims forced down a pullet's egg of nerves lodged in his throat. Of course she was, he said. How many Anarchas with fistula could there possibly be? he joked.

The younger Maury—Sims never caught his name—revealed not only that Anarcha was alive but that she was somehow married. It was difficult to imagine Anarcha married after all the work that Sims and others had done on her. The recent foreshortening he'd performed in New York to hold her bladder in place was likely to have failed by now. The operation had been experimental; he'd improved on the procedure since then. What sort of marriage would have been possible with what was left of her? The younger Maury announced that Anarcha had been leased to a man named Charles Mason in King George, Virginia. Mason was a good man, and he had married well, taking as his second bride a great-granddaughter of Thomas Jefferson. Maurys and Jeffersons, the younger Maury explained, had common roots in Charlottesville.

The elder Maury sensed Sims's discomfort. He said something about how Anarcha was like a comet or meteor, shooting through the universe.

Less like a comet, Sims thought, than a phantom. Anarcha was still alive, but she was like a curse placed upon him—a ghost who taunted him with ruin, haunting him from the other side of the world.

He hurriedly excused himself and made a point of not bidding the Maurys goodnight.

In France, the war culminated—and produced tragedy for Sims—when the infamous *Alabama* docked at Cherbourg and drew the interest of the USS *Kearsage*. The *Kearsage* had been hunting the *Alabama* for more than a year. The Union ship anchored off the coast, waiting for the rebels to leave port. Granville and Tom Pratt traveled to Cherbourg to watch the battle in June 1864. It ended in a little more than an hour, with the *Alabama* reduced to a wreck and sunk. Sims visited the Louvre to view Édouard Manet's *The Battle of the Kearsage and the Alabama*, hung within a month.

Days later, he traveled to Bad Kissingen. He promptly received a letter from Granville, who was determined to fight in the war, against his father's expressed wishes. Outraged by the dishonorable tactics used against the *Alabama*, Granville wrote that he would think and act for himself, for once. He would not accept any suggestion that he return to New York; to live among Yankees again would spell only trouble. He and his now brother-in-law Thomas Pratt had accepted a gentleman's offer of free passage from Liverpool to Galveston. He apologized for his strong language—but he had been dependent long enough.

Granville left France immediately. By the time his ship arrived in Cuba he was unwell. He sailed for Galveston but quickly grew very ill. He died of yellow fever a day after he arrived in Texas. Sims's oldest son was buried in a cemetery there.

* * *

The young McClellan, relieved of his military duties, was nominated as a compromise candidate among factions of the Democratic Party to oppose Lincoln in the 1864 presidential election.

By then, Sims was splitting his time between France and England. It was time to leave Paris. A contact in London had arranged for him to be named an honorary member of that city's obstetrical society, and he was promised publications—excerpts of his book—that would help him establish a presence in the English medical community. McClellan lost the election, badly—and just days later, Sims received the heartbreaking letter that revealed Granville's fate. Two months after that, McClellan left America to recover from his loss. When he visited Paris with his family, he reunited with Sims, also bereaved. The two men had not seen one another in three decades.

Seemingly by design, McClellan wore Napoléon's same imperial goatee. The French press treated him well, announcing him as a wise, humane, civilized man, hard on his enemies but magnanimous in defeat. In truth, he was bittersweet. McClellan had agreed to run for president, he told Sims—to the extent that he ran at all, having appeared in public only twice during the campaign—on the belief that most people wanted peace above all else. Wouldn't the soldiers he had formerly commanded rally to his candidacy? He'd wished to preserve the Union, but in doing so he would have offered concessions to the South. Its institutions would not be destroyed and it would not be required to accept negro equality. He had always felt more at home among southerners, he said. Several Confederate generals had attended his wedding, just months before South Carolina seceded. The Confederacy had attempted to lure him to the southern cause, just as Ohio, Pennsylvania, and New York had done—that much was true. But it was a malicious falsehood that he had permitted Lee to retreat and claim victory at Antietam. Nor had he had any awareness of an uncovered plot to assassinate Lincoln, set in motion by men who called themselves "Friends of McClellan." In the end, sensing imminent victory in the war, Union soldiers did not rally to McClellan's side with their votes—quite the opposite, in fact. Now, at thirty-nine, McClellan was planning to stay abroad for several years, just as Sims had done.

Broken by the loss of his son, Sims let McClellan regale him with his adventures and disappointments and then bade the young man good-night. Within days, it seemed, Lee surrendered and Lincoln was murdered, and a war and an era were over. All had been lost. Sims would survive unscathed, his covert mission undetected. All he needed now was to complete his book and observe from afar as the new Woman's Hospital rose on Fourth Avenue. When it was complete, he would return home.

* * *

From England, it was easier to respond forcefully to his critics. A Dr. Gream kicked back against a claim that Sims made about the dangers of dilating the cervical canal for painful menses and sterility. It had been many years, Gream wrote, since certain practitioners had proposed incision of the cervix as an artificial alternative to dilation. But now those practitioners had abandoned the procedure. It seemed that Dr. Sims and his compatriot Dr. Emmet were alone in continuing to advocate for the incision of the cervix.

In thirty years, Gream wrote, he had never seen a successful pregnancy result from the artificial procedure. By contrast, plugs and bougies worked frequently. What possible danger could there be in dilating the cervical canal? Was it not the most dilatable part of the human body, stretching as it did to permit passage of the fetal head? The case that compelled Gream to reply to Sims was that of a lady, desperate for an heir, incised six years earlier. She sought Gream's attendance when she was four months pregnant, and in examining her he discovered that her cervix had been left little more than a gaping, open cavity. He easily passed his finger into her gravid uterus and was able to touch the membranes of the ovum. He predicted that abortion would soon follow—the organ would be unable to retain its contents—and the woman soon miscarried.

In effect, she had been sterilized by the procedure performed to cure her sterility.

Sims replied in fine style. First, he noted that there could be no surer method of inducing abortion than by thrusting a finger into the uterus to explore its contents! Next, he seized on the opportunity to advertise the fact that the only incisions he had seen were those performed by himself and Emmet—more than five hundred of them. They had never had a case of the cervix opened too largely. He argued that it was a mistake to condemn an operation because of the singular failure of a clumsy practitioner. Should the procedure for vesico-vaginal fistula be abandoned simply because someone may have died in consequence of it? Lastly, Sims twisted Gream's criticisms to suggest that they applied more to his own procedure than to Sims's. In the future, he advised, Gream should endeavor to adjust the evils of his own teachings and correct the blunders of his followers.

Sims's book *Clinical Notes on Uterine Surgery* was published the following year. Notices and advertisements appeared in all the major journals.

Attention did not prevent further criticism in England, however. The *Medical Times and Gazette* acknowledged the widespread anticipation of Sims's work, but its reviewer fretted that his approach was too purely surgical. His discussion of vaginismus was faulted for his matter-of-fact acceptance of colleagues' use of ether to enable coitus. In addition, his work to confirm the presence of spermatozoa at increasingly briefer intervals after the marital act was rudely mocked. How would such a bargain be struck between husband and physician? Would the two men pass one another in a vestibule while the anxious, palpitating wife awaited examination? Or would the husband slip away via one door while the good doctor entered by another to transact his delicate business?

Sims's claim that there was an undiscovered muscle that caused the uterus to perform a sucking action to aid conception was similarly ridiculed. If such a muscle existed and suction was necessary, wouldn't it most certainly be a false philosophy to advocate for incising the cervix, like slitting the neck of a balloon? The review stooped even to criticizing

Sims's language, taunting him for a confusion of shoulds and woulds and wills and shalls. It concluded that a better book would have been produced by someone more at home with a pen.

Even more troubling was Dr. E. J. Tilt's paper "On Extreme Surgical Tendencies of Uterine Pathologists." Tilt criticized Sims for believing the knife was the omnipotent means of curing all the diseases of women. But that was not the worst of it. Rather, what loomed dangerously was the fact that Tilt reviewed *Clinical Notes on Uterine Surgery* alongside Isaac Baker Brown's now finished clitoridectomy book, *On the Curability of Certain Forms of Insanity, Epilepsy, Catalepsy, and Hysteria in Females.*

* * *

In 1867, the backlash against the surgeries performed at Brown's London Surgical Home culminated in the distribution of a biting, satiric pamphlet produced in the spirit of Jonathan Swift.

The pamphlet did not cite clitoridectomy directly. Rather, the satirist lauded Brown in grandiose language, praising him for several procedures he had devised to cure women of afflictions that struck at the very heart of feminine grace. To stem an epidemic of high-bred young ladies succumbing to a compulsion to steal away bits of cashmere and pearl at the shops, Brown had improved upon the barbarous but effective practice of severing the limbs of thieves. Surely, no civilized nation would consider such a treatment today! Hence, Brown's brilliant kleptodectomic operation, which limited itself to the division of certain palmar and digital muscles by use of a fine, small knife passed under the skin. Women afflicted with this shameful disease, fortunate enough to have wound up in Brown's care, were left with a reduced muscular ability that protected them from their most unladylike impulses. The treatment's propriety was not a concern, as palmar dexterity was not required of ladies—after all, what did any refined man expect of a woman's hand other than that it wave gracefully and glove well?

Similarly, Brown had turned his genius to yet another pathological tendency common to women of high breeding—the impulse toward excessive talk. The affliction of a too-long tongue, as the condition was crassly known, was easily remedied with the quick pass of a fine blade, severing certain muscular fibers. The mobility of the offensive organ was thereby reduced.

Last, the ever-innovative Brown had found the most merciful solution to gyromania, the disordered passion that refined women suffered for waltzing. Presented with a curious case of a woman who, whenever she was put to three-four time and her waist was encircled by a male arm, would dance herself to death's door, Brown devised the most gentle and lifesaving of treatments—the division of the gluteus and gastrocnemius muscles.

Nonbelievers were invited to visit the London Surgical Home in Ladbroke Grove, Notting Hill, to see for themselves the pale, female forms— now serene and tranquil—emerging after their cures from the most unpretentious building in all of Kensington Park!

Mockery aside, Brown's fall from grace began with the *British Medical Journal*'s review of his book, which appeared just two months after the *Medical Times and Gazette*'s unjust review of Sims. Cold rather than satiric, the reviewer chastised Brown for a claim that clitoridectomy was a procedure long practiced. Rather, as a cure for insanity, it was a thing wholly new under the sun. Brown had conflated masturbation and insanity, the reviewer wrote, and while no one would decry the established fact that masturbation caused nervous conditions, Brown's work went too far in suggesting that an operation to limit the former necessarily cured the latter. The book in question offered no proof that the effects of a dubious surgery were permanent. The medical men of London were well acquainted with hysteria cures that had been achieved without the elimination of an organ whose precise purpose remained elusive. What was clear was that Brown had considerably exaggerated the value of his operation.

Sims's book, in all likelihood, had been rescued from harsher treatment by the scandal that quickly attached itself to Brown. Sims remained loyal, as Brown had been among the first to champion his fistula procedure— but he was almost alone. When the first call came for Brown's censure and removal from the Obstetrical Society of London, he responded forcefully— as Sims would have done—by publicly naming those gentlemen who had been in support of his methods. The calls for his removal multiplied.

Former friends openly denied any association with him. Journals published vicious anonymous attacks. Doctors told stories of women subjected to Brown's procedure without consent and in complete ignorance of its nature. In January 1867, Brown was reduced to calling for a scientific investigation, agreeing to give up the procedure if it was found to be ineffective. It was too late. The expulsion process began in late February. On April 3, Sims attended the meeting that would determine Brown's fate.

The gathering was set for eight o'clock. Doctors began to arrive soon after seven, and the seats and standing areas were soon overflowing with medical men. The man himself arrived solemnly, content to wait for his turn to speak. Sims did not greet him; he did not mix with anyone he knew. He feared for his own reputation in America. His mission that evening was to anticipate the sort of public humiliation that might be visited upon himself. There were always dangers for the brave men who steered the ship of science directly into waters that less manly sailors avoided.

There was no sort of order from the start. A meeting that was supposed to last an hour extended until well past midnight.

Cries of *No!* and *Chair!* and *Order!* and *Sit down!* began as soon as one of Brown's few stray defenders attempted to interrupt the proceedings with a question. There were speeches by the physician who had made the motion to censure and by the man who had seconded it. There was jeering when Brown was mocked, and laughter when he was forced to admit that Dr. Brown-Séquard had insisted his name be removed from advertisements for the London Surgical Home. Calls of *Hear, hear!* encouraged speakers who articulated the grave ethical faults of which Brown was accused. It was well known, one speaker opined, how institutions such as the London Surgical Home came about: Some practitioner would make a claim to having discovered a cure for a class of female suffering hitherto regarded as hopeless. Circulars would be distributed in an appeal for patrons, and boards would be formed. A small house would be taken and labeled a "hospital for women" or a "home." The plan would be completed with an assurance to its patients that nothing was incurable so long as the hand of God's great goodness was recognized in the search for the proper remedy.

Much laughter! Applause.

The specifics of the London Surgical Home were particularly troubling, the speakers went on—not only because there had been credible reports of women operated on without consent. *Great uproar!* Brown had been accused of secreting women into his operating theater, while their husbands or fathers waited in a separate room of the house. When the dire process was complete, the good doctor cornered his patient's caregivers for his payment. *No! No!* If a check for two hundred guineas was not produced, they were told, both the disgraceful mutilation the woman had undergone and the disgraceful practice that had resulted in her seeking treatment would be revealed to the public. *No! Order! Order!*

When Brown was at last given a chance to speak, his words were mostly drowned out by hoots and laughter. He claimed that the fellows of the society had not studied clitoridectomy as scientific men. *Question!* He insisted that it was nothing more than circumcision. *Oh! Oh!* He argued that the movement against him had been launched by a scurrilous professional rival. *Roars of laughter.*

The raucous circus continued. Many speakers contributed to the proceeding, both in favor of Brown and against him. The display lingered until at last the time came to cast ballots. A group of twelve scrutineers left the room to tally the votes. They returned to a hall still crowded, despite the hour. A quiet pall took the space as the verdict was read. Votes for the removal of Isaac Baker Brown: 194. Against removal: 38. Nonvotes: 5.

Brown disappeared from public view for five years. The *British Medical Journal* refused to make mention of either him or clitoridectomy. In 1872, Brown suffered a series of strokes that left him an invalid. He couldn't stand, dress, or feed himself. He required the attendance of a full-time nurse.

On February 1, 1873, he was attacked with a violent case of vomiting and headache. He died two days later, at age sixty-one.

By then, Sims had been back in New York for five years.

Twenty-Eight

Lydia Maria Child—Maria Mason—Child-Mason feud—
Anarcha and Lorenzo—News of Delia—
The Battle of Fredericksburg—The northern lights

In 1844, ABOLITIONIST AUTHOR LYDIA MARIA CHILD PUBLISHED A POEM entitled "The New England Boy's Song." It began:

Over the river, and through the wood,
To grandfather's house we go . . .

Child self-published her first book—featuring a controversial depiction of an interracial love affair—when she was twenty-two years old. The book was ignored until she sought the patronage of critic George Ticknor, who shepherded her into Boston's intellectual community. In 1825, Child met Lafayette on his tour through America and thrilled when the old French general kissed her hand.

Additional books, including the highly successful *The Frugal Housewife*, soon followed. In 1830, abolitionist William Lloyd Garrison inspired Child to undertake three years of study of slavery and emancipation. In 1833, she published the country's first book-length abolitionist tract, *An Appeal in Favor of That Class of Americans Called Africans*. By the time Child wrote "The New England Boy's Song," she had become an influential and fervent champion of abolition.

On October 26, 1859, a week after John Brown and twenty-one others raided the arsenal at Harper's Ferry, Child wrote to Virginia governor

Henry Wise. She wished to visit Brown in prison, she said, to nurse his wounds. Wise took the bait. He wrote back to say that Child was a citizen of the United States—he could not stop her from visiting Brown. He regretted that abolitionists such as Child had whetted Brown's knives for the butchery of mothers and babes, but he promised to protect her rights if she traveled to Virginia.

Wise's letter and Child's subsequent response were printed in the *New York Daily Herald*.

How could she believe, Child wrote, that her rights would be enforced when the slave power so casually denied the rights of persons with brown and black skin? Had not Governor Wise publicly stated that his intention was to break with the Union? How could she trust a promise from a premeditated traitor? As to Brown's violence, Child wrote that she did not prefer it. However, the raid had been prefigured by ruffians sent to Kansas to drive from the polls northern emigrants who wished only to till that territory's soil. Governor Wise might grieve the babes of Virginia, but in no way could it be denied that the wind recklessly sowed by slave owners in Kansas had reaped a whirlwind at Harper's Ferry.

On November 11, two days after the exchange was printed, a letter in response appeared from the woman who would become Anarcha's final owner, Maria Jefferson Carr Mason (née Randolph). Maria Mason was a great-granddaughter of Thomas Jefferson and the wife of Charles Mason of the Alto plantation in King George, Virginia.

Had Mrs. Child read her Bible? Mason asked. A twofold damnation was prepared for those who failed to heed the Book of Matthew's warning against hypocrisy. Child wished to soothe a hoary-headed murderer, a leader of the earth's offscourings. But had she ever stood beside the bed of a dying negro? Had she softened the pangs of maternity of slave mothers? *We* do that for our servants, Mason wrote, in order to fulfill the duty which it has pleased God to bestow on us. None deserving of the name of woman should read a word Child wrote, Mason concluded, or purchase a magazine that bore her name.

Child responded two weeks after John Brown was executed, on December 2. In 1860, her reply along with the original Wise and Mason letters were printed as a pamphlet more than three hundred thousand times and distributed across the country by the American Anti-Slavery Society.

Child began with eighteen biblical quotations (Hebrews: "Remember those that are in bonds as bound with them") and provided a series of anecdotes to indicate the leading features of the system Mason cherished. In South Carolina, a slave was punished with a thousand lashes. He escaped, and was caught and lashed five hundred times more, and died. In Alabama, a slave was tied up and beaten all day with a paddle full of holes, leaving his flesh pounded to mash. In Virginia, Judge St. George Tucker wrote that even as white men had fought to live free or die, they had imposed on others a slavery ten thousand times worse than the oppressions they had complained of.

As to the pangs of maternity, Child wrote, no woman in the North failed to meet with the required assistance. The only difference was that after a northern woman gave birth her baby was not sold away.

Child asserted, in conclusion, that money alone could not end a despotism. Such systems ought to come to an end by moral means, but if they resist they must come to an end by violence. The civilized world had proclaimed slavery an outlaw. The best intellects of the age were active in hunting it down.

* * *

Anarcha was sent to King George, along with Fanny and her colt. Anarcha was leased, and the horse was sold, but Fanny got to keep her baby.

Bon Fanny & her colt have to go too; and Anarchy to be hired out.

Charles Mason was a wealthy farmer and a justice of the peace, and everyone knew that his wife, the missus, was a great-granddaughter of Thomas Jefferson. Maria Mason had sat on Thomas Jefferson's lap before he died, when she was a baby, and inside the Mason house there was a prominent old portrait of Jefferson. Also on display was a brass warming pan, like a covered fry pan on a stick, which Jefferson had used to warm his bed at Monticello in Charlottesville, putting embers inside it at night. When he died, it passed to his grandson, who also used it to warm his bed with embers, and when the grandson died, the warming pan came to the missus, who didn't put any embers in it and instead kept it beside the Jefferson portrait in the Mason home.

Anarcha lived with Lorenzo and his daughter Louisa in a cabin that was one of eleven slave cabins on the Alto plantation. Before the war began, there were forty-five slaves in the eleven cabins that were spaced

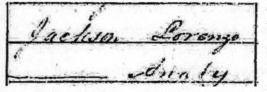

out in the dense woods above and behind the Mason home, which stood much closer to the Edge Hill road that ran all the way back south to Bowling Green and Old Mansion. The land where the slave cabins stood was too steep and hilly and too cut through with creeks to grow corn or tobacco or rye there, and too sheer to graze beefs or sheep, and behind the cabins the running waters gathered into a marshy lake, and the master and missus hoped to erect a mill there one day. After the war began, Yankees came streaming into Virginia, and some of the Mason slaves ran away, and the missus said that the Yankees had sneaked onto Alto and stolen slaves that didn't want to run away, and now the only slaves that remained were their favorites, William and Milly and Dilly and Diana. Some of the Mason slaves had taken last names, like white people—particularly men, such as Gusty Lee and Albert Grymes and young George Peyton, and it was only now that Anarcha learned that her husband had also taken a last name for himself—Jackson, his name was Lorenzo Jackson—and what that meant, because he was her husband, was that Anarcha too now had another name like a white person, Anarcha Jackson, though on the Alto plantation the master and missus and slaves didn't call her Anarcha or Ankey but something more like Anaky or Annacay, which was closer to what she had been called when she was a girl in Alabama.

Lorenzo wasn't an overseer or a slave driver. That was Uriah Inscoe, who lived nearby with his wife and four children. But Lorenzo was Charles Mason's favorite, trusted with many tasks and with looking after the whole farming operation of Alto, and when Anarcha arrived you could see why Lorenzo was favorite. He was half-white, as Anarcha herself may have been or probably was, but what she didn't know before she arrived was that none of the other Mason slaves were bright or yellow or mulatto, not one of them.

When Anarcha asked about it, because there were always bright or yellow slaves, she'd seen them everywhere, in cities and on plantations in Alabama and Richmond, and in Philadelphia and Washington City and New York City, there was always a mix of black and yellow, all Lorenzo would say was that he never knew who his parents were, never had a mother or a father. Master Mason had been a boy when Lorenzo was born, and Lorenzo had always been with him, they played the games that slave children and white children played together, and they were together before the master was married to his first wife, who died when she gave birth to Charles Mason Jr., who was now fighting the war in Richmond. They were together when Charles Mason came to King George in 1840. At that time he had his young son and fifteen slaves, and Lorenzo lived not with the slaves but in the house with both Charles Masons, senior and junior. They were together when the master bought the plantation called Forest Hill and changed the name to Alto, and when he married again, to the current missus, in 1849.

It was this missus, the great-granddaughter of Thomas Jefferson, who made Lorenzo go and live with the other slaves, even though it seemed likely that Lorenzo was more than just his master's slave, possibly they were half brothers, and Lorenzo was maybe not a slave at all but free. Even though Lorenzo now lived in a cabin, the master treated Lorenzo better than the other slaves, as when he permitted Lorenzo to ride south to Bowling Green for years to see his wife, and as when he agreed to lease Anarcha when Anarcha was of little value, while all the plantation owners in Virginia were suffering and either selling or hiding their slaves.

Because Lorenzo was the master's favorite and perhaps his brother, he always had very good news about the progress of the war. He heard stories told by both slaves and masters. In the early part of the war, when Anarcha did not hear from her husband for six months, Lorenzo and Gusty and William and Albert and young George worked the Alto plantation to make food for southern soldiers to the north, at Mathias Point on the Potomac River, where a respectable citizen one morning early in the war was shot off his horse on the riverbank. The master became active in the secret work of the Signal Corps, but he was also named assistant commissary of subsistence for King George County, and in the months after the war started, when Anarcha did not hear from her husband for six months, Lorenzo or Gusty or Albert would ride wagons of food to Mathias Point, at least until the Yankees streamed across the river.

The master's brother Wiley Roy Mason was also a successful lawyer in King George, with an even larger plantation nearby called Cleveland, a home that had been the site of many military weddings. Every one of Wiley Roy Mason's nine living children, five boys and four girls, was either a soldier in the Confederate army or married to one. The men of King George had mustered and trained in fields near the courthouse two miles from Alto. But then they left, and all that remained was women and old men, and then the Yankees crossed the Potomac, the swords of the officers clanking against the flanks of their horses as they pranced along the roads, and for a time Union soldiers occupied the King George courthouse and vandalized the clerk's office. They visited plantations to search homes for soldiers and ammunition, pulling apart beds and turning babies' cradles upside down and peeping inside every wardrobe. In the daytime, northern soldiers visited the homes to offer to pay for cakes and pies, but at night they stole turkeys and geese. They stole mules too, but the mules chewed through their halters and wandered home again in the dark.

The master told Lorenzo that the armies were gathering near Fredericksburg, fifteen miles to the west. He also told Lorenzo what every slave in northern Virginia had already heard on the grapevine. Abraham Lincoln was going to declare all the slaves free.

There was a physician who lived very close to Alto, but he had gone to war. And there was another doctor in King George who was killed by his neighbors when it was decided he was too friendly with the Yankees occupying the courthouse. When Charles Mason came down with gout, there was no local doctor to treat him. Lorenzo told the master of what Anarcha knew of herbs and cures, and Anarcha taught Louisa to search the dense, steep woods around the slave cabins for burdock root and mullein and pokeweed. Anarcha made her way down from the cluster of slave cabins to the Mason house to apply poultices made from the burdock root, and that didn't work, and then poultices from the leaves, the roots, and flowers of mullein plants, and those didn't work, and finally a poultice made from dried pokeweed and whiskey that could take the misery away but would not cure gout, and this worked. In this way, because the master needed repeated treatments, every other day, or every third day, Anarcha was able to glimpse the Jefferson portrait that was treasured even though it was flyspecked and had a crack down the middle, and the warming pan that looked like a giant piece of rock candy medicine on the end of a stick. She met the four children of the master and missus, also of Jefferson blood. There was Rannie, who was thirteen years old and already starting to look like a master. There was Lucy, who was eleven and thought croquet was the most exciting game. Jack was eight, and he liked Lorenzo very much. And Wilson was six and sickly, and Anarcha took pains to avoid Wilson because she didn't want to be called upon to care for any more white children who died and caused her to be sent away.

The pokeweed was how Anarcha learned news of Delia.

As she wrapped up the master's white, naked feet and toes, he explained that there was soon going to be a piece of paper that said she no longer belonged to Lieutenant Colonel Maury but to a man named James T. White, who was buying all of the lieutenant colonel's land and slaves for $1,200—greenbacks to be safe. The piece of paper didn't exist yet, but even when it did, she would still belong to Mason, because he had an agreement with James T. White. An agreement was equal to a piece of paper,

The wishes of Anthy's owners,

Anarcha knew. It represented paper money that Mason was paying every year as a favor to Lorenzo, because Anarcha was sickly with her limp and her cough, which was now more like strained breathing, and sometimes there was blood, and nothing she had tried, not goldenrod, not rabbit foot weed, not heart leaf, not lobelia (also called Indian tea), had made her breathing or her cough any better or any worse.

When the master wasn't talking he was listening to the missus, who for two years had watched the letter she had written in an enraged flush— the letter to Lydia Maria Child—appear in pamphlets distributed in every city in the country. The missus didn't have any house slaves. She wasn't any kind of housekeeper. It was said that her Jefferson people in Albemarle felt sorry for her because she was so far from home, and because she was an intellect reduced to menial labor, and not even traveling to convocations in Port Royal could succeed in making her happy. It was true: the missus was not good at keeping house. You knew this as soon as you entered the Mason house, which was not a tidy plantation house, despite the fact that Charles Mason was wealthier than most.

The missus had long, thin hair that parted in the middle and pressed down on the sides of her head like a tightly wrapped package. When she sat in a chair, she sat upright like a pine tree. Her back never touched the chair. This was how she sat to read letters to the master as Anarcha applied poke-weed to his feet. The letters were from his son at war in Richmond, or they were from commanders who needed food for their armies, or they were from members of the Signal Corps, and the missus complained that these letters made no sense or were written in code, and the master told her it was fine, he understood, just keep reading and throw them in the fire when you're done. Occasionally the letters were from Maurys, or from the man who was and was not Anarcha's owner, James T. White, and it was in these letters that there was sometimes a hint about Delia. A spinning wheel had been bought for her so that she could make pantaloons for Maury boy children. She was already starting to act like a mammy, even though she was only twelve years old. She had taken the young Maurys to see exhibitions of tableaux to benefit the Soldiers' Aid Society. Anarcha hid her fear when the letters hinted that Delia might need to be hired out, away from Milton, North Carolina. And she hid her sadness when it was said that Delia was the most suffering member of the Maury household, because all the moving about made her feel like a shooting star.

After Anarcha arrived in King George, rumors came through the master that a northern army general who was afraid to fight had been replaced with another general who wasn't afraid to fight, and who was a friend of the Mason family. This general had attended weddings at the Cleveland plantation of the master's brother. For some months after this particular general began overseeing the northern army, Yankee guards were placed at the gates of the Cleveland and Alto plantations to protect them from

Yankee soldiers. Both armies, camped far off, prepared for battle with reg-imental drills and dress parades and brigade reviews and target practice. For a time, life went on as though there wasn't a war at all. Hog-killing time came and went, and many more hogs were killed and cooked and the meat sent to the soldiers. Then, early one morning in December 1862, two immense balloons appeared on the western horizon, above Fredericksburg. When the light was clear enough to see at a distance, the sound of two cannon shots traveled all the way to King George, and then the dawn was filled with a thunder of guns and a splatter of rifles like a thousand packs of Chinese firecrackers. Thin lines of smoke curled into the sky above the trees and spread out like a black curtain, hiding the balloons.

The sounds of battle continued for two days. A wounded Confederate straggler, dressed in Yankee clothes, wandered onto the Alto property. Anarcha was sent for, to work at the boy's holes and scrapes with soot and cobwebs, needle and thread. The master questioned him about the Fredericksburg battle. On the battlefield, the young soldier said, there were acres of dead Federals, men killed and twisted into a common jelly. The remains of individual Yankees were strung out over a distance of five yards. Once he quit the battle, he came across forty-seven dead northern men lying on a road. He stole a uniform and a fine pair of low, quarter-sewed shoes. He killed a Yankee straggler he met, and he saw another man pay eight dollars for five biscuits. The Confederate soldier didn't have any money, and he almost perished when he risked eating a spoiled beef liver that he cooked on an open spit.

On the night of December 14, just after dusk, a ruddy glow appeared in the western sky. The lights were not followed by the concussion of artillery rifles. At first, the master and missus and the Mason slaves thought it must be stables burning. Then the lights began to move toward them. There were fiery lances of yellow and red darting toward the mid-heavens, columns of pearly luminescence, and waving garlands of gold in the sky. When the display manifested overhead, there was a crackling sound. The northern lights, the missus said, signaled the deaths of kings and heroes. They imag-ined the bodies of men in Fredericksburg, wounded in the field but killed by the cold, frozen now into ghastly shapes lit by the night's heavenly light.

Shortly before the new year, Anarcha was pregnant again.

Twenty-Nine

*A desolate winter—Black soldiers—Emancipation—The burning
of the Mason home—Seventh and eighth pregnancies—
A saddle of mutton—Delia returns*

THE WAR ENDED FOR THE WINTER. THE ARMIES FELLED THE LARGER
trees to build small cabins in the woods, roofed with sailcloth. Every
fence was pulled down for firewood, and when there was no more fence
to burn, the soldiers sneaked into towns to dismantle sheds and lumber
houses. Luxuriant weeds took over the rich fields. Sometimes there was a
grazing beef, but there was no sound of roosters, no sound of crows. All
was still as death for miles under the winter sun.

In the spring, slaves made underthings from the duck tents that the
armies left behind when they moved on to fight elsewhere. There were
clothes to salvage, packages of food, sometimes an old horse the soldiers
didn't eat and didn't have any more use for.

The northern general who had placed guards at Alto and Cleveland
was gone. There were no guards now. Sometimes Alto lay in land held
by the South and sometimes it was Yankeedom. A skirmish was fought
near the Cleveland plantation. They heard the musket fire and smelled
gunpowder sifting through the trees. That was as close as the war ever
came, though the master sometimes received instructions from the Signal Corps to steer Confederate soldiers through the marshy parts of the
plantation. Late at night, he arrived at Lorenzo and Anarcha's cabin with a
lantern and a small company of dirty, gray soldiers, and Lorenzo left with

them to coax their wagons along the spring path in the dark, a trail the Yankees couldn't follow or even see without assistance.

On April 11, 1863, four Yankee cavalry officers appeared on the Edge Hill road. The horses turned and trotted onto the Alto property. They were followed by a company of foot soldiers, blue-coated men who spread out to search the plantation. From the slave cabins, the Mason slaves watched as the horseback men gathered down near the porch of the Mason home. The master and missus appeared, with their children, and a Yankee soldier read something to them out loud from a piece of paper.

Albert Grymes pointed off at some of the soldiers searching the outbuildings. Now, look at that, he said.

Black soldiers. A huddle of black men worked separate from the white foot soldiers, some of them wearing the same blue uniform and kepi cap as the Yankee men, some in raggedy slave clothes, all carrying long guns. Several of the black soldiers hiked up to speak with the Mason slaves. Lorenzo and the other men formed a clutch to meet them, and the women and children and babies watched from behind. One of the black soldiers spoke directly to Lorenzo. He talked in a full, confident voice, like a man who didn't need a war to be free.

One of your master's friends betrayed him, the black soldier said.

It was known that the master's son was fighting in the war. It was also known that there had been unsavory characters on the Alto plantation. The master had been accused of general disloyalty. He would be taken away to be questioned, but probably he would return.

The black soldier asked Lorenzo if he knew anything about unsavory characters. Lorenzo said that sometimes he or one of the others helped the master steer southern soldiers through the plantation. And yes, there were people who came and stayed at the Mason house, but Lorenzo didn't know anything about whether they were savory.

The black soldier thought for a moment, squinting up at the bright sky. You know you're free?

It was early spring and cold still. But the words touched the Mason slaves like a pleasant breeze. A delicate thrill landed on Anarcha's shoulder: *Your baby will be born free.*

We heard it was coming, Lorenzo said. We didn't know it come.

You don't have to stay here. You can come with us. You can fight.

The Mason slaves looked amongst themselves. Anarcha stepped up closer to Lorenzo. She was five months pregnant, and already the weight of her baby was pulling on her lame leg, making it sting. She talked now only when she had to, because of her breathing. She nestled in beside her husband.

I reckon those that wanted it, Lorenzo said, have already run off.

It's better in the north, the black soldier said. He nodded toward the quarters behind them. It's better than this.

A bugle sounded from down near the Mason house. Voices called out commands for the soldiers to prepare to leave. For the white soldiers, there was one command. For the black soldiers there was another, harsher command, screamed out by a Yankee man. This white man used the same word for the black soldiers that masters and overseers used for slaves— the word that was pain itself, like the lick of a whip.

This is the land we know, Lorenzo said.

The black soldier frowned and nodded. He gestured off to the Mason house. Do any of you work down there?

Lorenzo shook his head.

Best to stay away from the house, the black soldier said. Then he turned with his fellows and ran down to the rear of the column as it began a weary march toward the Edge Hill road. The master was among them, on a horse, his hands bound behind his back.

He returned a day later, but only for a night. He assured the missus that everything would be fine. The master's brother Wiley Roy Mason and several others had been arrested along with him, and they would be held in the Old Capitol Prison in Washington City for a short time, and then they would be on parole in the city until he could reach General Burnside and Secretary of War Stanton and organize an investigation. He ordered Lorenzo and the others to keep caring for the animals and to work the fields until he returned.

Two days later, the missus received company. She and the children and her company went out on a long walk. Lorenzo and the others were far off, working the fields. The other working women were doing the housekeeping at the quarters, the work that Anarcha couldn't do any-more. She was the first to see the curls of smoke rising up from the roof of the Mason house, when there wasn't anyone in it. She could see the tiny figures of the missus and her company, more than a mile off, gathered under the big apple tree at the far end of the fields. Rather than call out, which made her cough, Anarcha beat on a pan to gather together Milly and Dilly. They rushed toward the Mason house, as fast as Anarcha could move. She told Milly to run off to the big apple tree for the missus, and she told Dilly to run ahead and go inside the house, if the parlor wasn't a furnace yet, and save the portrait of Thomas Jefferson and his warming pan too, if that could be saved, because if they weren't saved the missus would think it was the slaves that set fire to the house instead of a sneaky Yankee that crept in from the woods when no one was looking. The girls ran ahead.

By the time Anarcha caned her way to the house, Dilly had saved the portrait and the pan, and Milly had reached the missus and they were hurrying back across the fields. The plumes of smoke rose up from the house as thick and dark as storm clouds. The fire had been set in the roof to make it difficult to extinguish with buckets of water. Shingles popped in the air from the heat and thunked onto the ground. Mary and Diana arrived from the quarters, along with the boys Ben and Jonathan, and as they ran into the house Anarcha told them what to save: the bedding, the master's papers from his bureau and bedstead, clothes. The missus arrived half crazy, and she went rushing into the house to save things that she had hidden so that the slaves didn't steal them, but in her panic she forgot where they were hid. Everyone was screaming. Rannie ran into the house after his mother, pulling out mattresses and the china he could carry in his arms. The fire consumed the upper floor, ran downstairs, and strolled down into the cellar. By then all they could do was watch and stop the flames from jumping to the barn and the stables, both of which were empty, anyway.

The missus left the next day. She rode off in a carriage for her Jeffer-son people at Albemarle, along with her children and the portrait and the warming pan. The next months were the happiest that Anarcha could recall. The Mason slaves were no longer slaves, but the war raged on. They lived alone in the woods with no white people nearby and barely

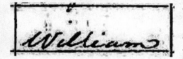

a white home occupied between Richmond and Culpeper. When her time came, she told Milly and Dilly what to expect because most of her babies were large, but this one was not large, and she came out easy compared to the babies she had lost and the babies who died before they arrived.

Anarcha was surprised it was a girl. And she was surprised too when Milly asked what her name was and there wasn't someone there to name her. She named the girl Elizabeth, to be called Lizzie, and in another year, she had another child, a boy this time. She called him William, for the way the name spilled out of your mouth, like a whisper: William, her boy William.

* * *

In Arkansas, after the war, a white man went out to the field where Eda Harper's mother-in-law was working and told her she was free. She dropped her hoe and ran up to the master's parlor so fast a bird could have perched on her dress tail. She gathered all her neighbors, and they danced all night long.

Frank Bell, from Louisiana, was a slave in his master's saloon until after the war. His master kept bad women and killed men in shooting scrapes, and when freedom came, he told Frank Bell he would pay him one dollar per week, and if he ran off, he would kill him or kill another black man in his place. Frank Bell was paid one dollar per month, not per week, until his master was killed in a scrape. Then Frank Bell bounced from place to place, and he almost starved before he worked up the nerve to leave New Orleans.

When freedom came to Texas, a master gave all his slaves $500 in Confederate money, bills with pictures of bosses on it. The children took the money and played store with it.

Some were like turtles and terrapins after freedom came. They only poked their heads out of their shells. Preachers quit their slavery wives after emancipation, and many slaves got sick and died of consumption in the years that followed, mostly children and old folks. What caused it was all the mixing in the quarters when they didn't have any resistance.

A master from North Carolina didn't want to give up his slaves, and his slaves didn't want to give up their master, so they put up their wagon and drove their cows fifteen miles a day to Arkansas, but slaves were free in Arkansas too. The master and three slaves got sick and died. They buried the slaves in Arkansas and took the body of the master back to North Carolina. Then the missus got sick and died. She too was taken back to North Carolina. The others stayed in Arkansas, but they weren't slaves anymore.

In the first years after freedom, freed slaves hunted in the woods for hickory nuts, acorns, cane roots, and artichokes. Plums, mulberries, and blackberries in spring. They ate cornmeal mush and salt water during the week, and mush and vinegar for Sunday dinner.

Some said slavery was one kind of bad thing, and another bad thing was the kind of freedom they got: nothing to live on. The first was a snake full of poison with its head pointed south, and the other was a poison snake with its head pointed north. Both bit the slave. Others said freedom was like putting a goat's skin on a sheep. A goat is smart and he comes running out of the rain because the rain makes him cold. The sheep has no sense, but he has a woolly jacket that turns off the water. He doesn't need any brains. Slaves were like sheep, and the master's protection was like the woolly coat. The end of slavery was like taking the woolly coat off the sheep, leaving him in the rain with only a goat skin for protection.

Many left their plantations on a strong notion to see what it was like to own your own body. Sometimes, those traveling north up the Edge Hill road stopped at Alto. Lorenzo and Anarcha and Albert Grymes and Gusty Lee and the others shared the food they had, always plentiful on the Alto plantation. The traveling former slaves told stories of people dying because they didn't have any food. They packed up and traveled on, and others came along behind them.

Master Mason returned after two months of parole in Washington City. The gout had gone to his kidneys. He had seen a white doctor, and after he got well he gathered the Mason slaves together and designed a new home to be built up around the chimney of the old home, still standing inside the charred ruins. For the months it took to clear the plot and build a new house, the Mason family lived in the old schoolhouse and in the cabin of an old slave named Mahala who had died before Anarcha arrived. During that time, the men did nothing but cut trees and hew boards and build walls, and the women worked a large garden so that they would all have food. The Alto fields lay fallow. The master knew the war was lost. Still, at the end of 1864, he ordered Lorenzo to carry a saddle of mutton, the best cut of the best killed sheep on Alto, to none other than General Robert E. Lee at his camp near Richmond. In addition, Lorenzo would travel through the war with a wagonful of provisions for Mr. Mason's son, including three racks of spare ribs, four balls of sausage meat, six pounds of coffee, a half pound of green tea, and one bag each of apples and meal. His orders were to deliver the mutton and a letter to General Lee, wait for a reply, and return home. Lorenzo confessed to concern about driving a wagonful of food through land that had once been prosperous. Now, it seemed that all of Virginia was a barren, wilderness frontier filled with wild deserters and stragglers with guns, men as desperate for meat as Raw Head and Bloody Bones.

A warm spell changed the mutton gift from a Christmas Eve dinner meal to a New Year's dinner meal. Anyway, it needed time to ripen. When Lorenzo left, he didn't tell Anarcha that he'd arranged a gift for her too. He was gone eight days. She didn't know what the gift was, or even that 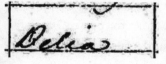 a gift was coming, until 1864 passed into 1865, and several days more passed because a snowstorm followed the warm spell, and there wasn't any traveling for a time. At last, the master's wagon appeared on the Edge Hill road, and from a long ways off you could see someone riding beside Lorenzo as he approached. The wagon inched through the snow. It was long minutes before Anarcha could even be sure it was Lorenzo holding the reins, and it wasn't until the person beside him stood up and waved that Anarcha saw it was her daughter Delia returned to her.

Thirty

*W*OMEN WERE DYING.

In the early days, Woman's Hospital had boasted of one of the lowest fatality rates in the city—in part because Sims had succeeded in hiding the death of Bridget Headley, the unfortunate girl with an ovarian tumor whom Sims had attempted to cure shortly after the hospital opened. Officially, the old hospital had a single death, in 1856; there were no others Sims could recall from before the war. He returned from Europe in September 1868. The new hospital opened in October, and in its first year six women died—so many they were obliged to construct a deadhouse for the purpose of storing the bodies and performing autopsies.

Even Sims was having deaths. Shortly after he returned, he saw in private practice a young woman who had been told that her failure to produce issue after five years of marriage was the result of painful cramps. Sims found her uterus anteflexed and her cervix abnormally formed in the vagina. It was a classic case of sterility by mechanical obstruction. He told her the only cure was to incise the cervix. Wary, she inquired as to the dangers. There was risk, Sims admitted, but he assured her that he had never seen a fatal result.

The operation went so well that Sims opted not to perform the vigorous tamponing of the vagina that tended to prevent the bleeding that had put Simpson and so many others off the operation. That night, feeling well enough to rise from her bed to urinate, the young woman climbed to her feet, triggering a hemorrhage that nearly killed her before Sims arrived at 3:00 a.m. After a few hours, the woman caught a fever and began to decline. Sims called on Josiah Nott in consultation.

Nott was a broken man. During the war, he had worked to organize hospitals for the Confederacy, and after the cause was lost, a hospital he had established in Mobile was converted into a school for former slaves. Seven of Nott's eight children were dead; four had died of yellow fever in the span of a single week. In the wake of the success of his books on racial theory, Nott had taken an interest in women's health. He publicly praised Sims for having made a true science of gynecology. He set out for New York, he said, because it was without morals, religion, and negroes. Sims approached Emmet on his old friend's behalf, and Nott was put on the staff of Woman's Hospital.

Sims believed the young woman was suffering from pelvic cellulitis, not a life-threatening condition. Nott's diagnosis was less sanguine: peritonitis. The woman died on the seventh day after surgery. An autopsy showed that Nott had been correct.

Not long after, Sims lost another woman to his incision of the cervix—an abscess of the fallopian tube burst into her abdomen. Peritonitis soon followed.

* * *

It would take time for Sims to find a place for himself again in the New York medical world. Emmet had secured a $200,000 donation for Woman's Hospital in New York, giving him a firm grip on the medical board. Sims was offered a title and became a member of the governing board, but he was not among the twenty-two doctors who saw patients at Woman's Hospital in 1868.

Fistula surgery was ruined for him. Woman's Hospital had almost closed when he'd been abroad, but Emmet and the Board of Lady Managers, despite having imposed a complete prohibition on cancer cases, had managed to save it. Emmet had been improving the fistula cure for years, and he had published a book on the subject. Furthermore, a young gynecologist in Germany, Dr. Gustav Simon, was endeavoring to show—by soaking slabs of raw meat in tubs of pus-and-blood-filled urine harvested from fistula cases—that it was alkaline and not acidic urine that affected the suture lines of fistula cures. In other words, both Sims's S-shaped silver catheter and the silver sutures were completely unnecessary.

Even the Sims speculum was under attack. Dr. Moritz Schuppert of New Orleans had been hostile to Sims ever since his lecture at the New York Academy of Medicine. Now, Schuppert was claiming to have found a better version of the Sims speculum in an 1846 paper from Prague. In addition, Schuppert produced a long list of those who had used wire sutures before Sims. How could any serious surgeon, Schuppert asked, continue to maintain the opinions that Sims represented?

Josiah Nott vigorously defended Sims with a claim that the Sims speculum did everything other specula did, and did it better. But even Nott was forced to admit that fistula treatment was no longer a wonder of the world.

Sims's income was being augmented by endorsements for various curative waters, for Darby's Prophylactic Fluid and for Peter Möller's cod liver oil. His book was selling well too. Word, however, appeared to have spread about the dangers of cervical incision; he now had to outright browbeat husbands who were too timid to provide consent for their wives. His vaginismus surgery came under fire as well. Cancer looked to be his best hope for continued success.

MOLLER'S
NORWEGIAN COD LIVER OIL.
Abbots Smith, M. D., M. R. C. P., &c., &c., late Physician to the North London Consumptive Hospital, says:—" Möller's Oil is less objectionable to the taste and smell, it is more readily taken by delicate persons and children, is more easily assimilated, and is productive of more immediate benefit than any other kinds of oil are."
Dr. J. Marion Sims says:—" For some years I had given up the use of Cod Liver Oil altogether; but since my attention has been called by Dr. Sayre to Peter Möller's Cod Liver Oil, I have prescribed it almost daily, and have every reason to be perfectly satisfied with it."
Sold by druggists   mh3t 3mTuTh&S

In 1868, a case confirmed what he had long suspected about silver wire and abdominal surgery.

A fifty-three-year-old woman from Philadelphia had an enlargement on her left side. Her physician diagnosed an ovarian tumor but advised it was too dangerous to remove it. The tumor grew until it was larger than a human head. Sims quickly scheduled an operation.

He used an experimental anesthesia—she vomited only once in the twenty minutes it took for her to be completely narcotized. A three-and-a-half-inch incision was enough to enable Sims to dig past a two-inch layer of fat and tap half a dozen cysts growing out of the firmer body of the tumor. He expanded the incision to snap the growth's many adhesions, strangulate its stalk, and heft it out of her body. The tumor weighed sixty-seven and a half pounds.

The interest of the case lay in what he did with the severed stalk. It was the plan he had envisioned years before, when he stitched closed the intestines of the doomed, stabbed slave in Alabama. He used three silver sutures to close the stalk and let it fall back into the woman's body. Eight more sutures sealed the external wound. The woman recovered in a week, and Sims published the good news in the *British Medical Journal*: abdominal surgery was no longer a warrant of death.

Cancer was even better than fistula—the fact that it threatened life made for more agreeable patients. For the next several years, Sims had no shortage of patients with growths attached to the cervix, but apart from successes like that of the woman from Philadelphia, what he mostly found was that he did not cut enough at the site where growths attached to healthy tissue. The disease burst forth again in a few weeks' time, and the women died.

What he needed was patients upon whom he could experiment with deeper cuts. Silver sutures, he was certain, would be more effective in digging out the cancer than the electro-cautery. The dilemma was that the women he saw in private practice came from too high a station, and Woman's Hospital had barred all cancer surgeries.

The new pavilion was a marvel. As with the old hospital, there were free beds on the top floor, and now there were dozens of them. The second and third floors offered accommodation for six dollars per week, and the ground floor offered private rooms for fifteen dollars per week, with partitions that stretched all the way to the ceiling. A new outdoor clinic on the hospital grounds—moved into the basement in the winter months—was available for patients who did not require direct surgical treatment. The operating room was a lofty space divided into two separate theaters, both well lit, capable of accommodating dozens of visitors. A modern ventilating apparatus aerated the entire building. Nurses had a separate space reserved as a dressing room. The new laundry and coal house offered vast improvements over the old hospital. There were plans to build an icehouse and vapor baths. They would connect a telegraph line to the matron's room and add a galvanic doctor to the staff.

Growth was critical. Asked to speak at the first anniversary gala held after the war—Sims and Theresa had dutifully attended the dry annual affairs before leaving for Europe—he offered the usual praise for the galaxy of surgical talent gathered at Woman's Hospital. He made a standard appeal that medical men should be idolized as soldiers and inventors were. He also tried a sly tack: he reminded the gathered governors and lady managers that the original plan for Woman's Hospital had aimed at advancing science and curing diseases beyond that which had afflicted the institution's earliest inmates. In this, a light touch was called for. A new generation of lady managers had come into ascendency during the war. Ostensibly, Mrs. Doremus was still the first directress, but she was frail now. The true leader of the group was Mrs. David Lane—Caroline Lane. Mrs. Lane's formidability was demonstrated even before Sims returned to New York, when she set in motion a series of administrative maneuverings. It was argued that because certain lady managers—including Lane herself—had acquired experience in hospital management during the war, the Board of Lady Managers should be granted total managerial powers over the medical staff of Woman's Hospital. Amazingly, the board of governors accepted the change.

Everyone at Woman's Hospital had been affected by the war. From washerwomen to house surgeons, all recalled the draft riots in New York in 1863, when red-shirted mobs wandered the streets wielding clubs and firing pistols. There were battles between military men and rioters. Gangs of Irishmen hunted door to door for black men, dragging house servants out into the streets to be beaten and hanged. The city was illuminated by fires at night. Lynched black servants dangled from lampposts on Lexington Avenue.

Among Sims's regrets from the war was the fact that he still had not had the chance to test a theory on soldiers wounded in combat. It was not, he believed, the introduction of bloody serum in the abdomen that resulted in peritonitis. Rather, it was the inability of the serum to drain from the cavity. Also, he regretted missing the raw experience of war. Younger doctors than himself regaled him with stories of great piles of men, dead of fever—they were rolled in tar, smoked, and buried in mass graves. A house surgeon had witnessed a large group of Confederate boys, caught in a chasm, massacred with balls and shells. There were accounts of sharpshooter duels, doctors tattooing the chests of deserters, and hardtack so full of maggots it had to be baked before it could be eaten. Medical curiosities abounded. A doctor recalled a man who'd had a ball enter his head at the apex of his nose and pass through it; he survived without a symptom. Another tended to a soldier whose forehead had been penetrated by a ball that broke the skin but not his skull. It rolled around to the back of his neck and exited again.

It was the lady managers who were most transformed.

Caroline Lane had raised four children before she'd been made manager of the Employment Society, to aid poor women. When the war started, she was recruited into the US Sanitary Commission, and a number of the women who worked on the commission's hospital ships later followed Lane to Woman's Hospital. Lane was a kind, steady Unitarian, but by the end of the war it was said that she had acquired the mien of a general. Her temper could not be ruffled. When Sims came home, she had a reputation for knowing all the workings of Woman's Hospital, the details of every inmate.

Josiah Nott did not last long—he couldn't hide the role he'd played in the war and the books that made him famous. The Board of Lady Managers claimed that he was poorly mannered with patients and lacked a true surgeon's dexterity with implements. They were concerned with a case in which Nott operated on a woman for torn perineum without realizing she was pregnant. She miscarried two months later. Sims created a series of diagrams to illustrate Nott's value for the ladies, but how could one bridge the gulf between Nott's views on race and those of the managers who had fought opposite him in a conflict only lately resolved? Sims kept his own views close. He wrote to friends of the dreadful mistake it had been to permit black men to vote, and in private company he complained that the South was now being degraded below the level of the meanest slave that ever wore a shackle.

Still, something would need to be done about the managers. Worse than the humiliation they inflicted on Nott was what they were attempting to do to the narrative of Sims's career. He had come to learn from the new chairman of the board of governors that a story had taken hold while he'd been in Europe. It was not Sims who had saved women with Woman's Hospital—rather, it was women who had saved Sims.

* * *

He didn't see the harm in it. Truly, there was no harm, unless you were one of the doctors stuck in the thrall of medical ethics.

Charlotte Cushman was a global celebrity, the day's leading actress. She was as famous for her portrayal of Lady Macbeth as she was for playing the gypsy crone Meg Merrilies in the stage adaptation of Scott's *Guy Mannering*. She was exactly the sort of figure who could transform public opinion—or the opinion of squeamish lady managers.

Cushman had a lump in her breast. Sims had seen her in Paris, visiting on the sly, as the slightest variation in her schedule could trigger a snowstorm of news. She had tried a variety of remedies: tincture of hydrastis, water cures (on Sims's recommendation), pig's blood. Sims returned to America, and Cushman traveled to Edinburgh to be seen by James Simpson. Simpson told her it was a malignant tumor. It could not be dispersed by waters or tinctures. That was Sims's opportunity. He wrote to Cushman to tell her that surgery was her only option for life—she should return to America at once. A successful cancer operation on the famous Charlotte Cushman would overwhelm the anxieties of the lady managers who were now keeping Emmet and the rest of the Woman's Hospital doctors on a short lead.

In the end, Cushman opted for Simpson as her surgeon. As predicted, her mysterious convalescence produced a great deal of public speculation. Sims didn't give a second thought to exploiting the situation to his advantage, but over time it would seem as though this small, innocent act was the beginning of his undoing.

In response to an article in the *New York Times*—an unfortunately accurate one, at least as to the nature of Miss Cushman's illness—Sims hurried off a few lines in reply. His goal was to attach his name to Cushman and do her the favor of disguising a complaint that could derail her career. Miss Cushman had sought out his opinion in France, Sims wrote. She had been distressed about nothing more than a small hardened gland. It posed no threat to life. He had advised no surgical interference and sent her to Malvern for the season.

Unfortunately, he went on, another surgeon had seized the opportunity to take credit for operating on Miss Cushman. If she was now unwell in any way, it was likely that either the conditions of her procedure or the practices of her doctor had resulted in a skin infection. The fact that news of Miss Cushman's death had not already arrived from Europe was a clear indication that she had averted danger.

Although Sims had many admirers across America, there had survived in New York a hidden coven of antagonists. The zealots of ethics were jealous of his fame and skill; these diabolical men had nursed their spite in the years he was abroad. The Cushman notice was seized upon by Dr. T. C. Finnell, who was notable otherwise only for having performed an autopsy on the famous courtesan Fanny White.

In a month's time, Sims was served with charges from the Committee on Ethics at the New York Academy of Medicine, the same institution that had heralded his return from Europe with a claim that he had raised the character of American medical science to an eminence heretofore unattained.

The committee ambushed him. He was invited to the home of one of its members on the night of November 11, 1869. Four of the members, and Finnell—who also sat on the committee—waited somberly in a drawing room. He was offered a seat and a cigar. He refused. After an awkward pause, one of the members took up a sheaf of documents and began reading aloud with the title: "Charges Against a Fellow."

The document included the entirety of what he had published in the *Times*. It was claimed that Sims's description of Miss Cushman's condition violated the code of ethics: particularly in peculiar circumstances, physicians should opt for strict secrecy and delicacy. Furthermore, it was charged that Sims's disparagement of the work of a trusted colleague violated a prohibition on expressing conflicting opinions. Last, he was accused of having provided support to media attention that had been given to him in Europe, and since his return. This breached the code's proscription of activity that affected the character of the profession.

Sims took it all in silently, calculating a response. He couldn't very well tell them that his article about Cushman was a lie, as well. By the time the speaker had finished, he had decided on a course of action. First, to leave no sense of hesitation, he announced unequivocally that the charges against him were false. He demanded a copy—one had been prepared for him—and he left in a rush with a promise of a prompt reply.

By morning, Sims had composed a brief notice for the newspapers, written as though it were authored by an offended observer. It was to be telegraphed to Europe and printed there. He wrote to Dr. Johnston in Paris as well, to request a note offering assurance that "Malakoff" had in no instance written at Sims's request, direct or otherwise.

He sent for Henri Stuart. Not only had Stuart survived the war, his influence had arguably grown as a function of negotiating the rights of gunmakers. He was now attaching a "Dr." to the front of his name, in honor of his association with the Eclectic Medical College of New York. Sims cared little that Stuart had mostly been a Union man. He was useful regardless, and his need for discreet medical services for women seemed unabated. Since Sims's arrival home, the two men had been plotting his return to medical duties at Woman's Hospital. It was unclear what Sims would be able to achieve medically—if anything—without access to experimental fodder.

Stuart agreed with Sims's plan for European newspapers. He pocketed the story Sims had scribbled out and promised it would appear in London the following morning. They agreed that the printed story would be useful to cite when Sims wrote his reply to the Committee on Ethics. Stuart advised delaying the reply, however. Make them wait, he said. Don't respond until you are about to leave the country. Your absence will muffle the effect of their judgment, whatever it is.

At first, Sims put off the committee's request for a hasty response with claims that the holidays had prevented him from composing a proper answer to the charges. After the new year, he simply ignored their entreaties. He delivered his reply, by hand, to one of the committee's members, on the eve of his departure for London in April 1870. As planned, he quoted from the self-authored defense that had been printed abroad. He claimed his only wish was that every member of the New York Academy of Medicine might be as guiltless of the charges as he was.

The committee rendered its judgment in June. He was guilty of violating the profession's code of ethics, and he was formally reprimanded. The reprimand mattered little, but in time it would come to seem like the tiny push that set the rest of his collapse in motion.

Thirty-One

Tempel and Tuttle—The return of the falling stars—A contract—
Ninth and tenth pregnancies—A huge ball of fire

WILHELM TEMPEL DEVELOPED A PASSION FOR THE STARS AS A BOY, observing them from the top of a bell tower where he worked as a ringer.

In 1856, Tempel paid four hundred florins for a 10.8 cm refractor scope, and he made his first discovery on April 2, 1859—a comet spied from the top of a famous staircase in Vienna. He made further discoveries from the balcony of his home in Marseille: asteroids, galaxies, the Pleiades nebula. Tempel's most important observation came on the night of December 19, 1865, when he sighted a comet whose return had been predicted for some time.

In America, Horace Tuttle was the younger brother of Harvard astronomer Charles Tuttle, the first to observe the dusky inner rings of Saturn. Horace Tuttle was eight years younger, a common laborer not noted for his studies. Nevertheless, Tuttle succeeded his brother at the Harvard College Observatory. Tuttle created detailed images of Jupiter and participated in the hunt for the phantom planet Vulcan. However, he was best known as a comet seeker, recording more than a dozen comets between 1858 and 1862.

After the Civil War ended, Tuttle began work at the Naval Observatory in Washington City, in the same building where Matthew Fontaine Maury showed Anarcha the slow fall of a star through the firmament. On January 5, 1866, Tuttle observed a comet inside the constellation Leo, the same comet that Wilhelm Tempel had recorded in France two weeks earlier.

The body would be named 55P/ Tempel-Tuttle, a comet with an orbital period of thirty-three years. It was the "parent" of the Leonid meteor showers, so named because the shooting stars appeared to emerge from the constellation Leo. The Leonids had produced the night the stars fell, on November 13, 1833. After a thirty-three-year absence, Comet Tempel-Tuttle had returned to Earth.

Comets and meteors were far better understood in 1866. Meteorites remained in space; aerolites fell to the ground. Star jelly was still mysterious, but shooting stars were not rocks shot into space by lunar volcanoes. Rather, the light showers were chips of diffuse matter, traveling at high speed, ignited by friction in the atmosphere.

As early as 1837, it was predicted that the Earth would once again pass through a dense swarm of Leonid meteors. After the identification of Tempel-Tuttle, it was calculated that a meteor shower similar to that of 1833 would occur on the night of November 13 or 14, 1866. An uptick in shooting stars on that date had been noticed ever since 1860.

News of the pending miracle passed around the globe. As the date finally approached, reporters complained that the public had developed a case of falling stars on the brain. Nothing was dreamed or read of but meteors. Shoemakers, tailors, bartenders—all had become as well versed in heavenly action as Galileo or Humboldt. The expectation was of a vision that would make one's hairs stand on end like the quills of a fretful porcupine.

* * *

The news traveled even to the Alto plantation in Virginia where, the year before, Lorenzo, Albert, William, Gusty and his son Joseph, and the young George Peyton signed a contract with Charles Mason to work the Alto land. Shortly after the war ended, a provost judge rode his horse onto the Alto property and informed the former Mason slaves that under no circumstances should they work for anyone, not even their master, without pay. The judge was shortly followed by a northern preacher who came around offering to marry slaves that hadn't already been married in a church or at a Freedman's Bureau office. Anarcha and Lorenzo said no thank you. They were already confessed to each other, they told the preacher. That was married enough. But Lorenzo did go to Charles Mason, and he told him that it was time to start running the plantation again, and Mason thought and gave a slow nod, and he still said nothing about whether Lorenzo was his kin or not. Instead, he said that Lorenzo and Gusty and the others should come to the house the following morning, and they would all ride to the King George courthouse to make it official.

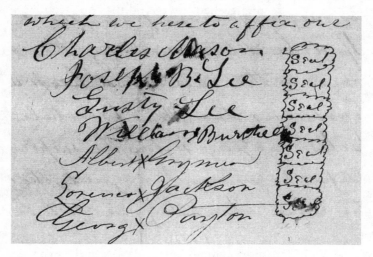

Mason had the contract prepared in the morning. They rode the wagon quietly into town, where the document was read out loud by the court-house clerk.

For the cultivation of the one hundred acres of the Mason estate known as the mill field, the said Charles Mason would furnish six mules and the necessary implements, and he would grant access to the stables and the corncribs. In return, the said former slaves would bind themselves to work the land when it was in order, in a thorough and farm-like manner, and they would deliver the crops prepared for market on board a vessel, the proceeds to be divided, after deducting for expenses, equally among the parties: one-half part to the said Mason, and one-half part to the said former slaves. The said men would further bind themselves to furnish firewood for Mason's family, to keep the fences in order, and to supply the Mason family with milk, cream, and butter. For their compensation, they would have equal use of the icehouse, and they would receive a one-half part of the sale of dairy, and a one-half part of the calves, pigs, and lambs that would come during the year.

Gusty signed for himself and his son, and William scribbled his name. Lorenzo, Albert, and George each put an "X" where the clerk told them to.

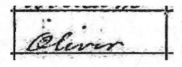

Not long after, Anarcha got pregnant again. A boy, Oliver, was born several months before the night when it was said the stars would fall again. For a time, Anarcha was able to nurse two babies at once, sitting in a chair outside the cabin, which she did most of the time now. She had opened up again, inside. She could feel it. Sitting or lying down was the easiest way to stay dry and to keep the loose parts inside. In the morning, Lorenzo carried her out to the chair and served her real coffee, which they now had regularly. He brought water up from the creek every day and left a jug by her chair before he went off to the fields and animals. She spent her days nursing and looking down at the Mason house, where the master's sickly son Wilson died in 1866, as she had thought he might. She watched as the family dressed in fine clothes and rode off to bury him. Only the Mason boy Jack came up to the cabins now, to play with Ben and Jonathan in the woods. In the evenings, Delia taught Louisa to cook.

On November 13, taverns stayed open late into the night so that people could drink their fill before going outside to watch the display of lights. Fire-bell ringers planned to ring their bells as soon as the show began, to wake up the whole world. Anarcha sat up into the night with the others. But just as she had known as a girl that the stars weren't really falling because you could see other fixed stars behind them, she knew now that the stars would not fall again as they had when she was woken by flashes through cracks in the roof of her family's cabin. It was like having babies, she thought. The first was the biggest show, and you thought the world was ending. Then it got easier. Now, the sky was tired, she thought—tired of the generations of fear and anguish it had silently witnessed, tired of the war it had watched over, mostly without comment. Life was now drained from it. Anarcha kept quiet in her chair, holding Oliver. A crescent moon hung low on the western horizon. Very few stars fell that night. There was much disappointment. But Anarcha was not disappointed, and after that night she felt her own life begin to drain away. It was not painful, and it was not sudden, but it was coming like bad news, or a bad story, and it was incorruptible.

She got pregnant again, her final pregnancy, a baby girl, but she died. They buried her in the woods.

It was another year before the sky summoned enough strength for a show. It wasn't as vivid or as frightening as the night the stars fell, and no one collapsed to their knees in prayer. A few of the electric tenants of the heavens shot madly from their places, printing the hues of the rainbow across a clear, dark night. One star in particular appeared as a huge ball of fire. It traced overhead in fifteen seconds, from horizon to horizon. Blinding in brilliance, vanishing into distant heavens, it left behind it a tail of light that curled and twisted into magical shapes and lingered in the sky.

Thirty-Two

Joseph Lister—Thomas Evans—The Battle of Sedan—
Surgical mortality—Beck's case—Battey's operation—
The lady managers rebel—An epidemic—The gala

BACK IN LONDON, SIMS VISITED THE LABORATORY OF DR. JOSEPH LISTER, who had achieved renown with his theories about antiseptic conditions for surgery. Sims generally agreed with Lister, but he didn't think, as Emmet was fond of saying, that the death warrant of every patient was carried under the fingernails of her physician. He wondered whether the same results that Lister was achieving with carbolic acid could be got with the fastidious use of cotton swabs.

He didn't stay in London long. War was looming again. For some time, France and Prussia had been listing toward conflict. It would be Louis Napoléon's final stand. At last, Sims had the chance of savoring firsthand experiences of battle, and he could employ its casualties to discover the true nature of abdominal wounds.

The only difficulty was that the work to assemble an ambulance corps to establish a hospital at the front was being conducted by a committee designed along the lines of the Sanitary Commission in New York—the same organization that had wound up causing so much mischief among the lady managers of Woman's Hospital. Worse, the committee was headed up by dentist Thomas Evans, Sims's counterpart in the secret exchange of messages with Napoléon during the war. The two men had met only briefly, when Evans administered anesthesia during two of Sims's operations. Sims was unsure whether Evans was even aware that they had carried out opposite covert missions. On traveling to Paris, Sims learned that he had been accepted as the man to head up the hospital at the front. He was invited to a meeting at Evans's home to decide when the gathered personnel and supplies would be dispatched to Metz and Sedan.

Evans lived between the opera house and Place Vendôme, on the Rue de la Paix. Sims arrived early, and when he shook Evans's hand, he could see in the man's expression that he had already concluded that Sims's motives were opportunistic. They most certainly were. What a sad loss it had been that men of Evans's ilk—like the Kappa Lambda men, the cautious sort—had come to hold sway over the medical world. What honors of advancement might have been possible had men who were truly men won the battle to seize every opportunity, however ugly, to promote science? Always, it was ethics that slowed progress. Always, it was ethics that stood in the way of knowledge and personal gain.

The meeting progressed at the pace of a throbbing ache. When at last the timing of the contingent's departure was raised, Sims argued that they should leave immediately. Evans opposed him. He offered a weak claim that the departure should be delayed until it was clear that their contribution would be helpful. An initial poll of the four-man panel found the vote deadlocked at 2–2. Sims and a colleague attempted a feint. They raised a motion to nominate Sims as a member of the board, effective immediately. Again, Evans spoke in opposition. It was clear, he said, that Dr. Sims did not genuinely wish to serve as a member of the board. Rather, he wished only to vote on the matter at hand. The motion was denied, and the deadlocked vote deferred to the wishes of the chairman.

Surely, Sims could not be blamed for what came next. He felt a galvanic pulse surge through his body. The censure he had received from the New York Academy of Medicine—handed down only when he was distant from the men who slapped his face—now wove itself together with fury that rose up toward Thomas Evans. Only a short time before, Evans had been Sims's enemy. Had Sims encountered him in the street during the war, honor would have compelled him to strike the man down, perhaps kill him. Given this, Sims's action as the meeting adjourned would likely be judged by history to be an act of honorable temperance. He approached while Evans still sat in his chair. Then, in a swift motion, Sims seized the man's throat and dealt his head a fierce blow. He let Evans's limp form fall to the floor.

He found his way to the front with a British group instead. A batch of sterilized catgut arrived from Lister just before they left. In the years to come, Sims would take guiltless pleasure in imagining the palpitations of Dr. Finnell in New York at reading the many newspaper accounts that chronicled his heroic march off to war. At Sedan, Sims assumed control of a large barrack close to the castle wall. The battle raged all around the makeshift hospital. The armies' new machine guns sounded from all sides; the sputtering of musketry and cannon was timid music compared to it. The hospital was hit with several shells during the worst of the fighting—two nurses were killed in blasts—and when the stream of casualties began to arrive, Sims and the doctors he brought with him, his son and son-in-law among them, couldn't amputate quickly enough. Others died before a saw was available for them.

He had ample opportunity to survey wounds of the abdomen. Men shot through the pelvis almost always survived. He found one young man so grievously butchered that for a time he defecated through one artificial hole and urinated through another. Still, he recovered. By contrast, nearly all of the men wounded in the abdomen died. Yet Sims was correct: wounds to the abdomen were fatal when men were struck above the brim of the pelvis. In such cases, the bloody serum was left trapped in the peritoneum. But in those cases where the wound was lower, the ball itself created a passage for drainage from the gut, and the man survived.

Sims saw Louis Napoléon at the front. His face was rouged to hide the effects of bladder stones. The war was going to be the end for him. He would soon surrender, and before long he would flee to London.

After the battle, Sims returned to Paris. He was put on trial for the gross and wanton assault of Dr. Thomas Evans. He was convicted and fined one hundred francs for violating the law of Napoléon, and three hundred more for damages to his countryman.

* * *

Back in New York several years later, on a morning in the middle of 1874, Sims encountered a flustered woman in the street, emerging from

Woman's Hospital. She had been examined by Emmet in regard to a large growth in her abdomen. Emmet explained that rather than an ovarian tumor, the growth was a fibro-cyst. It wouldn't kill her, he said. The dangers of removing it outweighed whatever inconvenience it posed in life. The poor woman was left in tears.

Sims could hardly have left the woman sobbing as she climbed into a hansom. He invited her into his office and examined her himself. Emmet was wrong: it was a tumor. A difficult one, to be sure, but precisely the sort of procedure the hospital needed, regardless of what the lady managers said. It was a case that could advance the cause of a cancer cure.

Sims sent for Emmet. They examined the woman once more. Initially, Emmet said, he had been able to work a probe seven inches deep into her uterus. Now, he could manage less than three. He relented in his diagnosis. They agreed that before an operation, the woman should be examined by Dr. Gaillard Thomas and Dr. Edmund Peaslee, the physicians who rounded out Woman's Hospital's new medical board, established two years before.

Emmet's control over the hospital had begun to slip almost as soon as Sims returned from the Battle of Sedan. Emmet had taken the loss of the Civil War hard. He was thrown by President Grant's suggestion that he would remain in office as long as "his army" was willing to keep him there. Even worse was the Board of Lady Managers. Emmet had never been particularly good—as Sims had—at manipulating the ladies, and after the war, their more hostile chatter had infuriated him. He was reduced to proposing a change to the bylaws that would impose a limit at formal meetings of one lady manager speaking at a time. When the managers were out of earshot, Emmet complained of his helplessness. He threatened to resign. Women lacked reasoning power, he said. As a rule, they were not fitted by nature for the trust of the management of an institution such as Woman's Hospital.

By 1871, Emmet was at a breaking point. The final stroke was an effort he made to appoint his nephew as a house surgeon. The Board of Lady Managers refused to accept the nomination. Emmet was left on the brink of collapse. That summer, when the hospital was mostly idle, he took an extended leave of absence. He traveled to Russia.

Henri Stuart agreed: it was the chance they'd been waiting for. It was time to insert Sims back into the medical workings of Woman's Hospital. He began by attending the lady managers' meetings, offering the argument that with the conflicts of the nation now resolved, and a new hospital that, thanks to the managers' efforts, was nothing less than a grand palace, the time was ripe for a thorough change, for growth in services, and for promotion to a larger staff. It wasn't difficult to imply that Emmet, a man whose frailty had compelled him to abandon his post and his patients—to leisurely explore eastern Europe—could no longer be trusted with shouldering alone the profound responsibilities of an institution the managers had taken great pains to create. Sims was particularly effective at molding the perspective of Mrs. Doremus, who had been with the hospital, and with Sims, even longer than Emmet had.

Stuart and Sims conspired to compose amendments to the bylaws radically transforming the composition of the medical board. Emmet was supplanted as sole leader. A four-man team was installed in his place, composed of Emmet, Sims, and two others. It mattered little that the others had already served as Emmet's lieutenants. The crux was that Sims was back in. With a hospital busier by a factor of four, there would be no way that any single lady manager—not even Caroline Lane—could keep track of every patient and every surgery that was performed at the hospital.

Gaillard Thomas and Edmund Peaslee had begun working for Emmet during the war. Thomas had South Carolina in common with Sims: he was from Charleston and attended the South Carolina Medical College. However, he had worked with Emmet at the Ward's Island Emigrant Refuge Hospital, and in 1868 he published a well-received book, *A Practical Treatise on the Diseases of Women.*

Peaslee was a New Englander and an altogether tougher case. He had been on the Committee on Ethics that censured Sims; Sims could feel the man's loathing whenever they shared a room. Before Woman's Hospital, Peaslee worked at New York University, and in 1872 he published the definitive work on female cancers, *Ovarian Tumors: Their Pathology, Diagnosis, and Treatment, Especially by Ovariotomy.*

In 1874, called upon to examine the woman whom Sims had found crying in the street, Thomas and Peaslee agreed: Sims was right, her condition was an ovarian tumor.

All four men—an alignment of the leading gynecological stars in America—attended the operation. From the first cut, an extensive cobweb of cancerous adhesions made it impossible to tell whether Emmet's or Sims's diagnosis had been correct. The tapping of the growth revealed it to be firmly attached to the bladder. They succeeded in separating it only to find another broad adhesion high up in the rectum. It was only by passing a double ligature around the base of the mass and removing it that they were able to recognize that Emmet's diagnosis had been the correct one. In error, they had removed the woman's uterus above the vaginal junction.

She never rallied and died in a few hours' time.

* * *

Even as the lady managers accepted Sims back into the hospital, he could feel the difference in their attitude toward him now—a lack of deference. The managers were aware that Sims had made enemies. Early in the hospital's history, they had not only ignored the voices that rose in criticism of him, they helped tamp them down. Now, a different atmosphere prevailed.

The initial months of the four-man medical board at Woman's Hospital was a largely harmonious time. All four surgeons were of a single mind about the importance of admitting cancer patients. The lady managers could hardly enforce their foolish prohibition when the entire medical board stood in opposition to it. Sims now had the chance to put what he had learned at Sedan into action. If it could be shown that the cul-de-sac of a woman's vagina could be punctured, and the vagina itself turned into a tube of evacuation for dangerous peritoneal serums, then gains might be realized not only in cancers peculiar to women. All cancers could be found to be curable. More broadly, it might be possible to show that abdominal surgery in men and women both could be rendered safe.

There were other promising developments for Sims as well. First, Dr. Joseph Beck of Indiana had answered Sims's decade-old call to search for a mysterious and elusive vaginal muscle. Beck's report began with a fervent defense of Sims. He was like a crusader of old: the only difference was that his pen was a readier and more trenchant weapon than the swords of long-forgotten warriors.

Beck had found a case that made Sims's claim that the cervix sucked seminal fluid into the uterus a testable proposition. He had taken into his care a woman suffering from prolapse; her cervix was now situated immediately behind the curtain of her labia. In Beck's initial examination, he was surprised when the woman experienced a profound orgasm at the first moment he touched her. Embarrassed, she rushed from his office. He did not see her again until the following day, when he visited her domicile. This time, the woman offered a warning that the spasm might happen again. She explained that she was capable of causing orgasm in herself with only the slightest of digital examinations.

Beck saw it at once: her prolapsed organ, combined with predictable contractions, afforded a unique opportunity. He arranged to examine the woman in sunlit conditions. Gently, he spread apart her labia so that he had an unobstructed view of her os uteri. It took only four swipes of his forefinger to trigger the contractions. Just as Sims predicted, the cervical opening turned a bright purple color. It then spread open, making in twelve seconds a number of pulsing gasps, like the mouth of a carp. Beck was certain that the passage of spermatic fluid into the uterus had been explained. Sims's theory had been proved true.

Even better than Beck, the potential for surgery to address illness of the female brain had quickly become a lucrative frontier for gynecology. Despite the sad fate of Isaac Baker Brown, Horatio Storer—Sims's old friend—had several years before completed a one-hundred-page study for the American Medical Association entitled "The Cause, Course, and Treatment of Insanity in Women." Gone were the days, Storer wrote, when it was believed that women's mental illness stemmed from worms of loathsome diversity or reptiles armed with fangs. The treatments then available to ladies suffering from mental maladies were indistinguishable from horrors inflicted on criminals. Insane women were locked into dungeons slowly filled with water to give the impression of imminent death. They were fastened into suspended swings and spun at one hundred revolutions per minute. They were tied down for hours at a time, subjected to abuses applied in the name of treatment.

Surely, Storer wrote, the ingenuity of modern medicine could improve on the tortures of the past. Women offered the most instructive of cases. Who could not take note of the maidenly reserve that emerged when healthy women came of age? Or of the troubles that formed when puberty went awry, or when women returned to their second sexual childhood? What was obvious to any observer was that mental disturbances emanated from a source outside the brain—often or perhaps generally in association with the reproductive organs. What the case of women clearly illustrated, Storer concluded, was that the organ of the mind was thrown into diseased action by its sympathy with other organs that were injured or diseased. Hence, treatment of mental illness in women should be of a surgical character.

The full potential of psychological surgery was unlocked, Sims thought, when a young doctor from Georgia made a manly effort to rise to the last of Storer's challenges. What might result, Dr. Robert Battey boldly asked in 1872, if we did not wait to find diseased organs in the bodies of women suffering miserably from epilepsy or hysteria, but instead removed her healthy ovaries to artificially induce menopause? Battey called his unsexing operation "normal ovariotomy." Sims thought it a misnomer. How could ovaries be considered normal if surgery was called for to remove them? Regardless, he felt a kind of paternal kinship toward Battey. The young man had come from an obscure village practice, just as Sims had. He encouraged Battey to name the procedure for himself, to seize the credit for "Battey's operation" and thereby ensure the worldwide fame that would be his just reward. Sims resolved to do what he could in the periodicals to ensure that Battey's operation would be properly embalmed for future generations.

* * *

The troubles at Woman's Hospital reached a boiling point precisely at the moment when the future of gynecology looked brightest. The distribution of power among the city's four great gynecologists had turned Woman's Hospital into a thriving hive of activity. Each of the surgeons enjoyed a following of physicians and medical students. The exponential increase in traffic made for a buzzing metropolis of innovation.

For upward of a year, Caroline Lane and the harried flock of lady managers could do little to control the new proliferation of cancer cases, which officially remained prohibited. They were equally alarmed by the hallways stuffed with physicians who regarded the hospital as a private club for men. One of Gaillard Thomas's surgeries drew more than seventy observers, and it was widely known that Sims's performances were so crowded that attendees risked suffocation to witness operations executed with such lightning-quick finesse that they were of little teaching value. Sims rejoiced at this. The hospital had become exactly what he had first envisioned. By contrast, the lady managers persisted in thinking of it—it was what he had tricked them into believing—as a dedicated fistula clinic, a place of retreat. Fistula treatment was supposed to be free of the horrors of hospitals, where death was a regular occurrence.

Trouble loomed in the summer of 1873. Inside a single month, more patients died than had perished in the entire previous year. This statistic included a woman who, in grief, threw herself out a fourth-floor window. The first sign of challenge to the medical board was the lady managers' decision to hire a full-time pathologist, and to equip the pathologist with a book to keep careful record of deaths. And then there were logistical complaints: under the onslaught of cancer patients, the nurses couldn't possibly perform all of their duties.

One of Sims's cases from December 1873 proved pivotal. In operating on a fibroid tumor, Sims accidentally broke the mass, resulting in the woman's entire vagina flooding with pus. The stench was unbearable. For the difficult period in which she might either recover or die, there was nowhere to put her but in one of the public wards. The woman spent a delirious six hours with a fever of 106 and a pulse of 160. This case, and others who died in their ward beds—the same wards where inmates took their meals—was turning Woman's Hospital into exactly the thing the lady managers had never supposed it to be.

Rumors began to circulate through the city that Woman's Hospital killed more than it cured.

In January 1874, the lady managers fired a doctor without the permission of either the medical or governance boards. At approximately the same time, they issued an ultimatum to the governors. They wanted a complete ban on cancer patients. In addition, they wished to impose a limit of fifteen observers to any surgery. Last, they called for a full investigation of rates of mortality at the hospital.

Sims and the medical board resolved to meet. The gathering was contentious from the start. Rather than respond to the ladies' demands with force and vigor, the other surgeons proposed a policy of weakness and capitulation. The managers had already convinced the governors, Sims's colleagues noted. The argument that ovarian tumor was a disease peculiar to women no longer worked. In this, the managers had made an apt inference—women were being experimented upon to further medical research that would yield benefits to both sexes. "Suffering womanhood" now appeared to mean that women should suffer so that a cure might be found for men. Even the governors had concluded that it was an insult to common intelligence to suggest that cancer cases fell under the classification of infirmities peculiar to women.

Furthermore, Emmet noted, Mrs. John Jacob Astor was both a manager and a major donor to the hospital. She believed Woman's Hospital was ill fitted to cancer cases. However, she had proposed a donation for a new building—to be called the Emmet Pavilion—that would be entirely dedicated to cancer. Why not wait until the new wing of the hospital could be constructed?

Sims harrumphed. Like the new hospital itself, he said, such a structure might take a decade or more to be completed. He offered a cogent and manly argument that giving in to the lady managers would embolden them to stage more radical interventions. They should insist on admitting cancer patients.

It was futile. Emmet, Thomas, and Peaslee united in the view that if they took the course Sims suggested, all four of them would be turned out into the street. They passed a measure to accept the cancer prohibition but requested twenty-five visitors rather than fifteen. Sims remained silent.

The managers rejected twenty-five visitors; the number stayed at fifteen.

However, the managers permitted cancer patients to be admitted with the permission of the governors' board. Unappeased, Sims resolved to continue with his cancer patients and his packed surgical theater.

* * *

It got worse. An epidemic of puerperal peritonitis—spread from Bellevue— laid siege to Woman's Hospital in the spring of 1874. Ten women died in the first half of the year. Then Sims botched another diagnosis. The patient was Thomas's. A woman of good health and morals presented with an immature tumor that gave her great distress. Sims advised proceeding—if Woman's Hospital could not operate when conditions were perfect, he argued, then what profitable services could they hope to provide? Peaslee responded that he would never operate on a case where the tumor was so small. Thomas proceeded with the operation, and the woman died four days later.

In the middle of the year, Sims learned that the Board of Lady Managers knew he had persisted with cancer surgeries. It seemed he had been betrayed, by a disgruntled doctor or a nurse loyal to Emmet. He tried throwing them off his trail by installing patients in beds reserved for other surgeons.

After the hospital slipped into its summer slumber, Sims used the annual meeting of the American Medical Association, held in Detroit, to staunch the bleeding of the wound the lady managers had inflicted on his career. In the conference's public discussion on ovariotomy, Sims diverted conversation from chloroform to the various experiments conducted at Woman's Hospital. As to deaths, he boldly asserted that the institution's doctors made no secret of their failed cases. To be sure, a physician's opinions were better formed by his work on the autopsy table than by his successes. And as to the patients themselves, he boldly announced, it was nothing but just that a woman who has received the kind benefit of a doctor's attendance should repay her debt, in death, by the use of her body to search out means for the relief of all humanity.

For this, Sims received loud and sustained applause.

* * *

When Woman's Hospital opened again in the fall, Mrs. Doremus resigned from the Board of Lady Managers. The remaining managers persisted with meddling actions. They proposed that the icehouse be converted to a special ward for cancer patients, complete with its own surgical theater. And they engaged the hospital engineer to act as a spy. The poor man's duties now included counting the heads of visitors at operations. No other surgeons in the city were compelled to obey such radical strictures.

Surgically, the fall was a time of mixed results. Sims performed a final operation on Woman's Hospital's patient-turned-nurse Mary Smith. Over the years, Smith had been subjected to as many as thirty-three surgeries. Before the war, Sims had managed to secure her bladder in place, using the procedure he tested on Anarcha. Emmet created a new urethra for her, rendering her dry. Now she had a bladder stone. Emmet advised against Sims's plan of dilating the artificial urethra to remove the stone. He did it anyway. Mary Smith was left with no power of retention, and she lost her position as nurse. She was reduced to begging in the streets near the hospital.

By way of contrast, Sims stumbled across a perfect candidate for Battey's operation. He took into his care a thirty-five-year-old missionary from Choofoo, China. Suffering from a variety of mysterious maladies over several years, the woman was ideal for normal ovariotomy. Hopeful of a cure, Sims scheduled the procedure for just after the new year, shortly before the woman's intended return to the Orient.

It would be at the year's annual gala that tensions stretching back as far as Sims's censure at the New York Academy of Medicine became unbearable. The night before the event, it took a great act of will to remain calm. Gaillard Thomas presented himself at Sims's home to secure his approval for the annual report of the medical board; Sims claimed his eyes were too tired to read. Thomas read aloud the board's cowardly capitulation to the injustices being visited upon them. Sims would have to stand alone in defense of the profession, he realized. The time to strike was now, he thought, when the ranks of the lady managers had grown thin. His colleagues were unwilling to marshal an attack even against that weakened foe. No matter—he would do what needed to be done.

He had a surgery in the morning—a difficult one. He was attempting an abdominal removal of a uterus afflicted with large fibroids, employing a method recently in vogue in Europe. It was his second attempt with the procedure. The woman in the first case had died not forty minutes after the operation—the capsule of the tumor broke, the woman lost a pound of blood in a moment's time, and she never rallied.

The woman in the second operation, performed on the morning of November 19, 1874, had already lost a great deal of blood. Sims resolved to operate anyway. The uterus and its tumor came away easily, but he sensed a looseness of the tissue as he secured the stalk with silver sutures. He feared sloughing along the entire line of the incision. He did what he could, went home, and began to prepare for the gala. He read over his prepared remarks. His patient, he knew, lay dying at the hospital. He wasn't sure how long it would take. A day, perhaps two or three—but she would fade and fail. He would not again attempt the fashionable European surgery.

The tradition of the gala—the mindlessly lavished praise, the dreary invited speakers, the pithy metaphors of brilliant comets and streaking shooting stars—it was now all two decades old. The callous display went on, every year, despite the rot that had infected the hospital's foundation from the very start.

Perhaps he should deliver his remarks in the usual desultory way. Perhaps he ought not speak at all.

No. An hour before Sims and Theresa were to depart, their son Harry arrived home with troubling news. For the first time, a visiting doctor at Woman's Hospital had been denied access to the surgical theater. He was late, and there were already fifteen doctors in attendance. Sims felt rage flush through him like a scratch of virus. If indeed a man hoped to be remembered for having stood for honor and progress, this was far more than he should be expected to endure without action in return. He spent a precious twenty minutes adjusting his remarks, and then he and Theresa climbed into a hansom.

Once again, the ground floor of the hospital had been completely transformed: the beds removed, their occupants temporarily installed in crowded rooms upstairs, the curtains drawn. There were flowers every-where, but no amount of masking could fully eclipse the odor of the fistula and cancer patients, the stink of piss and pus that had sunk deep into the wooden wainscoting and the rope-matting carpets that the managers had insisted on, to give the wards a faint feel of home.

The report of the Board of Lady Managers came first. Their secretary read a prim recounting of the paint job the hospital had received over the summer and a new charity bed that had been preserved in perpetuity thanks to the generosity of Mrs. John Jacob Astor. The secretary offered thanks for past mercies and asked for well wishes for worn and weary sisters in their hour of need.

The report from the board of governors was mercifully short, touching on details of the new pavilion—it would not, in the end, be named for Emmet. Next, Thomas hurried through the report of the medical board that Sims had already heard: the 264 women admitted during the course of the year, the 233 cured or improved, the 2,000 women seen at the outdoor clinics, and 10,000 more in consultations. In a year's time, fifteen women had died at the hospital.

As speaker succeeded speaker, Sims felt himself begin to slip away from the evening's dull thrum. When the invited guest took the podium—Sims would come next—he felt his mind begin to detach from that crowded, converted ward for the infirm. Something similar had happened whenever his most penetrating medical insights had come to him—they arrived as though delivered by some entity calling from a precinct far outside himself.

The invited speaker groaned on about women who had a particular aptitude for curing the evils of hospital life. The women of Woman's Hospital had done what was necessary to protect the sick from the exhaustive, inhumane inquisitiveness of the medical profession. Ignorant of the festering infections destroying the hospital from the inside, the man regaled the room with the diversity of Woman's Hospital's boards. This varied sort of representation was born in the very fiber of the American character, he said. The lack of same could lead to decay and weakness. He looked forward to the day when representatives of the lady managers, the governors, and the medical men could all gather at a single table and make their decisions together.

Sims was hardly listening. His imagination had lurched forward in time. The speaker concluded with words for the inmates, for the assistance rendered to rescued sisters sent forth with fresh, noble hope. For those who could not be saved, there was granted them an awareness that it is not all of life to live, nor death to die.

By the time the dutiful applause for the man's speech faded, Sims had fully separated from the moment. It was less as though he was outside of his body, as in a dream, than that he was outside his particular instant in time. He perceived himself as though he was looking into the past, as though he was recalling the moment he was living, recollecting it with the faculty that one would employ to take stock of one's own legacy. He watched himself rise from his seat on the dais and step to the podium. He listened to himself begin with a typical flourish about the tranquil, assured progress of the hospital. Then he turned, in pique and tone. He offered a bold complaint about the ad nauseam exercise in self-compliment that the annual gala had become. Would it not be worth the risk, he heard himself say, of rudely marring the harmony of the occasion to take advantage of the only evening of the year when members of all of Woman's Hospital's boards were gathered under a single roof?

Perched in the future, Sims saw how the fragility of the boards' relations was laid bare by his quick destruction of the room's festive mood. It served them right. All they could do was stare at him, blank and helpless. From the dais, it looked as though they were regarding a version of him that had already been cast in bronze.

From there, he proceeded in a way that was surely offensive to some, lashing out at the lady managers' exclusion of cancer cases, even in their mildest, early stages. He asked why fifteen visitors at the surgeons' operations was better than seventeen, or eighteen, or twenty. Sims listened to his own voice rise as he suggested that the better course of action would have been to leave judgments of the surgical theater to the doctors. The lady managers had no right to interfere in its doings. Yet that was what they had done! They had blasphemed on the sanctity of the operating room in order to dictate to surgeons, who were its true masters. Every invasion of that sacred territory was a moment when the doctors' authority was not respected and when the ladies had failed to confine themselves to their God-granted sphere.

As his speech gathered momentum, rising in tone and thrill, Sims read the faces of his audience. The governors regarded him as conceited, the lady managers thought him a monster, and his fellow surgeons believed that his outburst was the offspring of an insatiable craving for professional éclat. The last was the closest to correct. What they did not understand was that he fought for prestige so that he could use it to wage a valiant war on behalf of a profession under siege. Unless he kept control over the story of his career, unless the narratives of his case studies and papers ended with cures and tools emblazoned with his name, he would be left weaponless in the battles that would come. As P. T. Barnum had told him, now two decades before, a story is the most potent form of power. His entire career was built on a story. So far, he had succeeded in controlling Anarcha's story—just as he had once controlled her body. That narrative had sometimes been wounded under challenges, but he had kept it alive, stitching closed its fissures, cutting away its infected tissue. Now, the actions of the lady managers threatened to trespass into other carefully tended tales. They were attempting to crack a facade he had been erecting to himself for many years, with all noble purpose.

What he needed now was a bold, manly gesture—a line in the sand. He must insist that he be the one to write his own final chapter.

He delivered his final remarks in a froth of tempered rage. The imposition of a spy in the hospital to count the heads of visitors was an injurious breach of etiquette, he said. It was unworthy of any governance or managerial board. No doctor could thrive when suffering under tyrannical decisions. I have never heeded your edicts, he told them—he was nearly spitting his words now—and I never will. I will not remain at an institution where I am not treated as a gentleman. I will not remain at a hospital where my medical friends are rejected at the door. I demand that these heinous rules be rescinded. If you are aggrieved, my resignation is at your disposal.

Epilogue

IN ADDITION TO THE ONE HUNDRED ACRES OF TILLED LAND, THEY HAD A beef, five swine, and three horses worth $175 altogether. There was five hundred acres of woodland, and every year they made a few dollars from products pulled from the forest, nuts and medicines that Anarcha instructed the children to retrieve. These were sold to the dispensary in King George.

Anarcha told Lorenzo to bury her in those woods, when the time came, near the spot up high, where they had buried their baby that didn't live.

The census counter came to Alto in the middle of 1869. It was the first and only time Anarcha was counted as a person. The man asked her name and wrote it in a book along with those of Lorenzo, Delia, Elizabeth, and her two young boys.

She died a short time later. Lorenzo found her in her chair when he returned from the fields. He put her in the ground where she asked him to and then rode to town to tell the man at the courthouse that she had passed. When the man asked what she died of, he said Anarcha had trouble breathing, and a bloody cough.

Lorenzo never left Alto, and he never remarried. He died fifteen years later. John E. Mason, great-great-grandson of Thomas Jefferson and soon to be a member of the Virginia House of Delegates and a circuit court judge,

signed Lorenzo's will as a witness. Lorenzo
left ninety dollars to Oliver, fifty dollars to
Delia and Louisa. Lizzie died in 1880, at age seventeen.
William was alive when his father died, but is not mentioned in the will.

Lorenzo left
instructions that he be buried
alongside his wife.

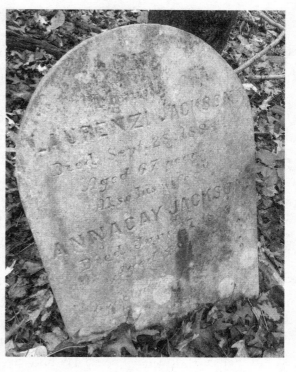

* * *

Sims immediately regretted
his speech at the Woman's
Hospital annual gala. He was
duty-bound, however, to send
a letter to the chairman of the
board of governors. He apologized for broaching private
disputes at a festive public
event. He repeated his offer to
resign.

In the days following the
gala, the study on the Woman's Hospital mortality rate
commissioned by the Board
of Lady Managers was forwarded to the board of governors. The study
showed that Sims had a significantly higher rate of fatal operations than
his colleagues.

His offer to resign was unanimously accepted. News of Sims's expulsion from his own hospital traveled across the country.

The following year, in a nationwide rebuke of the actions of the Board
of Lady Managers, Sims was elected to a one-year term as president of the
American Medical Association. In his speech to the AMA convention in
June 1876, he spoke at length about medical ethics. Had it ever occurred
to the men present, he asked, that the code of ethics could be used as an

engine of torture and oppression to blacken the character of noble practitioners?

By the late 1870s, most of the surgeries Sims devised or imagined had been abandoned or debunked. His vaginismus cure was only rarely performed. The incision of the cervix was being hotly debated and would soon vanish. There was no special muscle in the vagina that enabled the uterus to suck up semen. In a few years' time, infant lockjaw would be shown to be an infection that was not susceptible to surgical cure.

From 1875 to the end of his life, Sims remained an avid advocate of Battey's operation. He called the procedure the most important advance ever made in peritoneal surgery. He performed the operation at least twelve times. Three women he counted as cured. Two were improved, and three were left worse than he found them. Two died.

The operation was soon shunned by the medical profession.

On November 13, 1883, fifty years to the day after the night of the falling stars and his first day of medical school, Dr. J. Marion Sims died at his home in New York, in his bed, with Theresa beside him.

Five years earlier, at the third annual meeting of the American Gynecological Society, Sims's paper "On the Surgical Treatment of Stenosis of the Cervix Uteri" was read out loud to members by the secretary. Sims was in Paris. His paper was a defense of the incision of the cervix. He had continued to perform the operation even after acknowledging that many of his own procedures might have been unnecessary—and after English doctors Gream and Tilt publicly condemned the operation. The purpose of Sims's paper was to distinguish his methodology from that of James Simpson, and to ensure that he was not robbed of credit for the "antero-posterior incision." Credit for this incision belonged to himself alone, Sims wrote—not to Simpson, not to Thomas Addis Emmet, nor to anyone else. He claimed that he had incised the cervices of perhaps as many as a thousand women.

When the secretary finished reading the paper, several doctors remained in the room to discuss it. Emmet was there, along with Fordyce Barker, who had championed Sims when he first arrived in New York City.

Barker spoke first. As a surgical procedure, he noted, the incision of the cervix was falling out of favor. He wondered what could explain the fact that other doctors now performed the procedure only one-fifth as often as J. Marion Sims. Not only had many incision operations proved to be injurious, a mania for incising the cervix had taken hold among general practitioners and charlatans. What this illustrated, Barker said, was that Sims's reputation for greatness was the best argument for the scrutiny of his ideas. For far too long, it had been the habit of the profession to accept the dicta of great men without question.

Initially, Emmet refused to speak. He and Sims had feuded the year before. After several more speakers chimed in, Emmet was again prompted by the chair of the meeting. At last, he relented.

Even though he himself had performed the incision of the cervix many times, Emmet said, he now believed painful cramps due to mechanical obstruction to be a myth. The entire phenomenon might be the result of doctors having once enthusiastically employed nitrate of silver, which reduced the cervical opening to a pinpoint. In other words, Sims and Emmet had been using blades to cut open a hole that other doctors had closed with caustic agents. Now that nitrate of silver was used only infrequently, Emmet concluded, it was likely that the cutting operation would pass out of sight.

Worse came the following day. Dr. A. Reeves Jackson, surgeon in chief of the Woman's Hospital of the State of Illinois, read a paper called "On Some Points in Connection with the Treatment of Sterility." Sims's teachings, Jackson wrote, had proved themselves to be fraught with incalculable mischief. The work of his imitators had resulted in widespread uterine deformity. The total quantity of ruined health—and loss of life—fully offset whatever good had been accomplished by Sims and his disciples.

Despite these criticisms, the American Gynecological Society elected Sims as its president for the year 1880. By then, he had received the Legion of Honor he was awarded in Belgium, along with similar awards from a number of other countries.

Days after Sims died in 1883, Dr. William Baldwin, Sims's old nemesis from Alabama, offered a tribute at a memorial meeting of the Medical and Surgical Society of Montgomery. After a three-decades-long dispute, Sims and Baldwin had reconciled. By then, Baldwin too had served a term as president of the American Medical Association—he was the first southerner elected to the position after the Civil War—and Sims had lent Baldwin his fame and influence in the form of effusive public praise of Baldwin's work on quinine.

At the memorial, Baldwin offered the first enthused astronomical metaphor to describe Sims's career. The Sims speculum, Baldwin said, had caused his "name to flash over the medical world like a meteor in the night." A shower of melodramatic praise continued for decades. In 1894, the young medical student Edmond, whom Sims had employed as a translator in Paris, recalled Sims as "the guiding star I strove to follow." In 1937, Sims's eventual biographer Dr. Seale Harris described Sims as the "brightest star that shines in the firmament of America's brilliant and distinguished surgeons."

Even Sims's critics could not quit him. After warning that Sims's reputation had caused others to accept dangerous theories without scrutiny, Fordyce Barker chaired a committee to commission a Central Park monument to Sims. More than $8,000 was raised, the overwhelming majority coming from his colleagues—white, male doctors. The statue was raised in 1894.

Afterword

The Modern Legacy of the Alabama Fistula Experiments

JOY VILLAGE—ETHIOPIA

HER MOTHER TATTOOED HER FOREHEAD WHEN SHE WAS SIX, TO MAKE HER more beautiful. The girl refused when her mother wanted to tattoo her neck as well.

She was very young, seven, when she was given to a man as a future wife. Until she was old enough to marry, she worked as a servant in the home of her in-laws. She was perhaps twelve on her wedding day. She stood four feet nine, and she would never stand much taller. Her name was Asrebeb. She was from a small community in west central Ethiopia. It was, approximately, the year 2002.

She was sexually active for two years before her period came. She became pregnant that first month. When labor began, she was taken alone to her mother's home to deliver, but the baby would not come. It was said that the sun should not set twice on a woman's labor, but in Asrebeb's case it set twice, and then a third time, and then a fourth time. Sporadically, her husband arrived to see whether his child and his wife were still alive—then he left again. No one knew what to do.

On the fifth day, the people of her community resolved to take Asrebeb, who was in a coma by then, to the nearest hospital. They put her on a wooden stretcher and left, her mother, her stepfather, and a sister. It was four days' journey on foot.

They met a couple on the road. The man believed Asrebeb was already dead, but the woman looked inside the girl and could see the baby partly emerged, long since perished, beginning to decompose but still too large and too hard for Asrebeb's small body. The woman knew what needed to be done. The baby was still inside of Asrebeb when the woman used a knife to reduce the child's size until it could be removed. The woman and her husband brought Asrebeb and her family to their home. These kind strangers allowed them to remain for ten days.

It was three days more back to their community. By the time they arrived, Asrebeb was leaking urine and feces from her vagina. No one knew that her condition had a name, or that her case was a particularly severe one: like Anarcha, Asrebeb had two fistulae, one hole between her vagina and her bladder, another between her vagina and her rectum.

Her husband divorced her.

Asrebeb's stepfather made inquiries to find a cure, but he needed to take care. The community had begun to wonder whether Asrebeb had been cursed, for a crime of her own—murder or adultery—or perhaps a crime committed by a member of her family. Nerve damage along her pelvic bone, another injury inflicted by the pressure of her baby's head inside her, soon resulted in foot drop. She was left bedridden.

She remained in bed for seven years.

What she missed most was human contact—it was only her mother who cared for her. She missed the smiles on people's faces. She missed the sounds of children playing. She ate and drank little, to avoid leaks and to welcome death. She grew smaller and smaller, until she weighed less than fifty pounds.

One day, a man from outside the community arrived on the occasion of a religious celebration. He was told of Asrebeb's condition, and somehow this man knew of a place, a kind of clinic—he didn't know much, but he'd heard rumors—where conditions like hers were sometimes cured. Inquiries were made, and a car was sent to bring Asrebeb first to a government health facility, and then to the Bahir Dar Fistula Hospital, near Lake

Tana in the north. It was the first time Asrebeb realized that she was not alone—there were other women with conditions like hers.

Her fistulae, not to mention the state of her body—wracked with the comorbidities of emaciation, skin lesions, and foot drop—were too severe for Bahir Dar. She remained only five days before she was transferred to the Addis Ababa Fistula Hospital, a much larger facility inside a walled compound filled with trees and clean buildings, bustling with women and girls from all over Ethiopia in various stages of recovery. In the main ward, there was a wall plaque prominently displayed behind the registration desk. It read, in part:

> On October 18th, 1971, the James Marion Sims Charter presented to Drs. Reginald and Catherine Hamlin a gift of $1,000.00 for the Addis Ababa Fistula Hospital, the founding of which was inspired by the historic and noble example set by J. Marion Sims, and thereby linking inseparably together the only two hospitals in the world founded for the same purpose, the cure of fistula in women.

* * *

In 1939, twenty-year-old Princess Tsehai Haile Selassie of Ethiopia graduated as a registered nurse from the Great Ormond Street Hospital for Sick Children in London. She dreamed of opening a hospital and a nursing school in Ethiopia. She worked briefly as a nurse in Dessie, then married and moved west to Welega Province. In due course she became pregnant, but she died in childbirth in 1942.

In London, Princess Tsehai had befriended the antifascist activist Sylvia Pankhurst, who launched a journal in support of Ethiopia when Italy invaded the country in 1936. After Ethiopia was liberated, Pankhurst took up the princess's dream of a hospital and nursing school in Addis Ababa. The Princess Tsehai Hospital opened in 1951. Several years later, a plan was launched to add a school of midwifery. An advertisement for a gynecologist to establish the school was placed in the nearly two-hundred-year-old medical journal the *Lancet*.

The ad was answered by not one gynecologist but two. Reginald and

Catherine Hamlin, from New Zealand and Australia, respectively, were both descended from families with missionary traditions that ran generations deep and were anxious to spend a few years—as they first thought of their plans—in a country short on doctors. They were hired and arrived in May 1959.

On one of their first nights in the country, they heard the truth: Ethiopia, and nations across Africa, were plagued by obstetric suffering the likes of which hadn't been seen in the developed world in generations. Their work began. Women arrived at the hospital barely alive, with babies that had burst into their abdominal cavities. The decomposing infants grew germs that produced gas, which produced septicemia—which produced death. Early on, the biggest problem was blood. They lost one woman because they had only two pints in her type for a condition that required thirty. They saved others by finagling a way to catch the flow of a bad hemorrhage and pump a woman's own blood back into her.

Particularly challenging were the fistula patients. The Hamlins had read about obstetric fistula, but they had never encountered one—it wasn't the sort of thing a Western gynecologist saw anymore. After a week, they received their first fistula case and were struck by the double tragedy of the woman's injury and the manner in which she'd been forced to live. Several years later, the Hamlins coauthored a paper that included a description of the plight of fistula sufferers that stands out from many such descriptions that have come since for its brevity and pathos.

> Constantly in pain, incontinent of urine or feces, bearing a heavy burden of sadness in discovering their child stillborn, ashamed of a rank personal offensiveness, abandoned therefore by their husbands, outcasts of society, unemployable except in the fields, they live, they exist, without friends and without hope.

The Hamlins balked at the extent of the damage done to that first fistula sufferer. They weren't ready. They sent her to another hospital, but they recognized that if the woman had had access to the sort of midwife they'd been hired to supply, she might not have developed a fistula at all.

They began the planning for their school but also sought guidance for the treatment of existing fistula sufferers. Who could say how many more were hiding in the countryside? They contacted famed Egyptian gynecologist Naguib Mahfouz, who had achieved renown for performing hundreds of fistula surgeries over twenty years and succeeding more than 80 percent of the time. In addition to the books and articles Mahfouz sent them, the Hamlins ordered from England what was then the unquestioned creation story of the cure of fistula and of gynecology itself: Dr. J. Marion Sims's *The Story of My Life*.

They sat up at night and read—uncritically—of Sims's initial experiments, of the enslaved women Anarcha, Lucy, and Betsey, who became his assistants and nurses. They did not question the struggles that Sims claimed to have endured after he moved to New York and opened Woman's Hospital, which the Hamlins would come to regard as the world's first fistula clinic. What quickly became apparent to them was that fistula in Africa in the twentieth century was at least as bad as it had been in America in the nineteenth century—perhaps it was even worse.

Thus prepared, they admitted their first fistula case, applied the techniques they'd read about—not Sims's method, but those of others who had followed him—and waited anxiously for the days it took for the wound to heal. It worked; the girl was cured. They cured two more, and word began to spread. Women, dressed in rags, smelling horribly, arrived from distant communities. One mother brought her daughter to Addis Ababa, having walked for fifteen days. Another woman walked 450 kilometers. One girl arrived at the hospital in the afternoon, after it had closed for the day. Desperate, she hanged herself near the gate. She was discovered in time, cut down, and cured. In the years to come, there would be many more such stories. The woman who begged for seven years to afford bus fare; the woman who, after her divorce, was left with only a calf and had to wait for it to grow to adulthood before she could sell it and travel to the capital.

In 1962, the Hamlins opened a hostel for fistula patients alone—twenty beds at first, then thirty, then women sleeping two to a bed. None of them could pay. Hospital resources grew strained. Even in those early days, fistula patients began to do some of the work of the ward, just as Anarcha, Betsey, and Lucy had done. The connection to the Alabama fistula experiments would never be explicitly drawn, but patients in Addis Ababa were taught to make beds properly, then to clean examination couches, then to test urine and boil gloves and even to assist in the surgical theater. Before long, a dozen former fistula patients were trained as nurses.

By then, the Hamlins had realized that they would never leave Addis Ababa.

It was a dangerous time in Ethiopia. They lived through a failed coup and walked past the bodies of lynched plotters left hanging for days, one just outside the hospital. One of their matrons was raped and murdered in her home. The Hamlins took to sleeping with a gun beside their bed. Medically speaking, they saw no shortage of daunting emergencies. There was a case of stillborn conjoined twins, just one of the babies' heads protruding from the vagina: the head had to be severed, and the rest extracted through an abdominal incision. There was a woman who had been attacked by hyenas during birth: her child was eaten, and her thighs and buttocks were badly mauled. And there was the fistula case that was caused not by prolonged labor but by the imperfect cuttings of a traditional doctor attempting to treat an imperforate hymen—a surgical deflowering, to prepare her for her husband.

The fistula work began to take over, both because of the sheer volume of it and because it came to have the character of a mission. By the mid-sixties, the Hamlins were beginning to have success with innovative operations, and they had increased the typical fistula cure rate of 70 percent to more than 90 percent. Doctors from other countries began traveling to Addis Ababa, first to assist in operations, then to perform their own. Surgical procedures came to include muscle, fat, and skin grafting, as well as repair to the entire lower urinary tract.

In the late sixties, the rate of fistulous women finding their way to the city was still increasing. Clearly, they needed a hospital of their own. The missions of fistula and a school of midwifery were really one, the Hamlins realized. The problem wasn't just medical: it was education, it was infrastructure, it was the tradition of child marriage. As well, there was the lingering question of what could be done for the small percentage of patients whose fistulae could not be closed.

Fundraising abroad had already become an essential part of the work. At crucial junctures, they received a plasma supply from Australia and a large donation from a man who'd made a fortune in shoe-repair shops. They traveled to America in 1971 to request funds for a new hospital. New York proved to be a bust: the charter of the Rockefeller Foundation didn't go farther north than Uganda. American doctors brushed them off with advice to control fistula with birth control and forced sterilization. They came away with a small check from what was left of J. Marion Sims's Woman's Hospital. They were given a brick from Woman's Hospital's original 1855 location, to be built into the walls of their ward if it was ever constructed.

Then, providence seemed to provide. Catherine Hamlin found an appropriate piece of land in Addis Ababa—and immediately thereafter the hospital received an infusion of £10,000. The only obstacles left were bureaucratic. It took more than a year to receive permission to build, and construction wasn't completed until Emperor Haile Selassie, father of Princess Tsehai, had been deposed and murdered. The Hamlins opened the Addis Ababa Fistula Hospital with a private ceremony on the night of May 24, 1975. The brick from Woman's Hospital had been mortared into the wall of the ward, and the commemorative plaque credited Dr. Sims but made no mention of Anarcha, Lucy, and Betsey.

The hospital grew throughout Ethiopia's protracted civil war, a struggle that saw suspected anticommunists shot in the streets, pregnant women among them. Medical advances offered hope to those with incurable fistulae: diversion of urine into the rectal tract and a safer procedure that installed a permanent colostomy bag. The results weren't perfect—the women would be stigmatized in their communities—but at least they were dry.

The former patients took training as nurses, just as Anarcha, Lucy, and Betsey had done more than a century before. They proved essential to the initial formation of the hospital. Many lived together in dormitories on the hospital grounds, and later some patients-turned-nurses saved money and bought small homes. One former patient, Mamitu Gashe—recognized by Reginald Hamlin for her intelligence and skill—was trained as a fistula surgeon herself.

The civil war ended in 1991. The following year, a film crew arrived to document the hospital's work. More funding soon followed. Reginald Hamlin died in 1993.

By 1995, Catherine Hamlin—working alongside teams of locally trained Ethiopian surgeons—was performing more than one thousand fistula surgeries annually. The hospital began to send surgical teams to other parts of the country. Many more fistulous women were discovered huddling in dilapidated huts, abandoned by their families, dying slowly in filth. These women produced a new impetus to imagine ways to spread the word that the condition was not a curse. Even today, after more than half a century of outreach, women emerge from the remotest corners of a nation of one hundred million people.

In the late nineties, donations began to grow—AusAID gave $50,000; a Rotary Award brought $100,000—and physicians who trained in Addis Ababa began taking the hospital's work abroad. New fistula clinics were established in Nigeria and Sudan, and still more doctors were at work in Malawi, Benin, Tanzania, India, New Guinea, Pakistan, Bangladesh, and Nepal. In 1999, the Addis Ababa Fistula Hospital reopened after an extended period of expansion and renovation. This time, a formal ceremony was attended by Ethiopian president Negasso Gidada, himself a physician married to a midwife. Catherine Hamlin took the opportunity to present the plight of women with incurable fistula. They now had surgical options, but what they needed was a sanctuary.

The president thought for a moment, and then said he had just such a place in mind.

* * *

Zewditu is less than forty but looks twenty years older, and wears a resigned expression characteristic of persons older still. She got her fistula at fourteen, in 1996. Her labor lasted five days before her husband took her to a hospital. She began to leak, and it was six years before her father heard someone on the radio saying there was a solution in Addis Ababa.

She was operated on twice, but her fistula could not be closed. Zewditu was among that small unlucky percentage, and eventually she consented to the procedure that cut a small hole into the flank of her body—a stoma. She was taught how to care for her stoma and how to change the colostomy bags herself. In 2018, Zewditu was plagued by gastric ulcers, hypertension, migraines, and imminent kidney failure. She lived at Desta

Mender—Joy Village—the compound that President Gidada promised to Catherine Hamlin in 1999.

Joy Village is a large compound on the outskirts of Addis Ababa with tall trees, stone paths, flowering gardens, and a lake with herons. For years, dozens of women who had undergone stoma procedures lived here, working at the campus's small café or in its injera kitchen or on its dairy farm. Long before then, it had been recognized that successful surgery was just the first step toward surviving fistula. Treatment became economic as well: during recovery, women trained in one of a variety of trades—fattening sheep, seamstressing, opening a sundry shop. When they left the hospital, they were provided with a small grant of seed money to begin independent lives in their communities. This has become the standard care for the dozens of fistula clinics that have opened throughout the developing world in the last two decades.

Joy Village is one of a number of expansions that the Addis Ababa Fistula Hospital undertook after the turn of the millennium. Five smaller hospitals able to treat simpler fistula cases were also established around Ethiopia; Bahir Dar, where Asrebeb was first sent, was among them. In 2007, the Hamlin College of Midwives was founded on the Joy Village campus. Today, dozens of highly trained midwives are at work throughout Ethiopia. In 2004, Oprah Winfrey made the first of two visits to Addis Ababa. Later, she lent her name to a dedicated clinic for stoma patients. As of 2018, the hospital managed the care of more than three hundred women who had undergone the procedure, with up to five additional cases being added every month.

When Asrebeb, emaciated and grievously injured, was first examined in Addis Ababa in 2009, the doctor was surprised she was even alive. It was four years—four years of painful physical therapy and recovery—before they could even attempt to operate for her fistulae. Then came the first of ten surgeries. The news was not good: Asrebeb's holes could not be closed; the damage was too severe. She would never be fully cured.

In 2015, Asrebeb underwent the stoma procedure. She has worn a bag ever since. On the day she finally stood up on her own two feet in Addis Ababa, everyone cheered. She no longer needed canes to walk. Her mother was very ill, and no one from her community came to see her—nevertheless, she recovered her self-confidence. Today, she knits and makes pottery, and a small structure dedicated to crafts has opened in Joy Village. It is called Asrebeb's Cottage.

Growing from the handful of women recruited as aides by the Hamlins, in imitation of Anarcha and the women from Sims's "Negro Hospital" in Montgomery, Alabama, the corps of fistula survivors now working as nurses in Addis Ababa numbers close to 150. These women share meals, celebrate holidays, and attend church and funerals together. Just as Anarcha and the others once did in accidentally pioneering a model of patient-centered care, they provide companionship to one another and tend to the medical needs of survivors such as Asrebeb and Zewditu. They know more about each other than their sisters and mothers do.

Almost fifty years after the work began, the number of fistula cases emerging in Ethiopia has finally begun to fall. The mission of Joy Village has changed. What quickly became apparent was that a pristine farm offered no true substitute for a woman's home and family. It was, as one patient described it, both a heaven and a hell. So the mission of Joy Village shifted—from being a permanent refuge for incurables to a staging area for women to prepare to contend with their condition from inside their communities. Sometimes, these women hide their bags even from those closest to them: a partial home is better than a cozy purgatory. A handful of women, Asrebeb and Zewditu among them, are too weak to go home alone. Of these, Zewditu is one of the lucky ones. Her husband visits once a year, though long ago she gave him permission to divorce her so that he could have children. He brings his children with him when he visits. Zewditu still wears her wedding ring.

RED ROOF—NIGERIA

In 2018, at the Evangel Vesico-Vaginal Fistula Center in Jos, Nigeria, Dr. Ene George began a procedure with a large, weighted speculum. Her patient, a small woman whose fistula had already been repaired, was reclined on her back with her ankles elevated in stirrups, situated in what's known as the lithotomy position. Every part of her was covered save that which George needed to access in order to clear her urethra and insert a large catheter to dilate it.

The weighted speculum looked like a clunky piece of a knight's suit of armor. Unlike the Sims speculum, which requires an assistant, the weighted speculum worked with the help of gravity. The operative portion of vaginal specula is inelegantly labeled a "blade" or "tongue." The protruding, curved shape of the blade is described as "duckbilled," though this term is sometimes mistakenly applied to double-bladed specula that vaguely resemble a duck's head in profile. In truth, the blade of a speculum is, in shape and action, more like a shoehorn. In a weighted speculum, the blade is inserted into the vagina, and a knob of metal hangs below and tugs the device down to afford the surgeon a clear field of view.

George inserted the weighted speculum, but she decided at once that her patient was too small for it. She removed it and asked an assistant named Cletus for something smaller. Cletus had been assisting surgeries at Evangel for more than twenty-five years.

The Sims? Cletus asked.

Yes, Sims, George said. Then she considered it. There's nothing you can do about that name, she said. It's just part of our world.

* * *

George was born in Jos, Nigeria, about five miles from the Evangel Vesico-Vaginal Fistula Center. She began her medical education at Jos University Teaching Hospital in the 1990s, and her training continued with a residency in obstetrics and gynecology in Ohio, followed by three years of work as a generalist. In 2007, she began a fellowship in urogynecology in Irvine, California, and later she established a practice in southern California as a specialist in female pelvic medicine and reconstructive surgery. It was during the fellowship that she came upon an article about fistula. George knew what obstetric fistula was, but it was only when she read the article that she learned of the full extent of the crisis in the country of her birth.

Fistula data is notoriously difficult to compile. The rate at which mothers die from complications during childbirth is easier to track. In the developed world, a handful of women per 100,000 deliveries die as a result of giving birth—5 women in Sweden, 6 women in Germany, 14 women in the United States. Various studies in Nigeria conducted between 1976 and 2011 found much higher rates of maternal mortality. In Jos, 740 women per 100,000 deliveries died during childbirth; in Zamfara, 1,732 women; in Nguru, 2,849 women; in Sokoto, 5,415 women. Nigeria registered 40,000 deaths from childbirth annually, more than any other African nation.

Rates of maternal mortality can be used to make informed estimates of annual rates of women who survive complications of childbirth. This information can then be used to infer—though the guesses become less and less precise at each level of inference—the total number of existing fistula cases in inaccessible regions of the country. In Nigeria, a nation of 200 million people, estimates of the total number of extant fistula sufferers—the exact condition Anarcha suffered from for her entire life— range from 150,000 to 800,000. At the lowest possible number of sufferers, and the highest reported rates of cure at Nigeria's seventeen fistula clinics, it would take three decades to clear the country's backlog of already existing cases.

Beginning in 2009, Dr. George began annual trips to Nigeria to learn fistula surgery, to perform procedures herself, and to provide aid in the form of a half dozen oversized duffel bags or storage containers stuffed with gowns and shoe covers, catheters and cannulas, surgical blades, epidural kits, spinal packs, and suction tubing.

* * *

To get to Jos, in Plateau State—a city that in 2014 experienced twin Boko Haram terrorist bombings that killed 118 people and wounded 56 more— drive northeast from Abuja. If you're lucky, you won't get stuck behind a money convoy carrying currency from the capital to banks across the country. Regardless, you'll be stopped at military roadblocks; at roadblocks operated by the Nigerian customs office, the drug task force, and the highway patrol; and at roadblocks dedicated to specific military initiatives: Operation Safe Haven and Operation Flush Out II. You'll drift through small cities where men walk the streets with scissors in hand, clicking them together to advertise nail-clipping services, and where small

cars with giant metal megaphones strapped to their roofs idle slowly forward, blasting announcements about the availability of traditional cures.
The acid rain of nascent capitalism is everywhere in small Nigerian cities:
discarded black plastic bags gathered into drifts like snow or ash. Bands
of children swarm every vehicle slowed by traffic, selling cheese balls, kola
nuts, bananas, sugarcane, live chickens, peanuts, dish towels, and water
sealed inside plastic bladders that are precisely the size of your bladder.
Among the sellers are young girls, nine and ten years old, garishly made
up with fluorescent streaks of color across their brows and lips. They are
trained for husband hunting with leers and smirks that they are not yet
old enough to understand. They offer no product other than themselves.

Between towns, the land is strewn with rock outcroppings like giant
cancers or carbuncles. Water is so scarce that even the baobabs are terri-
torial. With spindly canopies like root systems straining toward the sky,
the trees resemble nothing so much as anatomical drawings of the human
female reproductive system. Jos is at higher elevation than much of the
rest of Nigeria, and the road climbs past whole mountain ranges of stone,
boulders perched sometimes three and four high, as though stacked by a
god grown weary of communicating with mortals through twisters and
tempests. Closer to the city, small woodland ecosystems sit perched atop
boulders the size of small moons—stars or meteors that, centuries ago,
fell from the sky and half buried themselves in the earth.

* * *

Dr. George's half-African, half-American medical education stands as a
fair summary of the recent history of the Evangel Vesico-Vaginal Fistula
Center. Evangel began in 1959 as a facility associated with SIM—Sudan
Interior Mission—an evangelical missionary organization founded in
1893. For three decades, Evangel remained a general hospital and came
to be known locally for a quirk of its architecture: Jankwano—red roof.

In the late 1980s, a young urology student named Steve Arrowsmith
fell in love with a medical-school classmate intent on doing missionary work in Africa. In 1987, the couple spent a month in Liberia, and
Arrowsmith performed his first fistula surgery on a woman who had
been made to wait for the young doctor arriving from America. On his

second night in the country, Arrowsmith was woken at 4:00 a.m. to per-form the operation. As a urologist, he was better prepared for surgery than most medical officers and even most gynecologists, but his only pre-vious experience of fistula had been a random glance, a few weeks earlier, at a text illustrating abdominal surgery to cure fistulae caused by radia-tion treatment. The hospital was close to home, but Arrowsmith rode a motorcycle in the dark to avoid stepping on mambas warming themselves on the asphalt. Despite the hour and his ignorance of obstetric fistula, the woman was cured.

The young couple went home at the end of January 1987. Their return to Africa was delayed by Arrowsmith's obligation to the US Air Force and by the Liberian civil war, which broke out in 1989. Of the missionary organizations they applied to for a replacement posting in 1990, only SIM replied. They were sent to Red Roof in Jos, Nigeria.

It had always been a question: As a urologist, what would Arrowsmith do in Africa, exactly? The fistula case in Liberia had called on his surgical skill set, but it seemed like a one-off. As it happened, Evangel's only other surgeon quit a day before he arrived. Arrowsmith was instantly called upon to perform a host of procedures he only barely understood. Then a fistula patient arrived, and another, and another. Word spread that fistula was being cured in Jos.

Fistula surgeries had been happening in Nigeria for some time. Sister Ann Ward, an Irish doctor and nun of the Medical Missionaries of Mary, had arrived in far western Nigeria the same year that Catherine and Reg-inald Hamlin arrived in Ethiopia. Over a career of more than fifty years, Ward performed more than two thousand surgeries while establishing a reputation for golf and whiskey. Professor Una Lister had treated 250 fistula patients annually at the Ahmadu Bello University Hospital in Zaria, but she retired not long after Arrowsmith was assigned to Red Roof. A short time later, a van carrying sixteen of Lister's most difficult cases—women who had remained uncured after four or more surgeries—arrived in Jos to see if the new surgeon could make them stop leaking.

By then, Arrowsmith had traveled back and forth to the Hamlins' hos-pital in Addis Ababa, where fistula treatment was already twenty years old. He wasn't permitted to touch a patient during that initial visit, but in his first year in Nigeria he performed one hundred fistula surgeries. Over the next several years, as more and more fistula cases arrived to be treated, he began seeking donations from the United States. In the meantime, Jonathan Karshima, a Tiv transplant from eastern Nigeria, piqued the interest of the SIM missionary for whom he worked as a gardener. The missionary sponsored Karshima's training as a community health worker, and then his time in medical school. During his gynecological residency, Karshima worked alongside Arrowsmith at Red Roof.

In the mid-1990s, Arrowsmith moved to Ethiopia for several years. Karshima took over in Nigeria as medical director. As time passed, more and more of Red Roof's general services were eliminated to sustain the fistula mission. Since then, like Dr. Ene George's hybrid medical education, Red Roof has benefited from a unique blend of training and leadership. African doctors train Western-educated physicians who arrive with surgical skill but zero clinical experience in obstetric fistula, and in turn these doctors—some stay a week, some years—train new African nurses and gynecologists. Currently, the lead surgeon at Red Roof is Dr. Sunday Lengmang. Initially trained as a family physician, Lengmang took over as head of medicine at Red Roof in 2004, at age thirty-four. Like a number of native Ethiopian physicians trained in Addis Ababa, Lengmang is considered one of the world's leading fistula surgeons.

Today, the most innovative and experienced fistula doctors are African.

* * *

In February 2018, a month before Dr. Ene George made her annual journey to Red Roof, a sixteen-year-old girl arrived in the reception area of the Doctors Without Borders fistula clinic in Jahun, Jigawa State, in far northern Nigeria. The young woman had a recto-vaginal fistula, a hole between her vagina and her rectum. More pressing was the condition that had resulted from what her family had done in response to the uncontrollable flow of feces from the girl's vagina: they locked her in a room and didn't feed her for five weeks.

As with Asrebeb, in Ethiopia, it is not uncommon for fistula sufferers to present for treatment in advanced states of emaciation. Yet the Doctors Without Borders clinic in Jahun was unprepared to receive her. They didn't have the proper feeding packs that are given to people on the brink of starvation, nor did they have contacts inside of Nigeria that would have permitted them to transport the girl to a facility that was better prepared. The Jahun clinic had no surgeon on staff. Two general surgeons—only one of them an OB-GYN—arrived from Abuja biweekly to treat simple fistula cases. Twice per year, a Belgian surgeon arrived to treat difficult cases, though he was neither a urologist nor a gynecologist but a general surgeon with a specialty in combat trauma. The Jahun clinic was the only fistula clinic in the world run by Doctors Without Borders. It was not particularly well funded, and there were no plans to expand its mission.

The girl with the recto-vaginal fistula was admitted, but all the clinic could do was call around Jigawa State in an attempt to find a nearby nutritional clinic. There wasn't one.

The girl died.

The incident is symptomatic of a chronic problem in the ongoing efforts to curtail fistula in Africa and the broader developing world: a persistent belief that Western physicians and aid organizations offer the best option for fistula sufferers. In the 1970s and '80s, crusading nuns and lone operators struggled to offer at least one choice to women who had no other. Even then, however, the lure of a vulnerable population gave rise to what Reginald Hamlin in Ethiopia called "fistula tourism": doctors and medical students visiting Africa to give themselves surgical experience. Exuberant aid organizations trumpeted relief efforts that sounded good in press releases but were in fact underfunded and sometimes dangerous. In short, the opportunistic atmosphere that J. Marion Sims had enjoyed and exploited in America in the nineteenth century repeated in Africa in the twentieth century. The problem lingers even today.

* * *

Four years before Steve Arrowsmith performed his first fistula surgery, a Dutch surgeon named Kees Waaldijk traveled to Nigeria as part of a leprosy initiative. Dr. Waaldijk had some training in obstetrics and gynecology but, a little like Sims, he had found the prospect of "looking inside women for the rest of [his] life" to be distasteful. He opted to become a "real surgeon" instead. In Nigeria, Waaldijk encountered a fistula sufferer and recognized that fistula sufferers were even more marginalized than leprosy patients. He'd been a "war surgeon" in Cambodia, and he had done work in Kenya as well, but he had been aware of obstetric fistula at least since he had spent several weeks at a leprosy training center in Addis Ababa, not far from the Hamlins' Addis Ababa Fistula Hospital. He never saw the Hamlins perform surgery but, regardless, his life was transformed when he encountered a fistula patient in Nigeria. Today, he boasts of having performed more than twenty-five thousand fistula surgeries.

Waaldijk is a controversial figure. Some experienced fistula surgeons express concern that his methods do not include routine sanitary practices, and others reject claims that Waaldijk once made about anesthesia. For procedures that require only a single suture or are performed on the still-numb vaginas of women who have recently given birth, Waaldijk has argued, fistula surgery can be performed more simply and economically without anesthesia at all, as Sims once did. In addition, Waaldijk has sometimes championed the "camp model" of fistula care: Western doctors fly to Africa to perform surgery, assembly line–style, and leave the extended period of aftercare to others. In 2005, Waaldijk was the primary physician associated with an initiative called Fistula Fortnight, funded in part by Richard Branson's Virgin Group and Johnson & Johnson. Deaths in fistula surgery are extremely rare; not even Sims's experiments in Alabama produced a fatality. But of the five hundred women operated on during the two weeks of Fistula Fortnight, four died. No autopsies were performed, and the deaths were blamed on disease.

In the nineteenth century, J. Marion Sims benefited from radically different ethical standards and his own selective record keeping. A similarly lax atmosphere in Africa means that reports of abuses are anecdotal. Sometimes the abuse is stemmed before it occurs. A young missionary physician with extensive fistula experience was asked to give a lecture in Palm Springs, California. He had to dissuade his audience of mostly retired doctors from dropping everything to go to Africa to perform a procedure they didn't truly understand. An enthused would-be fistula doctor from Arkansas made inquiries into offering his services, and was stopped only when he was asked what his regular practice consisted of: small-animal surgery.

More often, the abuse occurs and vanishes without becoming a statistic. An inexperienced doctor didn't know what to do when part of a patient's ureter snapped and fell away. He tied it off, closed the incision, and flew home. The patient died three days later. A Turkish urology team encountered a simple fistula, but they had no idea how to close it. Instead, they performed a much more difficult urinary diversion, and now the still-fistulous woman urinates from her rectum. Organizations are no better. Medical-supply companies furnish doctors with kits for particular surgeries, along with instructions to employ them on women from the developing world before using them on patients back home. Inadequate funds provided for camp-model efforts result in fistula sufferers resorting to prostitution in order to eat while awaiting surgery or during their periods of aftercare.

* * *

Not long ago, a very experienced white, female surgeon and gynecologist from America visited Red Roof. She voiced concern when Drs. Sunday Lengmang and Ene George planned to perform a procedure that she didn't think was possible. A patient's ureters, the tubes that carry urine from the kidneys to the bladder, had sloughed away. Lengmang was going to repair the damage vaginally. As a rule, vaginal surgery is safer than abdominal surgery—but a vaginal procedure might fail because there is not enough room to work.

When Dr. George first returned to Nigeria to work on fistula, she was already an experienced surgeon; there were procedures she could perform even when she first arrived. It was the more difficult operations that she had to learn—procedures that Western-trained surgeons almost never saw, surgeries that called on skills they never had an opportunity to either practice or witness. George modestly thought of herself as a competent fistula surgeon, but she was the first to admit that she was not on the same level as Dr. Lengmang and other African fistula doctors. She would assist Lengmang in the ureter surgery.

The suspicious American watched. When it worked, she advised Dr. George not to bother telling anyone in the United States about it. No one would believe her.

In early 2018, a representative range of cases presented at Nigeria's fistula clinics. There was a patient whose fistula had spontaneously closed, but her urethra had been completely destroyed. She would require diversion surgery. There was a patient whose fistula was enlarged to facilitate the removal of a bad bladder stone—then her fistula was closed. There was a urethral prolapse in a two-year-old girl, and a twenty-five-year-old fistula in a woman who had suffered a botched cesarean section. A cesarean performed on another woman had come too late: she formed a fistula, and the incision where they cut her baby out became septic as well. There was a ten-year-old girl who had been leaking for nine years because the man who performed her circumcision had removed her urethra along with her clitoris. There was a two-and-a-half-year-old girl with a rectovaginal fistula that was the result of rape.

Dr. Sunday Lengmang operated on many of these cases, or he trained the surgeons who did. He performed 450 fistula surgeries at Red Roof every year—the most difficult cases from across Nigeria were sent to him—and perhaps a hundred more at hospitals in the south. In addition, Lengmang has authored or coauthored papers on a wide variety of fistula-related topics: marital disruption among fistula survivors, the use of slings to stem incontinence after successful repair, rare fistula caused by botched cesareans. Sometimes, Western medical journals have required Lengmang to provide more than the ordinary documentation in support of what he claimed to be able to do.

In 2018, on the first day of surgeries after Dr. Ene George arrived, Lengmang wore a T-shirt into the operating theater with a slogan on the back: Rebuilding Lives One Person at a Time. Chatting with an African gynecologist who was also visiting, Lengmang noted that southern Nigeria had more fistulas that resulted from out-of-wedlock pregnancies, and that women tended to go to churches to deliver their babies because they believed it would protect them from witchcraft.

Country music played in the surgical theater. Then gospel. Then African pop. When the power went out, the surgical teams continued work by cell-phone light. At one moment, Lengmang was doing some stitching and needed more room. He tried a large retractor. He couldn't get it to fit. Cletus, the assistant, found a Sims speculum in a tray and offered it.

Sims?

No. Lengmang scowled, and he went on.

TERREWODE—UGANDA

For hundreds of years, two kingdoms in what is now western Uganda, Bugunda and Bunyoro, remained completely isolated from the rest of the world. Flanked by volcanic land, impenetrable forests, and immense swamps, the region's undulating interior plains were entirely unknown to Portuguese traders. Scant influence from ancient Egypt survived, but for centuries the two cultures remained cut off, maintaining uneasy relations with each other and developing only under the guidance of long lines of kings.

Goods from the outside world began to circulate in the region in the middle of the eighteenth century. A soldier from Zanzibar visited Bugunda in 1852. He was followed by Arab traders, and then by European explorers who broke through tsetse-ridden swamps in the north.

Bunyoro remained unvisited until the 1860s. After the sequester was broken, the inhabitants of Bunyoro became known for hostility to outsiders. Missionaries dismissed Bunyoro medical men as witch doctors.

Englishman Robert Felkin studied medicine for two years in Edinburgh before he signed on as a medical missionary to Uganda in 1878. Little was known about African medicine. The Masai performed amputations. The patient took alcohol as skin and muscle was cut, and a hatchet was used to sever the bone. Hot butter staunched bleeding. Otherwise, indigenous medical practices had remained a mystery.

Over several years, Felkin made a study of African birthing practices, offering gifts of cloth and beads so that he could observe births in the districts of Madi and Moru and in Kidj country. In some places, pregnant women abstained from meat, and their nipples were drawn out in the days leading up to birth. During labor, women were fed millet-seed porridge, or they were given millet-seed beer through a drinking tube. At Kerrie, on the White Nile, women sat over a pot boiling with a decoction of herbs that was said to ease pains. The umbilicus was cut with a stone knife, or it was bitten, four inches from the infant's body. Cultures had a variety of strategies for pressing or kneading the abdomen if the placenta did not come away easily. In some places, the baby, mother, and placenta were all bathed after birth. In others, the placenta was buried, in one spot if the child was a boy, another if it was a girl.

In 1879, Felkin traveled to Bunyoro. Here, his offers of cloth and beads were refused.

The medicine of Bunyoro was notorious. As a culture, its people appeared ignorant of anatomy and had little insight into the nature of disease, but they were known—though the practice was disavowed by neighboring tribes—for infecting infants with endemic syphilis to render them immune to the disease in adulthood. It seemed that the kings of Bunyoro had empowered doctors to carry out vaccination experiments designed to mitigate the effects of illnesses that ravaged their people. In addition, Bunyoro surgeons punched holes in the chest to treat inflammation of the lung and pleurisy, and elevated bones in cases of depressed fracture. For penetrating war wounds, they used halved gourd shells to retain the bowels during abdominal surgery.

Despite the fact that his trinkets were refused, Felkin was granted permission to observe a Bunyoro doctor perform a cesarean section in the community of Kahura. The procedure was notably sophisticated, and it was the only time in Africa that Felkin saw a cesarean performed in an attempt to save the life of both the mother and the child.

A large group had assembled around a thatched hut. Inside, the Bunyoro doctor and several assistants attended a twenty-year-old woman, heavy with child, laid on an inclined cot made of wood and cowhide. She was secured in place with cuffs made of bark cloth, stretched across her chest and thighs. She was already inebriated on banana wine. She had been in labor—the baby was breech—for two days.

The doctor sharpened an elongated knife, reciting something like a prayer or incantation. When he was done, he uttered a sharp cry that was echoed a hundredfold by the group outside the hut. The woman's exposed belly was washed, first with banana wine, then with water.

Stretching from the top of the pubes to just below the navel, the cut was deep and precise, severing in a single stroke skin, fat, muscle, the sack of the peritoneum, and the wall of the uterus to permit amniotic fluid to escape in a sudden gush. There wasn't much bleeding. Assistants cauterized points of hemorrhage with a red-hot iron. The infant suffered only a slight nick in its shoulder.

The nurses pried apart the abdomen and the walls of the uterus. The child was removed, handed off to another assistant, and the cord was cut. The doctor cleaned the uterus of clots and the placenta as additional helpers struggled to keep the mother's intestines inside her body. The uterus was not sutured; the doctor squeezed until it contracted. The mother was tilted onto her side to permit the remaining fluids to drain from her body.

Her peritoneum and her exterior wound were brought into close apposition with material made of metal.

Seven thin, highly polished iron spikes—like acupressure needles—were used as sutures, bound together with bark cloth string. The wound was coated with a mash of pulped roots, then covered with a banana leaf and, finally, cloth dressing. One suture was removed after three days, three more on the fifth day, and the final three on the sixth day. A fresh dressing was applied each time.

Felkin left Bunyoro before the woman was fully healed. But he had seen enough to recognize that in complete isolation, the kingdom had formed complex medical practices that were wholly in line with the development of medicine in the West: cleaning the surgical surface with alcohol, not attempting to suture the uterus, draining the abdominal cavity of fluids, and the use of metal suture material. Who could say how many generations it had taken to develop these techniques, and to form teams of knowledgeable medical personnel who worked in calm, careful concert?

Felkin published his story five years later. By then, the arrival of Europeans in Africa—and European doctors—had supplanted the development and spread of indigenous medical practices in the region that would become modern Uganda.

* * *

In the 1980s, as a schoolgirl in Soroti, a small city in northern Uganda, Alice Emasu had six friends, all slightly older, young women who took under their wings the precocious girl who was destined to become a visionary.

Political unrest compelled Emasu's family to relocate. She completed her schooling in Kampala, to the south. After five years, negotiations brought peace to Soroti, and Emasu returned home to visit her friends. Four of them were dead. Two had died while giving birth, another died during labor, and one more died of complications of birth a short time later. The other two friends were a mystery. People referred to them using very rude terms—the women were "mad," or "dirty," or "cursed." They avoided other people, did not care for their bodies, ran off whenever they saw others. Eventually, Emasu learned that both women were suffering from obstetric fistula.

She was unable to locate her friends on that journey home, but it was the predicament of these women that inspired Emasu to investigation and action.

Fistula was described as an accident of childbirth, she learned. But it wasn't an "accident" at all. It was an inevitable outcome in a society like Uganda, plagued as it was by a host of factors associated with high incidence of prolonged obstructed labor. Prevalent child marriage, zero antenatal care, age-old traditional beliefs, unjust laws limiting the rights of women, poor medical facilities, ragged infrastructure, and so on. Furthermore, the simple cure of a fistula—the stitching closed of a hole—was only the beginning for women who were likely to suffer ongoing ostracization and stigmatization at home even if they were cured.

A glimmer of Emasu's vision sparked even then, in the early 1990s. She went on to become a journalist and activist, inspiration flickering all the while. In 1999, she founded the Association for the Rehabilitation and Re-Orientation of Women for Development (TERREWODE).

Terrewode identified fistula sufferers, assisted them in seeking out what medical treatment was available, and then, following in the footsteps of the Addis Ababa Fistula Hospital in Ethiopia, aided their reintegration into their home communities. By 2002, Emasu was working closely with what she called "flying doctors," borrowing the image from the Flying Doctors Society of Africa, which worked on the camp model championed by Dr. Kees Waaldijk, in Nigeria, and others. Emasu recognized that the camp model sometimes used fistulous women as fodder for surgical training, but there was no better option. The doctors flew into the country, did their work, and left behind no equipment. There was little follow-up for a procedure that required weeks of aftercare.

Emasu began to feel the call to a leadership role when she wrote a news story about child marriage, and her editor tore it up right in front of her. Few were willing even to consider the underlying causes of fistula.

In 2005, Emasu found her two old friends and arranged for them to be cured. By then, Terrewode had identified more than three hundred cases waiting for an opportunity for treatment. Over the next two years, foreign fistula aid in Uganda began to dry up. The government gave Terrewode six beds at a state-run hospital, but physicians complained that there was never enough money for treatment. Everyone from local leaders to fistula sufferers began to call for a hospital dedicated to obstetric fistula.

Emasu had once heard a rumor: fistula had first been cured in the United States, in the 1850s. She wondered if the strategies that had been used to eradicate fistula in the West could be replicated. To further this goal, a journalist colleague suggested that Emasu apply to study in the United States, at the Brown School of social work at Washington University, in Saint Louis.

Luckily, also in Saint Louis was Dr. Lewis Wall, founder of the Worldwide Fistula Fund. In spring 2008, transported to Missouri, Emasu found herself knocking on Wall's office door.

I am here, but I am bleeding, she told him. I left behind three hundred women in Uganda, and my country cannot help them.

* * *

Lewis Wall's father was an Oklahoma kid, from the panhandle. He was drafted into World War II to copilot a B-17, shot down, and lost seventy pounds as a POW. After the war, he studied obstetric medicine.

Lewis Wall bad-mouthed his father's choice of specialization for two decades—until his own career began to creep toward his father's footsteps.

Wall won a Rhodes Scholarship to pursue anthropology and ancient languages at Oxford. Frustrated with theory, he left to join a study organized by the Liverpool School of Tropical Medicine on remote medical dispensaries in Nigeria. He threw himself into preparations and was awarded a Fulbright-Hays Fellowship—then funding for the research project vanished.

He went to Nigeria anyway. It was here that he first learned of local women suffering from fistula. Less like Kees Waaldijk and more like the Irish nuns who had taken up the fistula crusade, Wall's first intimations of Africa's fistula crisis arrived even before he went to medical school.

He enrolled in 1978, and he was entirely surprised to find himself drawn toward gynecology. He completed a DPhil in social anthropology at the same time. Years later, he would earn an additional degree in bioethics.

The eighties passed in a flash. He was in Zaire for some months, then London studying urogynecology. There was a residency at Duke University and a series of academic postings.

In the early nineties, his career came into focus when he was recruited by a man launching the first OB-GYN training program in Ghana. Wall was now making several trips to Africa per year. In 1994, he visited Catherine Hamlin in Ethiopia. He became a surgeon. Heeding Reginald Hamlin's warnings about "fistula tourism," Wall focused his efforts on fundraising, training, and organization. The goal was not to create institutions to celebrate Western surgeons but to launch programs that would produce doctors in Africa whose skill level in fistula surgery would soon exceed that found in Western medicine.

He worked for a time alongside Steve Arrowsmith in Nigeria, at Red Roof. The Worldwide Fistula Fund was founded, raising money to build several new structures in Jos. Plans were drawn up for another fistula hospital, in northern Nigeria; unrest necessitated a move to neighboring Niger. A former leprosy facility would become another dedicated fistula hospital.

It was then that Alice Emasu from Uganda knocked on Wall's office door.

Her plan was twofold, she explained. In the short term, she was seeking funding for women receiving care in existing facilities in Uganda. In the long term, she wanted to build a hospital of her own.

The vision that Emasu had been nursing for years was more expansive than the model of care that had spread across Africa. What distinguished

Terrewode from the Addis Ababa Fistula Hospital was that it began with programs of reintegration and community activism and worked backward toward surgery. A line of sutures and a gift of a manual sewing machine might cure a single woman, Emasu thought, but it did little to bring about the eradication of fistula.

Before she traveled to the United States, she had implemented an additional layer of fistula survivorhood. Beyond shepherding sufferers to treatment, Terrewode invited women who had been cured to partici- pate in training programs to become community organizers and activists. Again echoing the work of Anarcha, Lucy, Betsey, and the others who had cared for one another during the Alabama fistula experiments, groups of survivors lived and trained together and then returned to their local communities to teach others of the underlying causes of obstructed labor. The true cure of fistula would require a radical transformation of culture.

Women in Uganda did so much, Emasu knew. Yet they were treated almost like slaves. The deaths of Emasu's friends had brought this inequal- ity home to her—made it *live* for her. Now, the final piece of the puzzle was a hospital for women, conceived by women, run entirely by women. She was extending the Addis Ababa model of fistula care, but what she couldn't have known was that it began as a variation on the model of care that had been championed by the Board of Lady Managers at Woman's Hospital, and which was itself a model of care that had been spontaneously pioneered by a group of enslaved teenagers in Alabama in the 1840s.

Lewis Wall was impressed. Alice Emasu was intelligent, determined. Her vision was ambitious. She burned with a passion that just might make it possible. Alice Emasu, he thought, could become the new leader in the battle against the fistula crisis for all of Africa.

* * *

It took more than a decade of work.

There were years of study, and then organization began in the early 2010s. A group in the United States, originally called Uganda Fistula Fund and later renamed Terrewode Women's Fund, spearheaded the planning and funding of a hospital. A plot of land was acquired outside Soroti, in northern Uganda. In the years to come, Emasu would work tirelessly to coordinate additional support from the International Fistula Alliance, the Addis Ababa Fistula Hospital, philanthropist Lynne Dobson, the government of Uganda, the Soroti District local government, and Lewis Wall's Worldwide Fistula Fund. In 2018, Emasu wasn't sure she would be able to succeed in hiring an all-female medical staff for what would come to be called the Terrewode Women's Community Hospital.

By early 2019, she had done exactly that. Dr. Josephine Namugenyi, a member of the College of Surgeons of East, Central and Southern Africa, was hired to oversee a staff of fifteen, including Chief Nurse Elizabeth Atiang and Deputy Chief Nurse Agnes Amidiong. The entire staff of the Terrewode Women's Community Hospital traveled to Ethiopia to study clinical methods at the Addis Ababa Fistula Hospital.

In August 2019, an audience of a thousand gathered at the newly constructed hospital to celebrate its opening. The guests included ministers and members of parliament, donor partners, district local council leaders, and many fistula survivors—women already cured by Terrewode.

After a long series of speakers and performances, Emasu took up a microphone. She thanked them all for treasuring her cause. The goal was not just a hospital, she said. It was a place of healing, of renewed hope. Once here, the women afflicted with the curse of fistula would be cared for by fellow women who understood them—survivors turned into sister friends.

The hospital opening today, Emasu said, was the baby born to the mother of Terrewode. Already, nine women had been cured. Soon, the hospital would cure six hundred per year. Emasu insisted that the focus would be on education, in addition to curing women. The Terrewode Community Women's Hospital was the realization of a dream, one that made them independent in every sense except money. She hoped for the day when her own government would cover bills now paid by foreign aid. Her dream was for her country to be free, too.

About the Author

J. C. Hallman is the author of five previous works of nonfiction and a book of short stories. His previous work on Anarcha has appeared in *Harper's Magazine* and the *Forum* (of the African American Policy Forum). He has received fellowships from the McKnight Foundation and the John Simon Guggenheim Foundation, in the general nonfiction category.